Acute stroke nursing

Edited by

Jane Williams
Portsmouth Hospitals NHS Trust, Portsmouth, Hampshire, UK

Lin Perry
University of Technology Sydney and the Northern Network Hospitals, South Eastern Sydney and Illawarra Health, Australia

Caroline Watkins
Clinical Practice Research Unit, School of Nursing and Caring Sciences, University of Central Lancashire, Preston, UK

WILEY-BLACKWELL

A John Wiley & Sons, Ltd., Publication

This edition first published 2010

© 2010 by Blackwell Publishing Ltd

Blackwell Publishing was acquired by John Wiley & Sons in February 2007. Blackwell's publishing programme has been merged with Wiley's global Scientific, Technical, and Medical business to form Wiley-Blackwell.

Registered office
John Wiley & Sons Ltd, The Atrium, Southern Gate, Chichester, West Sussex, PO19 8SQ, United Kingdom

Editorial offices
9600 Garsington Road, Oxford, OX4 2DQ, United Kingdom
2121 State Avenue, Ames, Iowa 50014-8300, USA

For details of our global editorial offices, for customer services and for information about how to apply for permission to reuse the copyright material in this book please see our website at www.wiley.com/wiley-blackwell.

The right of the author to be identified as the author of this work has been asserted in accordance with the UK Copyright, Designs and Patents Act 1988.

Library of Congress Cataloging-in-Publication Data

Acute stroke nursing / edited by Jane Williams, Lin Perry, Caroline Watkins.
    p. ; cm.
  Includes bibliographical references and index.
  ISBN 978-1-4051-6104-6 (pbk. : alk. paper) 1. Cerebrovascular disease–Nursing. 2. Evidence-based nursing. I. Williams, Jane (Jane E.) II. Perry, Lin. III. Watkins, Caroline.
  [DNLM: 1. Stroke–nursing. 2. Evidence-Based Nursing. WY 152.5 A1897 2010]
  RC388.5.A288 2010
  616.8′10231–dc22

                                                                    2009029833

A catalogue record for this book is available from the British Library.

Set in 10/12.5pt Sabon by Toppan Best-set Premedia Limited
Printed and bound in Malaysia by KHL Printing Co Sdn Bhd

1 2010

Contents

Foreword

Fifteen years ago, I was asked to assume responsibility for a clinically and financially 'failing' Stroke Service at a large academic medical centre in the south-central United States, for the purpose of clinical quality improvement and outcomes management. I accepted the job reluctantly; after all, there was no treatment available for acute stroke other than tradition-bound methods that focused on diagnosis, some degree of secondary prevention, and rehabilitation. Few resources existed at that time to support critical care and emergency nurses in the management of acute stroke patients. There were no textbooks that covered the full spectrum of stroke care, and papers authored by nurses that addressed acute management of stroke were relatively unheard of. But, within a year, things began to change with the onset of the NINDS' (National Institute of Neurological Disorders and Stroke) randomised controlled trial of tissue plasminogen activator for treatment of acute ischaemic stroke (National Institute of Neurological Disorders et al. 1995).

Today, acute stroke management is following closely in the footsteps of cardiology, supported by a growing arsenal of interventions that aim to reduce neurological disability and death, as well as prevent a first-ever or secondary stroke event. What used to be a clinical practice area deemed highly undesirable and difficult to recruit nurses to, is now viewed as exciting and attractive in centres that have adopted aggressive reperfusion therapies. Rehabilitative strategies have also expanded dramatically and now include exciting technologies such as robotics and a variety of approaches to support return to functional independence. Overall, evidence-based, cross-continuum strategies are being implemented in centres once plagued by traditional and often unscientific practices, supporting improved interdisciplinary health care and ultimately, enhanced patient and societal outcomes. In short, stroke nursing care has come of age.

This text provides a 360-degree orientation to stroke nursing. From the prehospital environment, to hyperacute/acute management, complication avoidance, secondary prevention, and neurological recovery, readers are provided with an evidence-based, holistic approach to the management and prevention of neurovascular disease. With the knowledge gained by reading this text, I challenge my nursing colleagues to continue to push their local practice paradigms to adopt an evidence-based approach to the interdisciplinary management of stroke, and to commit to questioning and studying new and evolving practices that aim to improve the lives of stroke survivors and their loved ones.

Nurses are the key drivers of health care quality throughout the world. As the most numerous of the health professions employed within all of the practice settings across the health continuum experienced by stroke patients, nurses must commit themselves to ensuring 'safe passage' of stroke survivors and their family through an increasingly complex and fast paced health care environment. Mastering the knowledge contained within this text is an important first-step in a journey toward attainment of stroke nursing excellence; pledging to continue that journey through formal education, knowledge generation and dissemination, as well as ongoing self-reflection are the next key steps to ensuring best nursing practices for stroke patients. I congratulate the editors and authors of this text for making this journey possible, and look forward to watching stroke nursing knowledge ignite and expand among our readers.

Anne W. Alexandrov

An Australian perspective

As elsewhere in the world, stroke is a leading cause of death and disability in Australia (Senes 2006); hence, optimal management is imperative. Results from the Cochrane systematic review of randomised controlled trials of organised stroke care provided compelling evidence for the effectiveness of stroke units (Stroke Unit Trialists' Collaboration 2003). In Chapter 1, Professor Watkins explains this evidence and the key features of stroke units. As a result, provision of care for stroke patients in dedicated units by coordinated, multidisciplinary teams is one of the pivotal strategies for improving patient outcomes internationally. This evidence has underpinned health reforms for hospitalised stroke patients throughout the world, including Australia.

As in the UK, stroke is a national health priority area in Australia. In 2006, a National Service Improvement Framework for Heart, Stroke and Vascular Disease was developed which outlined '*critical intervention points*' along the continuum of stroke care where it was likely that health gains and improvements to services could be made (National Health Priority Action Council (NHPAC) 2006). The Framework recommended as a priority that stroke unit care should be '*available to all Australians who suffer a stroke*'. The National Stroke Unit Program funded by the Commonwealth Government was undertaken by the National Stroke Foundation (NSF), a not-for-profit, non-government organisation, to promote optimal treatment of stroke patients (National Stroke Foundation 2002). The Program included a review of stroke service policy, development of acute stroke guidelines and performance indicators. In addition, a Stroke Services Model was developed to classify hospitals according to categories A to D, based on the structure and processes of care and the clinical profile of patients (Cadilhac et al. 2006c). Category A and B hospitals have access to comprehensive stroke services such as on-site computed tomography (CT) scanning and intensive care/high dependency beds with Category A hospitals also having on-site neurosurgery. Category C hospitals have access to CT scanning within 12 hours, usually off-site, whilst category D hospitals have neither CT scan access nor availability of other structural criteria. It is expected that all Category A and B hospitals have a stroke unit. However, a survey conducted in 2004 indicated that only 83% of Category A and 30% of Category B hospitals had such units (Cadilhac et al. 2006b). In total, only 19% of Australian public hospitals had a stroke unit. This figure did not compare favourably internationally, particularly with data from Norway and Sweden where 60% and 70% of hospitals respectively have stroke units (Rudd & Matchar 2004). Hence, whilst equity of access to stroke unit care is a health care policy issue for many countries, it is particularly so for Australia.

Provision of equitable stroke care within Australia remains a challenge. With the majority of the nation's population located along the eastern coastline, this is where most stroke services were initially established. Further, Australian stroke units are primarily located in metropolitan hospitals and/or in hospitals with 300 beds or more (Cadilhac et al. 2006b). This potentially disadvantages rural and non-metropolitan inhabitants. New South Wales (NSW) currently has the highest number of stroke units in Australia, as a direct result of the state government providing dedicated funding which increased their numbers from 7 to 23 in metropolitan areas over five years (Cadilhac et al. 2006b). Subsequent initiatives have established seven stroke services in rural NSW.

Encouragingly, Australian hospitals with stroke units have been shown to have greater adherence to important processes of clinical care when compared with either a mobile stroke service or general medical ward (Cadilhac et al. 2004). Processes of care were chosen because of association with improved outcomes, and included early CT-scanning, swallowing assessment, and regular neurological observations. The importance of this was reinforced by clinical audits, demonstrating significant reduction in death and disability for patients admitted to NSW metropolitan stroke units (Cadilhac et al. 2006a). As in other countries, 'best practice' guidance has been made available through development and publication of Australian clinical practice guidelines for the management of acute stroke, rehabilitation and recovery (National Stroke Foundation 2005, 2007).

To support practice and service development, a cohesive platform for training, education and implementation of collaborative, multidisciplinary stroke services including research is provided by Stroke Services NSW. Similar mechanisms for fostering clinician and health service management partnerships have been endorsed in the states of Victoria and Western Australia through state-based stroke strategies (Department of Health Services, Victoria (DoHSV) 2007; Department of Health Western Australia 2006). Other support initiatives include the Towards A Safer Culture (TASC) Clinical Support Systems Program and establishment of the Australian Stroke Clinical Registry (AuSCR). These have been implemented in several Australian states and territories, and aim to embed evidence-based clinical practice with clinical quality improvement activities by the use of online, web-based data acquisition and feedback systems for minimum and extended data sets for stroke patients. Establishment of formal liaison between acute stroke and ambulance services ensures that stroke patients receive appropriate pre-hospital care and are transported to hospitals with an acute stroke unit.

Professional networks such as the Stroke Society of Australasia and the Australian Stroke Unit Network, comprised of multidisciplinary clinicians, policy makers and researchers, work to improve delivery of evidence-based stroke care. In addition, a number of research teams are undertaking leading-edge stroke research from basic science through to public health research in collaboration with researchers around Australia and overseas. Further, many stroke units throughout the country are involved in multicentre national and international clinical trials and research aimed at improving stroke services. The National Stroke Foundation provides information for stroke patients and their carers and at state level, local stroke support associations play a vital role in raising community awareness and supporting stroke patients and their families.

Although coverage is not comprehensive, Australia has well-developed support for patients experiencing stroke. A proactive and growing stroke health care professional community is a crucial element, and the important contribution of nursing is recognised. Education and continuing professional development are key to this. This book sets out in detail what excellence in stroke nursing comprises, in an easy-to-read style. It makes a unique and essential contribution to dissemination of evidence-based practice and hence to improvement and enhancement of stroke nursing care services at all levels and internationally.

Sandy Middleton

References

Cadilhac, DA, Ibrahim, J, Pearce, DC, Ogden, KJ, McNeill, J et al. for the SCOPES Study Group, 2004, Multicenter comparison of processes of care between Stroke Units and conventional care wards in Australia, *Stroke*, vol. 35, no. 5, pp. 1035–1040.

Cadilhac, D, Pearce, D, Levi, C, & Donnan, G, 2006a, Preliminary audit results of a clinician driven, government funded program to implement 19 networked stroke care units (SCUs) in one Australian state, *Cerebrovascular Diseases*, vol. 21, p. 134.

Cadilhac, DA, Lalor, EE, Pearce, DC, Levi, CR, & Donnan, GA, 2006b, Access to stroke care units in Australian public hospitals: facts and temporal progress, *Internal Medicine Journal*, vol. 36, no. 11, pp. 700–704.

Cadilhac, DA, Mooie, ML, Lalor, EE, Bilnet, LE, & Donnan, GA on behalf of the National Stroke Foundation, 2006c, Improving access to evidence-based acute stroke services: development and evaluation of a health systems model to address equity of access issues, *Australian Health Review*, vol. 30, no. 1, pp. 109–118.

Department of Health Services, Victoria (DoHSV), 2007, *A state-wide stroke care strategy for acute and sub-acute stroke care*, Department of Human Services, Melbourne, Victoria.

Department of Health Western Australia, 2006, *Model of Stroke Care for Western Australia*, Department of Health, Perth, Western Australia.

National Health Priority Action Council (NHPAC), 2006, *National Service Improvement Framework for Heart, Stroke and Vascular Disease*, Australian Government Department of Health and Ageing, Canberra.

National Institute of Neurological Disorders, Stroke rt-PS Stroke Study Group (NIND, & Srt-PA SSG), 1995, Tissue plasminogen activator for acute ischaemic stroke, *New England Journal of Medicine*, vol. 333, no. 24, pp. 1581–1587.

National Stroke Foundation, 2002, *Stroke Services in Australia: National Stroke Unit Program Policy Document*, National Stroke Foundation, Melbourne.

National Stroke Foundation, 2005, *Clinical Guidelines for Stroke Rehabilitation and Recovery*, National Stroke Foundation, Melbourne.

National Stroke Foundation, 2007, *Clinical Guidelines for Acute Stroke Management*, National Stroke Foundation, Melbourne.

Rudd, AG, & Matchar, DB, 2004, Health policy and outcome research in stroke, *Stroke*, vol. 35, no. 2, pp. 397–400.

Senes, S, 2006, *How we manage stroke in Australia*, Australia Institute of Health and Welfare, Canberra.

Stroke Unit Trialists' Collaboration, 2003, *Organised inpatient (stroke unit) care for stroke (Cochrane Review)*, Issue 1: CD000197, Oxford.

Editors and Contributors

Dr Jane Williams

Jane Williams is Consultant Nurse in Stroke Care based in Portsmouth Hospitals NHS Trust, UK. This broad role covers expert clinical practice, education and training, professional consultancy and leadership and service development, evaluation, audit and research. The Portsmouth Stroke Service provides acute, inpatient rehabilitation and early supported discharge. She has many stroke-specific interests, including service redesign, clinical leadership and further developing the role of the nurse within stroke rehabilitation. Jane has been involved in many national working parties, including the National Stroke Strategy, UK Forum for Stroke Training, and UK Stroke Forum. Jane is a member of The Stroke Association research awards committee. A founder member of the National Stroke Nursing Forum, Jane undertook a term of office as chair.

Professor Lin Perry

Lin Perry is Professor of Nursing Research and Practice Development, University of Technology, Sydney and the Northern Hospitals Network, South Eastern Sydney and Illawarra Area Health Service. She has a special interest in chronic conditions, practice and service development, particularly in relation to knowledge translation and change management for front-line staff. A member of the Intercollegiate Stroke Working Party in the UK, the National Stroke Foundation Guidelines Working Party and Stroke Services New South Wales in Australia, she has extensive experience with national guideline development, benchmarking, service review and evaluation.

Professor Caroline Watkins

Caroline Watkins leads a multidisciplinary team of researchers with a large portfolio of clinically relevant research, which makes a significant contribution to stroke service development, at a local and national level. As a member of the Vascular Team at the Department of Health, she is working to implement the National Stroke Strategy, and leads the development of the new UK Forum for Stroke Training. She is a member of the Training and Development Group, and the Clinical Study Group for Rehabilitation, of the UK Stroke Research Network (SRN), and the Steering Group for the North West Local SRN. Caroline is President of the Society for Research in Rehabilitation (SRR) and on the Steering Group of the National Stroke Nursing Forum (NSNF), representing the NSNF on the Scientific Committee for the UK Stroke Forum.

Contributors

Anne W. Alexandrov, Professor, Acute & Critical Care, School of Nursing, University of Alabama at Birmingham, USA.

Elizabeth Boaden, Head of Adult Speech and Language Therapy Services (Chorley), NHS Central Lancashire, UK.

Louise Brereton, Lecturer in Adult Nursing, University of Nottingham, Nottingham, UK.

Wendy Brooks, Stroke Nurse Consultant, Epsom and St Helier NHS Trust, Carshalton, UK.

Christopher R. Burton, Senior Research Fellow, School of Healthcare Sciences, Bangor University, Bangor, UK.

Madeline Cruice, Senior Lecturer in Aphasiology, School of Community and Health Sciences, City University, London, UK.

Kathryn Getliffe, Visiting Professor of Nursing, School of Nursing and Midwifery, University of Southampton, Southampton, UK.

Jo Gibson, Senior Lecturer (Research), Clinical Practice Research Unit, School of Nursing and Caring Sciences, University of Central Lancashire, Preston, UK.

Aeron Ginnelly, Senior Speech Pathologist, Neurosciences, Royal Prince Alfred Hospital, Sydney, Australia.

Katerina Hilari, Joint Research Director, School of Community and Health Sciences, City University, London, UK.

Peter Humphrey, Consultant Neurologist, Walton Centre for Neurology and Neurosurgery, Liverpool, UK.

Stephanie Jones, Research Fellow, Clinical Practice Research Unit, School of Nursing and Caring Sciences, University of Central Lancashire, Preston, UK.

Cherry Kilbride, Physiotherapy Lecturer, School of Health Sciences and Social Care, Brunel University, London, UK.

Peter Knapp, Senior Lecturer, School of Healthcare, University of Leeds, Leeds, UK.

Rosie Kneafsey, Lecturer in Adult Nursing, University of Birmingham, Birmingham, UK.

Michael Leathley, Post-doctoral Research Fellow, Clinical Practice Research Unit, School of Nursing and Caring Sciences, University of Central Lancashire, Preston, UK.

Jill Manthorpe, Director, Social Care Workforce Research Unit, King's College, London, UK.

Jane Marshall, Joint Head of Department, School of Community and Health Sciences, City University, London, UK.

Sandy Middleton, Director, Nursing Research Institute, St Vincents and Mater Health Sydney; Professor of Nursing and Director National Centre for Clinical Outcomes Research (NaCCOR), Nursing and Midwifery, Australian Catholic University, Australia.

Sheila Payne, Help the Hospices Chair in Hospice Studies, International Observatory on End of Life Care, Lancaster University, Lancaster, UK.

Elaine Pierce, Principal Lecturer, Institute for Strategic Leadership and Further Improvement, London South Bank University, London UK.

Julie Pryor, Director, Rehabilitation Nursing Research Unit, Royal Rehabilitation Hospital, Sydney; Associate Professor at Flinders and at Charles Sturt Universities, Australia.

Graham Williamson, Lecturer in Adult Nursing, School of Nursing and Acute Care, University of Plymouth, Plymouth, UK.

Chapter 1

Setting the scene

Caroline Watkins and Michael Leathley

Key points

- Transforming stroke services is of paramount importance in the quest to save lives and reduce dependency.
- Translating research evidence into clinical practice is challenging but many examples show that this is both achievable and worthwhile.
- Continued development of stroke nursing through expansion of the stroke nursing knowledge base and demonstration of competence and skill is pivotal to the future of the specialism.
- Continued development of stroke nursing is essential for development of stroke services, locally, nationally and internationally.

Introduction

In the UK and internationally, stroke and its impact on people's lives is finally gaining the recognition it deserves both as an acute event and as chronic disease. The profile of stroke has been raised partly by the burden it places on an individual, their family, the health service and society but more recently because effective treatments have become available. However, to make these treatments available for everyone who might benefit, it is imperative that the public know about and have a heightened awareness of stroke symptoms. Public awareness campaigns are graphically driving home the message that if a stroke is suspected, contact the emergency medical services. Emergency services must respond rapidly and get patients to centres providing specialist acute-stage treatments, ongoing rehabilitation and long-term support. Throughout this care pathway, best-available treatment can only be provided if staff have stroke-specific knowledge and skills commensurate with their roles, and if all agencies involved work collaboratively, providing a seamless journey for the person affected by stroke. Nurses are the largest section of the workforce, and involved throughout the entire pathway. Consequently, nurses have the greatest opportunity to play a key role in providing leadership and delivery of evidence-based stroke services.

This chapter sets stroke nursing in the context of wider systems. Starting by identifying the extent of the problem of stroke, it illustrates why stroke has become a burning issue for health care and research. It discusses policy imperatives and the present and future stroke-specific infrastructure; it identifies the need to support stroke service developments, to put in place mechanisms to produce evidence for practice, as well as clarifying how evidence can be implemented into practice. Fundamental to delivery of this huge agenda is the development of a stroke-specialist workforce, such that those staff delivering care along the stroke pathway not only have the right knowledge, skills and experience in stroke, but achieve recognition for it. Suitable recognition for the specialism should ensure that the most able staff pursue careers in stroke care. This then should establish a virtuous circle, whereby able staff stay in the specialty and contribute further, delivering sustainable quality improvements into the future.

Stroke epidemiology

Stroke is a major cause of mortality and morbidity in adults. It is the third leading cause of death, and a major cause of adult neurological disability. In the UK, the incidence per annum of stroke is approximately 130000 people, with a further 20000 people per annum experiencing transient ischaemic attack (TIA) (National Audit Office 2005). In the UK, the incidence of first-ever stroke is approximately 200 per 100000 people per year (Sudlow & Warlow 1997), similar to other Western countries, including Australia. The case fatality of first-ever stroke has been reported as approximately 12% at 7 days, 20% at 30 days, 30% at 1 year, 60% at 5 years and 80% at 10 years (Dennis et al. 1993; Hankey et al. 2000; Hardie et al. 2003). There is a 10% risk of recurrent stroke within 7 days, 18% within the first 3 months (Coull et al. 2004; Hankey 2005; Hill et al. 2004).

Earlier estimates suggested that in the UK between 1983 and 2023 there would be a 30% increase in numbers of people experiencing a first-ever stroke, increasing the demand on stroke services. More recently, it has been suggested that the incidence of stroke is falling, but with increasing numbers of older people in the population, the overall burden of stroke is nonetheless likely to increase due to a rise in prevalence (Rothwell et al. 2005). Lifestyle issues, for example obesity and binge drinking, may also result in an increased risk of stroke (Reynolds et al. 2003; Zaninotto et al. 2006) and have become the focus of important public health messages. Currently, trends are unclear and further research is needed to understand what the future holds. Recent work, which is shown in Table 1.1, indicates trends of stroke incidence may not increase, and may even decrease (Dey et al. 2007). However, it is clear that more people are surviving stroke and living with the sequelae, which can have profound effects in all domains of life (Jagger et al. 2007). Whilst we want acute stroke interventions to improve survival rates, we also want them to ensure independent survival.

Table 1.1 Summary table of predictions. Reproduced with permission from Dey, P, Sutton, C, Marsden, J, Leathley, M, Burton, C, & Atkins, C, 2007, *Medium Term Stroke Projections for England 2006 to 2015*, Department of Health.

Disease definition	Number occurring in 2005	Number predicted to occur in 2015 by primary model	Model sensitivity analysis: range in predicted numbers for 2015
Stroke attacks	137917	83959	79263–116396
Stroke deaths	33428	20206	20138–28356
Cerebrovascular disease	47213	34429	34429–46538
Cerebrovascular disease with inflation factor applied	47213	34829	34829–42259

Stroke attacks = incidence.

Cerebrovascular disease = all International Classification of Diseases (ICD) stroke categories (160-19 under ICD-10).

Stroke policy

Developing stroke as a health care priority

Over the past decade stroke has received increasing attention from professional health care providers and the UK government. A similar situation has been seen in Australia (see Preface, Australian perspective). When the first National Sentinel Audit (NSA) was performed in 1998, it highlighted the poverty of stroke services. One of the biggest problems was the lack of stroke units and how few people were admitted to a stroke unit at some point during their hospital stay. This was particularly discouraging because the benefits of organised inpatient care had been known for over a decade (Indredavik et al. 1991; Langhorne et al. 1993). Not long after this first audit the first edition of the *National Clinical Guidelines for Stroke* (Intercollegiate Stroke Working Party 2000) was developed. From the start, guideline developers agreed that patients' views would be an important factor in determining how services should be run. Focus groups were used to elicit the experiences of those affected by stroke, their preferences and recommendations for service provision (Kelson et al. 1998). The guidelines give health care providers best practice recommendations, underpinned by evidence from research or expert consensus, and incorporate the views of those affected by stroke. Both the NSA and the clinical guidelines have been important levers in the improvement of stroke care, demonstrating the influence that stroke metrics (data collection points) and clinician-led practice standards can achieve. The success of this model has led to its replication in Australia and other countries.

Key components of stroke care are assessment, management and treatment, and evidence to underpin these have been used to produce and update UK *National Clinical Guidelines for Stroke* (Intercollegiate Stroke Working Party 2000, 2004a, 2008a). Concurrently, successive rounds of the National Sentinel Audit (Intercollegiate Stroke Working Party 2002, 2004b, 2007, 2008b) have revealed the relationship – and shortfalls – between evidence and practice.

Overall, the judgement has been that response to suspected stroke has not been fast enough, either in terms of actions taken for an individual experiencing a stroke or in implementing into practice what scientific literature indicates should be done (National Audit Office 2005). That is, scientific advances are not consistently or rapidly translated into clinical practice. It is precisely this which has led to current benchmarking of stroke services.

In 2001, the UK National Service Framework (NSF) for Older People was published (Department of Health 2001). The NSF set standards to provide person-centred care, remove age discrimination, and promote older people's health and independence. Standard Five in this document focused on stroke and set milestones (dates) for the provision of aspects of care, for example, that those affected by stroke would have access to a stroke unit. The NSA demonstrates these milestones still have not been fully met. Furthermore, it has taken time to ensure that all important milestones are recognised. For example, the second edition of the *National Clinical Guidelines for Stroke*, published in 2004, updated the evidence from the first edition, but still missed an important element of the stroke pathway – that between symptom onset and arrival at hospital. An addendum around early recognition and management of suspected stroke and TIA addressed this shortcoming (Jones et al. 2007).

A National Audit Office report in 2005 outlined advances in stroke care and made recommendations about future improvement (National Audit Office 2005). The following year, Professor Roger Boyle, National Director for Heart Disease and Stroke, published the *Mending Hearts and Brains* document. His aim was to encourage continued development and change in the way we think and act about stroke and heart disease. The document acknowledged the hard work and enthusiasm of NHS staff and set a challenge to improve services: 'we have to set the bar a lot higher in defining the level of service the public should be able to expect' (Department of Health 2006). This was followed by a consultation process with health care providers and service users, resulting in the National Stroke Strategy in 2007 (Department of Health 2007) – see below. The next round of updated guidelines saw initial management of acute stroke and TIA published by the National Institute for Health and Clinical Excellence (NICE) linked with the third edition of the *National Clinical Guidelines for Stroke* (Intercollegiate Stroke Working Party 2008a).

Between 2004 and 2005 the UK Stroke Association developed the 'FAST campaign', designed to raise public awareness of stroke through use of the 'Face, Arm, Speech, Test' (Harbison et al. 2003). Their campaign was revised in 2009, with the 'T' in FAST now standing for time rather than test, which emphasises the importance of rapid response. The campaign ran alongside a Department of Health public awareness campaign, also using FAST, through television and radio advertising. The potential value of such campaigns is great. Stroke has been calculated to cost the NHS £2.8 billion in direct costs; additionally £1.8 billion accrued due to lost productivity and disability, plus £2.4 billion in informal care costs (National Audit Office 2005). The National Audit Office report stated that response to stroke was not as fast and effective as it could be and that, with more efficient practice, there was scope for potential savings of £20 million annually, with 550 deaths avoided and over 1700 people recovering from their stroke each year who would not otherwise have done so (National Audit Office 2005).

UK stroke policy development

Throughout the world, countries are developing documents and guidelines to mandate the provision of quality stroke care. In England, for example, the National Stroke Strategy (NSS) was launched in 2007 (Department of Health 2007). The NSS is underpinned by substantial research evidence and expert consensus, and endeavours to clarify the components of guideline-concordant care, whilst acknowledging the current lack of comprehensive, integrated stroke care systems to deliver this. To assist in implementing NSS recommendations, an additional £105 million was identified for stroke care in the 2007 Public Spending Review. A commissioning framework was developed (Department of Health 2006) with guidance to Commissioners on key issues and resources to inform decision-making.

Nevertheless ensuring that 'the system provides patients with the precise interventions they need, delivered properly, precisely when they need them' (Woolf & Johnson 2005, p. 545) is challenging. Whilst the NSS can tell us what we need to do, we must determine how this can be delivered in local health care systems. Where there is evidence for effectiveness of interventions, we need to understand the design of the studies, underlying suppositions, and the context (organisational, geographical, demographic, etc.) in which the intervention was tested. Often, studies report the effectiveness of interventions with only an outline of the intervention; methods of testing are detailed, but processes (barriers, facilitators, etc.) of introducing the intervention are rarely considered. Without detailed knowledge of how to implement research evidence into practice, implementation is hampered, and potential benefits to patients not fully realised. Consequently, despite having effective treatments for stroke and TIA, unless we understand the health care delivery models that can ensure timely access to treatment and care, people with TIA will continue to go on to have completed stroke, and those with completed stroke will be more likely to die, or to survive with severe disability. However, implementation of NSS recommendations entails challenge; for example, emergency admission to hospital of high-risk patients may place increasing demands on acute stroke services (Figure 1.1).

The National Stroke Strategy

The UK National Stroke Strategy (NSS) was launched in December 2007, and provides a quality framework for the development of stroke services. Successful implementation of this strategy will save lives and reduce disability, decreasing health and social care costs, whilst limiting the devastating effects on people's lives. The strategy describes best practice in the form of Quality Markers (QMs), 16 throughout the whole pathway (see Figure 1.2), from recognising and acting upon suspected stroke through to long-term care. In

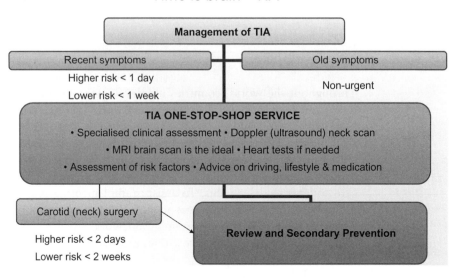

Figure 1.1 Management of transient ischaemic attack (TIA). Department of Health (2007). Reproduced with permission.

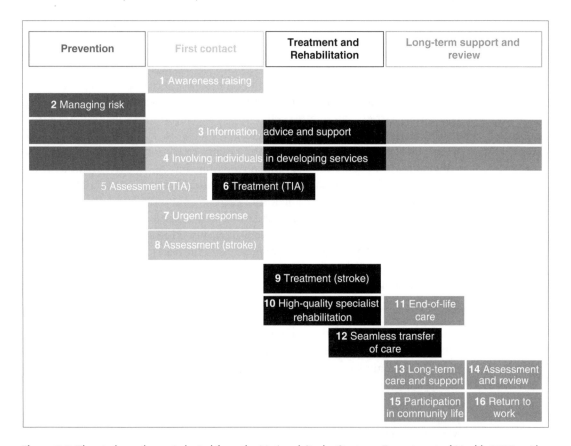

Figure 1.2 The stroke pathway (adapted from the National Stroke Strategy; Department of Health 2007, with permission).

addition, the QMs 17–20 signpost the need for staff to have stroke relevant knowledge, training and skills, together with an awareness of audit and research to support clinical practice.

Meeting the recommendations in the NSS will challenge not just the NHS but also other health, social and voluntary care services. To deliver this, the NSS proposed the establishment of Stroke Care Networks, supported by a national Stroke Improvement Programme (http://www.improvement.nhs.uk/ stroke). This mirrors methods for development of cardiac services, and is supported locally by Cardiac Networks, and nationally by the Heart Improvement Programme team. Local examples of stroke-specific care networks already exist, for example the North West Stroke Task Force (NWSTF). The NWSTF was established in 1999 and through review, guideline sharing, networking, etc., as well as the enthusiasm and efforts of local stroke teams, achieved a doubling of numbers of acute and rehabilitation units and stroke-specific beds over a five-year period (Watkins et al. 2001, 2003, 2006). Stroke Care Networks serve populations of between 500,000 and 2000000, with around 28 in total covering England, as for Cardiac Networks.

The purpose of these networks is to ensure equitable availability and review of progress towards comprehensive stroke services in keeping with the QMs of the NSS. As well as supporting development of stroke services per se, they work collaboratively to develop and deliver improvements in stroke care through:

- Social marketing (e.g. public and professional awareness)
- Workforce development (e.g. delivering competence through education, training and updating)
- Setting standards (e.g. for achievement of QMs)
- Coordinating monitoring of achievements (e.g. progress towards QMs, patient experiences and outcomes)

The Stroke Improvement Programme, working through these care networks and with teams within localities, is developing a series of nationally recognised and coordinated projects to cover the whole of the stroke care pathway.

In determining the service developments that are required and ways to implement these, evidence of effectiveness and evidence-based approaches to implementation must be employed. Currently, one of the biggest challenges to the effectiveness of the NSS is the implementation of existing research evidence (Tooke 2008). Implementation issues and potential tensions include consideration of:

- Organisational context and culture (research-focused, specialist teaching centres as compared with district general hospitals; teaching GPs as compared with non-teaching GPs; level and type of leadership; communication strategies, etc.)
- Geographical location (metropolitan, urban, suburban, rural and remote)
- Team structures (specialist, generalist, coordination, professional/discipline specific leadership)

- Professional roles (traditional, new ways of working)
- Research culture (competences for participation and utilisation)

Participation in clinical trials is promoted via the national Stroke Research Network (SRN: http://www.uksrn.ac.uk). Whilst trials provide evidence of what can work, it is imperative that applied health research undertakes the translational work to demonstrate how this evidence can be applied within routine clinical services. This requires close collaborative working between clinicians, stroke care networks, stroke research networks, and academics. For example, for people with suspected stroke, stroke care networks will facilitate the development of new pathways of care, including 'hub and spoke' models of hyper-acute stroke care. This might mean that within a geographical region one centre provides hyper-acute treatments, for example thrombolysis (within a stroke unit), with other centres offering specialist care in the form of stroke units. This process will need to be supported to enable accurate early identification of people with suspected stroke, optimal choice of destination, and effects on current local services, including ambulance services. This will require work to determine local feasibility, and later evaluation of cost-effectiveness.

Stroke management strategies

Stroke unit care

The mainstay of stroke services is stroke units. More than 15 years ago a statistical overview demonstrated the value of specialist stroke units (Langhorne et al. 1993). Much has been written since and a meta-analysis of outcomes of stroke unit care has been published as a Cochrane Review (Stroke Unit Trialists' Collaboration 1997). Stroke unit care has been shown to reduce mortality and dependency, with some evidence also pointing to a modest reduction in length of hospital stay (Stroke Unit Trialists' Collaboration 1997).

Outcomes from clinical trials may not directly reflect what can be achieved when trial interventions become routine clinical practice, but combined evidence from observational studies also demonstrates significant benefit from stroke unit care (Seenan et al. 2007). Given the range and strength of this evidence, admission of all stroke patients to stroke units is recommended in guidelines of many countries, for example Australia (National Stroke Foundation 2005, 2007), UK (Intercollegiate Stroke Working Party 2008a) and the US (Adams et al. 2007). As most stroke patients can potentially benefit by this model of care, it has been described as the most important treatment for stroke patients (Indredavik 2009).

Organised inpatient care is, by definition, not a single intervention. This, together with the fact that stroke unit trials have not systematically measured component interventions, has meant that the contents of the 'black box' of stroke unit care were unknown (Gladman et al. 1996). Consequently, researchers have aimed to unpack this 'black box' and identify the key components of organised inpatient care (Langhorne & Pollock 2002). In a survey of 11 stroke unit trials the following similar approaches were identified:

- Assessment procedures (medical, nursing and therapy assessment)
- Management policies such as early mobilisation and treating suspected infection
- Ongoing rehabilitation policies such as coordinated multidisciplinary team care (Langhorne & Pollock 2002)

The value of these approaches has been demonstrated by recent studies showing benefits to patients in terms of increasing mobilisation (Bernhardt et al. 2008) and preventing complications (Govan et al. 2007).

Nurses play a key role in identifying complications after an acute stroke through physiological monitoring. With their constant presence along the care continuum (Langhorne et al. 2002), particularly in the first 72 hours, nurses are best placed to be vigilant, and to detect and act on any physiological variations. However, simply connecting patients to monitoring equipment is only part of the process. Nurses must also respond to variations in physiological parameters, because up to one-third of stroke patients deteriorate neurologically during the first few days (mostly in the first 24 hours) and over 25% of patients suffer 'stroke progression' (significant, persisting neurological deterioration) after admission to hospital (Jorgensen et al. 1996). Stroke progression can dramatically worsen outcome; about half of those who die or are left with serious long-term disability have undergone stroke progression in the first 72 hours (Birschel et al. 2004). In some cases, progression is due to intracerebral processes such as the 'ischaemic cascade' (see Chapter 3), the prevention of which has been the focus of much pharmacological research (Davis & Donnan 2002). In many cases, progression is associated with systemic haemodynamic, biochemical or physiological disturbances that are potentially treatable (Davis & Barer 1999). Organised acute stroke care should therefore include intensive acute-stage monitoring and responsive interventions. Intensive management regimes do not currently have a research evidence base but expert consensus considers them clinical common sense; these patients are unstable physiologically and consequently require physiological support.

The underlying pathology of 85% of strokes is cerebral infarction, which implies that treatment directed at this group has the potential to make the greatest impact. Therefore, a key component of effective treatment for ischaemic stroke entails optimal uptake of thrombolysis in locations where delivery is safe. Practical barriers to local introduction of thrombolysis in the UK include:

- Lack of knowledge about thrombolysis for stroke
- Lack of necessary skill mix
- Nursing fears of the haemorrhagic side-effects, and
- Consent issues (Innes 2003)

Consequently, for safe delivery of thrombolysis, appropriate training is required, which must ensure capacity and competence within stroke services.

Safe delivery of acute and intensive interventions requires specialist training. To date in the UK, only medical staff have a (recently introduced) formal route to becoming a stroke specialist, although in the US stroke specialist credentialling is not limited by discipline. In the UK, nurses and allied health professionals need to develop standardised stroke specialist qualifications and training, which needs to be available and accessible to all (see later in this chapter for UK Forum for Stroke Training and the Stroke-Specific Education Framework).

Stroke as a medical emergency

Benefit can be gained by treating stroke as a medical emergency and ensuring that all patients receive effective treatment early. Effective short-term treatment brings long-term gain, including cost benefit. To achieve this, signs and symptoms of stroke need to be recognised, and acted on as a medical emergency by the public and health care providers. The ambulance service needs to react quickly to suspected stroke, which should be triaged to Category A response (currently, within eight minutes), with rapid arrival at the scene. Rapid action at the onset of stroke symptoms is a key issue within the NSS (Department of Health 2007) because stroke outcomes can be improved by timely care (Wojner-Alexandrov et al. 2005).

Once at the scene, ambulance personnel need to be able to recognise the symptoms of suspected stroke, triage and transport patients rapidly to the most appropriate hospital. Early presentation to an appropriate hospital provides greater opportunity for time-dependent stroke treatment, such as thrombolysis (Wojner-Alexandrov et al. 2005). Over time, advances in brain imaging technology and development of new interventions will increase the proportion of acute stroke patients eligible for treatments. More immediate access to organised stroke care will also positively impact on survival and dependency rates (Stroke Unit Trialists' Collaboration 1997). Therefore, rapid access has the potential to reduce severity of stroke, health service usage and length of stay, with overall reduction of the burden of stroke for individuals, carers and society as a whole.

In the UK a rapid ambulance protocol was established in 1997 to facilitate rapid transport of patients to an acute stroke unit (Harbison et al. 1999). A FAST assessment forms part of the process (see Chapter 4 for discussion of stroke identification tools). Paramedics using the FAST showed good agreement with physicians' ratings of stroke patients (Nor et al. 2004). Development of valid scales is only the first part of the process; local staff education and training is also required. Training is important for first-line paramedic staff; call handlers and ambulance dispatchers who receive the emergency calls also require this. A multilevel educational programme has been shown to improve rapid hospitalisation and paramedic diagnostic accuracy, and increased the number of patients presenting for evaluation within the three-hour time window for thrombolysis (Wojner-Alexandrov et al. 2005).

Research and education

Research plays an important part in service development: support and facilitation of research are national priorities around the world. Various strategies are employed to support research capacity development and to maximise engagement at the stroke unit level and recruitment of individual stroke patients. In the UK this has included establishment of the Stroke Research Network.

Stroke Research Network

The national Stroke Research Network (SRN), part of the UK Clinical Research Network, aims to facilitate clinical stroke research by enhancing NHS research infrastructure and exploring ways to remove barriers to conducting world-class research. This has entailed facilitation of collaborative working between academics, stroke clinicians, stroke service users and research funders. The SRN is comprised of a UK Coordinating Centre, Local (regional) Research Networks (LRNs), Research Networks in Scotland, Northern Ireland and Wales, a UK Steering Group and a number of national Clinical Studies Groups (CSGs, e.g. Acute, Rehabilitation, Biostatistics). CSGs have been tasked with promoting research portfolio development and advising on the suitability of studies for the portfolio. LRNs' role is to increase participation in stroke research studies, and involve people with stroke and their carers in network activities. They support the set-up and running of research studies within the SRN portfolio on local sites, development of the local research workforce and establishment of service user groups.

Specialist training

High-quality care and services for people with stroke need staff with appropriate knowledge and skills; there are presently no coordinated mechanisms to achieve this in the UK. In the wake of the NSS the UK Forum for Stroke Training has been established to work towards achievement of recognised, quality-assured and transferable education programmes in stroke. This Forum is responsible for linking training and education, workforce competences, professional development, and career pathways. A Steering Group and four Task Groups have been established, with representation from stroke-specific and stroke-relevant professional bodies, health and social care, voluntary organisations and service users. The Task Groups have developed a Stroke-Specific Education Framework, based around 16 of the QMs that cover the whole stroke care pathway (see Figure 1.2). QMs 17–20 form the basis of future plans for development of the infrastructure for further development, sustainability, accreditation and embedding of the Framework through delivery of a stroke-skilled workforce (see Box 1.1).

Box 1.1   Quality Markers (QMs) from the UK National Stroke Strategy. Department of Health 2007. Reproduced with permission.

1. Awareness raising: stroke as a medical emergency
2. Managing risk: primary and secondary prevention
3. Information, advice and support to those affected by stroke
4. User involvement in care and service planning
5. Assessment (TIA): assessment and management at time of event
6. Treatment (TIA): assessment and management at follow-up
7. Urgent response: pre-hospital assessment and management
8. Assessment (stroke): emergency assessment and management
9. Treatment (stroke): hyperacute assessment and management
10. High-quality specialist rehabilitation
11. End-of-life care
12. Seamless transfer of care
13. Long-term care and support
14. Review
15. Participation in community life
16. Return to work
17. Networks
18. Leadership and skills
19. Workforce review and development
20. Research and audit

The overall purpose of this Education Framework is to add stroke-specific knowledge and skills to the generic skills that health, social, voluntary and independent care staff already possess. To achieve this it will be fundamental to consider how to:

- Build on existing skills, knowledge and experience – *generic competences*
- Develop stroke-specific knowledge and skills – *stroke-specific competences*
- Develop the ability to implement knowledge and skills gained through education and training in practice – *work-based learning*

The relationship between these three aspects, essential to the provision of a stroke-skilled workforce, is detailed below and diagrammatically in Figure 1.3. In order to reinforce learning from participating in education and training opportunities, individuals reflect upon on how practice relates to new knowledge, and theoretical knowledge to practice. Ideally this utilises work-based practice opportunities, where clinical mentors facilitate such reflection.

Through engagement with the UK Forum for Stroke Training, the NHS, Social Services, voluntary and independent sector organisations can contribute to the development of a stroke-specialist workforce. Staff delivering care along the stroke pathway must have the right knowledge, skills and experience in stroke, and the opportunity to participate in clearly defined career pathways. Improving recognition of stroke as a prestigious specialism will ensure future quality improvement through investment in stroke-specific and stroke-relevant services, and the workforce required to deliver it.

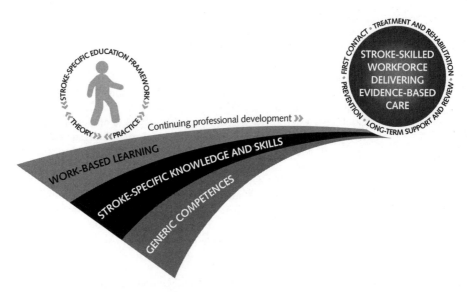

Figure 1.3 Stroke-specific education framework: delivering a stroke-skilled workforce (adapted from the National Stroke Strategy; Department of Health 2007, with permission).

Conclusion

This chapter describes the recent stroke service context in the UK, setting out how stroke has developed to become recognised as a policy priority, with a national strategy, service and management developments, and a Framework and Network to support education and research. Similar processes are underway in other countries. Altogether, these will ensure that stroke services achieve the best possible outcomes for patients and families affected by stroke. Stroke services can now provide staff with stimulating work environments, and educational and professional development within clear career pathways. From a hard-to-recruit-to clinical backwater stroke is maturing into an exciting, challenging and progressive specialism; the following chapters, which include anonymised case examples, set out in detail what this entails for stroke nurses.

Stroke nursing is now a rewarding specialism and provides opportunities for nurses to become active in exciting cutting-edge clinical practice, research and education. This book aims to inspire and enthuse nurses to become involved and drive the specialism forward.

References

Adams, HP, Jr, del Zoppo G, Alberts, MJ, Bhatt, DL, Brass, L et al., 2007, Guidelines for the early management of adults with ischemic stroke: a guideline from the American Heart Association/American Stroke Association Stroke Council, Clinical Cardiology Council, Cardiovascular Radiology and Intervention Council, and the Atherosclerotic Peripheral Vascular Disease and Quality of Care Outcomes in Research Interdisciplinary Working Groups: the American Academy of Neurology affirms the value of this guideline as an educational tool for neurologists, *Stroke*, vol. 38, no. 5, pp. 1655–1711.

Bernhardt, J, Chitravas, N, Meslo, IL, Thrift, AG, & Indredavik, B, 2008, Not all stroke units are the same: a comparison of physical activity patterns in Melbourne, Australia, and Trondheim, Norway, *Stroke*, vol. 39, no. 7, pp. 2059–2065.

Birschel, P, Ellul, J, & Barer, D, 2004, Progressing stroke: towards an internationally agreed definition, *Cerebrovascular Diseases*, vol. 17, no. 2–3, pp. 242–252.

Coull, AJ, Lovett, JK, & Rothwell, PM, 2004, Population based study of early risk of stroke after transient ischaemic attack or minor stroke: implications for public education and organisation of services, *British Medical Journal*, vol. 328, no. 7435, pp. 326–328.

Davis, M, & Barer, D, 1999, Neuroprotection in acute ischaemic stroke. II: Clinical potential, *Vascular Medicine*, vol. 4, no. 3, pp. 149–163.

Davis, SM, & Donnan, GA, 2002, Neuroprotection: establishing proof of concept in human stroke, *Stroke*, vol. 33, no. 1, pp. 309–310.

Dennis, MS, Burn, JP, Sandercock, PA, Bamford, JM, Wade, DT et al., 1993, Long-term survival after first-ever stroke: the Oxfordshire Community Stroke Project, *Stroke*, vol. 24, no. 6, pp. 796–800.

Department of Health, 2001, *The National Service Framework for Older People*, Department of Health, London.

Department of Health, 2006, *Mending Hearts and Brains*, Department of Health, London.

Department of Health, 2007, *National Stroke Strategy*, Department of Health, London.

Dey, P, Sutton, C, Marsden, J, Leathley, M, Burton, C, & Atkins, C, 2007, *Medium Term Stroke Projections for England 2006 to 2015*, Department of Health, London.

Gladman, J, Barer, D, & Langhorne, P, 1996, Specialist rehabilitation after stroke, *British Medical Journal*, vol. 312, no. 7047, pp. 1623–1624.

Govan, L, Langhorne, P, & Weir, CJ, 2007, Does the prevention of complications explain the survival benefit of organized inpatient (stroke unit) care?: further analysis of a systematic review, *Stroke*, vol. 38, no. 9, pp. 2536–2540.

Hankey, GJ, 2005, Secondary prevention of recurrent stroke, *Stroke*, vol. 36, no. 2, pp. 218–221.

Hankey, GJ, Jamrozik, K, Broadhurst, RJ, Forbes, S, Burvill, PW et al., 2000, Five-year survival after first-ever stroke and related prognostic factors in the Perth Community Stroke Study, *Stroke*, vol. 31, no. 9, pp. 2080–2086.

Harbison, J, Massey, A, Barnett, L, Hodge, D, & Ford, GA, 1999, Rapid ambulance protocol for acute stroke, *Lancet*, vol. 353, no. 9168, p. 1935.

Harbison, J, Hossain, O, Jenkinson, D, Davis, J, Louw, SJ et al., 2003, Diagnostic accuracy of stroke referrals from primary care, emergency room physicians, and ambulance staff using the face arm speech test, *Stroke*, vol. 34, no. 1, pp. 71–76.

Hardie, K, Hankey, GJ, Jamrozik, K, Broadhurst, RJ, & Anderson, C, 2003, Ten-year survival after first-ever stroke in the Perth community stroke study, *Stroke*, vol. 34, no. 8, pp. 1842–1846.

Hill, MD, Yiannakoulias, N, Jeerakathil, T, Tu, JV, Svenson, LW et al., 2004, The high risk of stroke immediately after transient ischemic attack: a population-based study, *Neurology*, vol. 62, no. 11, pp. 2015–2020.

Indredavik, B, 2009, Stroke unit care is beneficial both for the patient and for the health service and should be widely implemented, *Stroke*, vol. 40, no. 1, pp. 1–2.

Indredavik, B, Bakke, F, Solberg, R, Rokseth, R, Haaheim, LL et al., 1991, Benefit of a stroke unit: a randomized controlled trial, *Stroke*, vol. 22, no. 8, pp. 1026–1031.

Innes, K, 2003, Thrombolysis for acute ischaemic stroke: core nursing requirements, *British Journal of Nursing*, vol. 12, no. 7, pp. 416–424.

Intercollegiate Stroke Working Party, 2000, *National Clinical Guidelines for Stroke*, Royal College of Physicians, London.

Intercollegiate Stroke Working Party, 2002, *National Sentinel Stroke Audit*, ICWPS, London, Royal College of Physicians.

Intercollegiate Stroke Working Party, 2004a, *National Clinical Guidelines for Stroke*, ICWPS, Royal College of Physicians, London.

Intercollegiate Stroke Working Party, 2004b, *National Sentinel Stroke Audit*, Royal College of Physicians, London.

Intercollegiate Stroke Working Party, 2007, *National Sentinel Stroke Audit: Phase I (Organisational Audit) 2006: Phase II (Clinical audit) 2006*, Royal College of Physicians, London.

Intercollegiate Stroke Working Party, 2008a, *National Clinical Guidelines for Stroke*, 3rd edn, Royal College of Physicians, London.

Intercollegiate Stroke Working Party, 2008b, *National Sentinel Stroke Audit (organisational audit)*, Royal College of Physicians, London.

Jagger, C, Matthews, R, Spiers, N, Brayne, C, Comas-Herrera, A, Robinson, T, Lindesay, J, & Croft, P, 2007, *Compression or expansion of disability? Forecasting future disability levels under changing patterns of diseases*, University of Leicester.

Jones, SP, Jenkinson, MJ, Leathley, MJ, Rudd, AG, Ford, GA et al., 2007, The recognition and emergency management of suspected stroke and transient ischaemic attack, *Clinical Medicine*, vol. 7, no. 5, pp. 467–471.

Jorgensen, H, Nakama, H, Reith, J, Raaschou, H, & Olsen, T, 1996, Factors delaying hospital admission in acute stroke: the Copenhagen study, *Neurology*, vol. 47, pp. 383–387.

Kelson, M, Ford, C, & Rigge, M, 1998, *Stroke Rehabilitation: Patient and Carer Views. A Report by the College of Health for the Intercollegiate Working Party for Stroke*, Royal College of Physicians, London.

Langhorne, P, Pollock, A, 2002, What are the components of effective stroke unit care? *Age and Ageing*, vol. 31, no. 5, pp. 365–371.

Langhorne, P, Williams, BO, Gilchrist, W, & Howie, K, 1993, Do stroke units save lives? *Lancet*, vol. 342, no. 8868, pp. 395–398.

Langhorne, P, Cadilhac, D, Feigin, V, Grieve, R, & Liu, M, 2002, How should stroke services be organised? *Lancet Neurology*, vol. 1, no. 1, pp. 62–68.

National Audit Office, 2005, *Reducing Brain Damage – Faster Access to Better Stroke Care*, The Stationery Office, London.

National Stroke Foundation, 2005, *Clinical Guidelines for Stroke Rehabilitation and Recovery*, National Stroke Foundation, Melbourne.

National Stroke Foundation, 2007, *Clinical Guidelines for Acute Stroke Management*, National Stroke Foundation, Melbourne.

Nor, AM, McAllister, C, Louw, SJ, Dyker, AG, Davis, M et al., 2004, Agreement between ambulance paramedic and physician-recorded neurological signs with Face Arm Speech Test (FAST) in acute stroke patients, *Stroke*, vol. 35, no. 6, pp. 1355–1359.

Reynolds, K, Lewis, B, Nolen, JD, Kinney, GL, Sathya, B et al., 2003, Alcohol consumption and risk of stroke: a meta-analysis, *Journal of the American Medical Association*, vol. 289, no. 5, pp. 579–588.

Rothwell, PM, Coull, AJ, Silver, LE, Fairhead, JF, Giles, MF et al. 2005, Population-based study of event-rate, incidence, case fatality, and mortality for all acute vascular events in all arterial territories (Oxford Vascular Study), *Lancet*, vol. 366, no. 9499, pp. 1773–1783.

Seenan, P, Long, M, & Langhorne, P, 2007, Stroke units in their natural habitat: systematic review of observational studies, *Stroke*, vol. 38, no. 6, pp. 1886–1892.

Stroke Unit Trialists' Collaboration, 1997, Collaborative systematic review of the randomised controlled trials of organised inpatient (stroke unit) care after stroke, *British Medical Journal*, vol. 314, no. 7088, pp. 1151–1159.

Sudlow, CL, & Warlow, CP, 1997, Comparable studies of the incidence of stroke and its pathological types: results from an international collaboration. International Stroke Incidence Collaboration, *Stroke*, vol. 28, no. 3, pp. 491–499.

Tooke, J, 2008, *Aspiring to Excellence. Findings and Final Recommendations of the independent Inquiry Into Modernising Medical Careers*, Aldridge Press, London.

Watkins CL, Lightbody CE, & Auton MF, 2001, *Stroke Services in the North West*, University of Central Lancashire, Preston.

Watkins CL, Lightbody CE, & Auton MF, 2003, *Stroke Services in the North West*, University of Central Lancashire, Preston.

Watkins, CL, Lightbody, CE, Auton, MF, & Bamford, C, 2006, *North West Stroke Task Force Services Survey Volume 3*, University of Central Lancashire, Preston.

Wojner-Alexandrov, AW, Alexandrov, AV, Rodriguez, D, Persse, D, & Grotta, JC, 2005, Houston paramedic and emergency stroke treatment and outcomes study (HoPSTO), *Stroke*, vol. 36, no. 7, pp. 1512–1518.

Woolf, SH, & Johnson, RE, 2005, The break-even point: when medical advances are less important than improving the fidelity with which they are delivered, *Annals of Family Medicine*, vol. 3, no. 6, pp. 545–552.

Zaninotto, P, Wardle, H, Stamatakis, E, Mindell, J, & Head, J, 2006, *Forecasting Obesity to 2010*, Department of Health, London.

Chapter 2

Developing stroke services: a key role for nursing and nurses

Christopher R. Burton

Key points

- Stroke services are coming of age, being recognised internationally as a priority for practice and policy development.
- Nursing has a key contribution to make within this, at many levels.
- Stroke nursing role development is occurring within specialist and generalist dimensions.
- It is important that nursing remains in touch with its essentially patient-focused core.

Introduction

This chapter focuses on stroke service development and explores the potential that nursing can bring to this. After considering what is meant by service development, the different components of the nursing role in stroke care are explored, and new nursing roles such as specialist and consultant nurses are considered. This exploration provides the basis for identifying the knowledge, skills and expertise that nurses bring to stroke service development. A range of policy and professional initiatives that are driving changes in the configuration of services and clinical practice in the UK will then be considered.

Service development

Health services in general, and stroke services in particular, appear to be in a continual state of flux, responding to changes in health policy and new evidence for practice. However, it is clear that despite the dissemination of evidence through National Clinical Guidelines (Intercollegiate Stroke Working Party 2008a), translation of this evidence into improvements for patients has been limited.

With considerable political investment, the most recent audit of stroke services in England, Wales and Northern Ireland indicated modest improvement in the delivery of evidence-based stroke care (Intercollegiate Stroke Working Party 2008b, 2008c). For example, in 2006 62% of stroke patients were admitted to a stroke unit at some point in their stay in hospital, with only 54% spending more than half of their time in hospital in a stroke unit (Intercollegiate Stroke Working Party 2007). By 2008, on the day of audit with 6452 patients with either stroke or transient ischaemic attack (TIA) in hospitals, 1502 (23%) were not in a stroke unit bed (Intercollegiate Stroke Working Party 2008b). This audit report goes on to note numbers of non-stroke patients occupying stroke unit beds, a feature of bed shortages and admissions policies internationally. This means that substantial numbers of stroke patients still were not receiving this most basic component of effective stroke care, whilst stroke specialist nursing time is being spent caring for non-stroke patients. The authors note that, 'a little bit of common sense and simple management skills could make a major difference to patient outcomes'.

In addition, significant variations in access to stroke unit care appear to exist between the different countries of the UK, with patients in Wales at distinct disadvantage when compared to their counterparts in England and Northern Ireland. Other aspects of stroke care appear to change only slowly: for example 6% of all stroke admissions were catheterised because of urinary incontinence, a reduction from 10% in 2006 (Intercollegiate Stroke Working Party 2007, 2008b). Urinary catheterisation is associated with an increased number of medical complications and longer length of stay, and is therefore recommended for urinary incontinence only as a last resort after alternative methods of management have been considered, and after a full diagnosis has been made (see Chapter 6 for more details).

Many initiatives that aim to improve the implementation of evidence-based practice focus primarily on the individual professional and include education, local opinion leaders, patient-mediated interventions, and audit and feedback (Grimshaw et al. 2004). Other strategies to promote evidence-based practice, such as clinical audit and feedback of performance, may focus on either individual or team level performance (Jamtvedt et al. 2006). However, there is an increasing awareness of the organisational context in which the implementation of research findings occurs (or not). For example, a trial of two education and training strategies to enhance the use of research by speech and language therapists in the management of post-stroke dysphagia showed that the organisational contexts, characterised by staff participation in research projects and formal dissemination activities such as journal clubs, were a significant predictor of the success of education (Pennington et al. 2005).

Research implementation in health care is complex, with a number of potential barriers to the use of evidence in decision-making from a variety of perspectives. Addressing these barriers in stroke has focused primarily on the inter-relationship between the producers and users of research, and effective modes of communication between researchers and clinicians such as the synthesis of key research findings into the *National Clinical Guidelines for Stroke* (Intercollegiate Stroke Working Party 2008a). However, in stroke, evidence-based practice must also operate in a context that includes the contributions of a wide variety of professional groups with alternative practice paradigms, and a care pathway that spans numerous health settings and organisational boundaries. The organisational context of evidence-based practice in stroke care is significant, and must feature in the evidence-based development of stroke services.

Traditionally, evidence-based practice has placed considerable emphasis on knowledge generated from scientific knowledge. Whilst this approach has seen many successes, it is limited for two key reasons. Firstly, practitioners need advice and guidance even when the research has yet to be undertaken. For example, recommendations about palliative care in the National Clinical Guidelines are underpinned by consensus within the guideline development group, or extrapolated from the cancer literature. Secondly, there is an increasing awareness of the usefulness of other forms of knowledge such as patient experience, practical 'know-how' and information from the local context on which to base the development of services (Rycroft-Malone et al. 2004).

Whilst the implementation of research demonstrating clinical and economic effectiveness is a key issue for all health and social care professions, nursing has adopted a broad approach to service development. For example, 'technical practice development' has been associated with the uptake of scientific knowledge, and reflects a traditional evidence implementation model with close links between knowledge and practice; 'emancipatory practice development', on the other hand, is particularly interested in the transformation of organisational culture and context to sustain practice development, and to encourage innovation (Manley & McCormack 2003). The two approaches are underpinned by different values, assumptions and theories, and consequently, approaches to working. Existing approaches to the development of stroke services (such as the publication of the National Clinical Guidelines and evaluation of their uptake through national audits, as seen in both the UK and Australia) can be located within 'technical practice development'. The challenge is to ensure that this focus on evidence implementation does not stifle innovation and the development of organisational context and culture.

The development of stroke services must reflect the multidisciplinary nature of service delivery. All professional groups have the capacity to contribute knowledge and expertise to service development, although this will reflect differing theoretical perspectives and practice models.

The nursing contribution to stroke services

At first glance, asking what nurses do in stroke services may be obvious, and lists can be constructed which outline the components of nursing care. However, without any theoretical or research base to this list, this approach is problematic for a number of reasons.

- *Firstly*, there is a danger that important components of the nursing role are missed. Observational studies not underpinned by a theoretical framework that describes the nursing role may miss important, 'hidden' aspects of nursing practice that may be clinically effective. In this case, a theoretical framework will inform what is observed, and help to understand what is not observed, and why it is not observed.
- *Secondly*, the commissioning of stroke services requires that nurses can articulate the contribution they make, both in terms of what they do, the staffing and other resource requirements to deliver best practice, and the outcomes this contribution achieves.
- *Thirdly*, without an understanding of this nursing role, the implications of role expansion, such as the transfer of interventions between professional groups, cannot be studied in any meaningful way. For example, new standards for the management of stroke risk after TIA, and developments in thrombolysis have the potential to provide important opportunities for nurses to expand their contribution to stroke services for patient benefit, particularly in acute stroke care. These may help to enhance the perception of stroke as a specialist area of practice, and coupled with the opportunities for learning new skills that these developments bring, may improve the recruitment of staff to stroke services.

Clearly there is a need to ensure that patients have the opportunity to receive the interventions they need, when they need them. There is an increasing recognition, for example, that nurses can effectively reduce the amount of time patients spend with no oral intake while waiting for assessment of their swallowing function. From the patient perspective, however, it is important to consider what nursing interventions are not going to be done, or who else is going to do them, as professional resources are redistributed. When nurses take on additional aspects of nursing care, for example dysphagia, it is difficult to understand the true implications, because it may not be easy to discern those tasks that may not be being performed. If the focus of the evaluation is on the impact of dysphagia management, then the full impact will not be captured unless the whole range of nursing tasks was known.

Finally, if nursing aspires to professional status, then an ability to define our knowledge base for practice must be underpinned by a robust understanding of those aspects of health services that have special relevance for nurses.

What is the theoretical basis of this contribution?

In the UK literature, the nursing role in stroke mirrors the predominant service model that underpins UK stroke care: care of older people. Stroke services have typically emerged from this service model, reflected in the inclusion of stroke as Standard Five in the National Service Framework for Older People (Department of Health 2001). This is significantly different to Australia, the United States and some European countries, where stroke care has grown from neuroscience roots. As a consequence of the UK 'older adult care' derivation, there is significant attention paid to the rehabilitative component of the nursing role, with relatively less emphasis on the role within the acute phases of stroke. Other countries experience the reverse of this.

A comprehensive literature review specific to stroke (Kirkevold 1997) described two dimensions of the nursing role in stroke rehabilitation: the provision and management of the context for effective rehabilitation, and the provision of specific therapeutic interventions. Kirkevold's (1997) review was underpinned by an earlier study of experienced nurses working in a specialised stroke unit (Kirkevold 1992). Interviews and observation identified four therapeutic functions or domains in stroke rehabilitation nursing:

- An interpretive function that helped patients and families understand the implications of stroke
- A consoling function in providing emotional support
- A maintenance function to ensure that patients attain the best possible 'state' for therapy, and finally
- The integration or translation of therapy, where nurses help patients to assimilate discrete skills or activities learned in formal therapy into meaningful self-care or social activities

In an exploratory study in the North West of England, nurses tended to see themselves as the principal providers of care for stroke patients, with most citing the continual presence of nurses on the rehabilitation unit as evidence for this (Burton 2000). The major theme identified in this study related to nursing activities that were predominantly aimed at the completion of interventions where basic physical needs were provided for, patient safety was maintained and harm to the patient prevented. Often these activities were prescribed by other professional groups, or were related to nursing policies and procedures, and established practice regimens. Importantly, the nurses did not directly relate their activities to patient outcomes of rehabilitation.

The 24-hour presence of nurses for stroke patients can be responsible for the development of an environment that is conducive to rehabilitation (Waters 1987). However, a clear analysis of what nurses are actually doing within these 24 hours, and why, is essential. Nurses also undertake a range of care management activities designed to coordinate the input of other health care professionals, and to enable smooth transitions of care for patients. The case conference has been identified as the principal process by which important decisions regarding patient care are made (Burton 2000), where nurses provide information relating to patients' general progress, coping and emotional health, and social support. The managerial aspects of the nursing role imply the role is secondary to the roles of other professional groups because no specific function is delineated (O'Connor 1993). If, however, nurses do operate in stroke rehabilitation with a holistic awareness that is drawn from 'getting inside the patient's skin' (Henderson 1980), then this does imply a unique function. The nurse would indeed be best placed to coordinate and mediate the contributions of other professional groups to ensure that the patient's progress is maintained. However, the nursing contribution to the development of patient management strategies may be limited, and may only include putting into operation the decisions of others (Gibbon 1999).

Burton's (2003) description of therapeutic nursing in stroke requires a more meaningful degree of interaction between the patient and nurse, the key purpose of which is the development of coping strategies and the maintenance and improvement of well-being over time. This focus mirrors to some extent the interpretive nursing function identified by Kirkevold (1997). Although recognising this function is important in helping patients to come to terms with the consequences of stroke, the major focus on Kirkevold's analysis is restricted to the early stages of stroke, and does not include the development of coping skills for rebuilding life with stroke.

To date, theoretical descriptions of the nursing role in stroke appear to focus on the provision of interventions which are technical, managerial and therapeutic in nature. This care is aimed at a range of patient outcomes that include the maintenance and improvement of health and well-being, and the development of coping strategies. There is a core of well-established activities that attempt to prevent further deterioration in the patient's condition, to prevent harm, and to maintain safety that appear to be 'done for' a patient. Nursing also appears to have a patient management function which primarily facilitates the coordination of therapy and services. However, there would also appear to be a range of therapeutic activities that promote an active partnership between the patient and nurse. The focus of this partnership is the achievement of wider outcomes of recovery, including the development of effective strategies that enable patients to deal with the aftermath of stroke. Nursing interventions within this theme would appear to focus principally on education and emotional support.

In summary, nurses can bring a wealth of knowledge and expertise to the development of stroke services, underpinned by their experience in clinical practice. Synthesising theory on the nursing role in stroke services, and some of the policy and practice opportunities emerging in stroke care, identifies some core themes that represent the nursing contribution to stroke service development:

• Care provision to meet physical needs, and prevent harm
• Care management to ensure continuity and an appropriate care environment
• Education and emotional support to facilitate coping and adaptation to the consequences of stroke
• Family and carer engagement

This does not mean that nurses should not engage in other areas of service development, dependent on their individual skills and interests, and the needs of patients and services. However, it does provide a thematic framework to organise the nursing contribution to stroke care.

In recent years, advances in acute stroke care such as thrombolysis are providing opportunities to develop new nursing roles and skills in the early stages of stroke management. These include comprehensive assessment, monitoring and interventions to limit cerebral damage and to enable the administration of thrombolytic therapy where appropriate. An increasing emphasis on primary care has also provided important opportunities for the development of primary and secondary stroke prevention practice. However, there is a need to ensure that refocusing energies on the development of acute nursing care does not militate against sustaining or developing existing components of the nursing role. Studies have consistently demonstrated that practice may still have some way to go in ensuring patients have access to these fundamental aspects of the nursing role.

New nursing roles

The provision of stroke-specific post-registration educational opportunities is limited and variable across regions and between countries. Where these opportunities can be accessed by nurses, specialist qualifications can be obtained. The development of stroke services has, however, provided opportunities for nurses to develop new roles that support the implementation of policy and evidence, including stroke coordinators and nurse consultants. In England, for example, nurse consultants appear to have taken a lead role in the implementation of service models outlined in the National Service Framework for Older People (Burton et al. 2009).

In the UK, nurses operating at a consultant level have been charged with addressing four core role domains: expert clinical practice; leadership and consultancy; education and training; and service development, research and evaluation (Department of Health 1999). In stroke, health care policy has presented the opportunity for nurse consultants to focus on the development of stroke services. Whilst this is an important success, preoccupation with policy implementation may limit the scope for this role in development of professional nursing knowledge. Importantly, it would appear that reorganisation of stroke services has provided stroke nurse consultants with an opportunity to develop new components of the service, such as nutrition management, which build and expand the nursing role (Burton et al. 2009).

However, development of stroke-specific nursing roles is not uncontested: there may be an advantage for nurses in stroke care to be specialists but with generalist knowledge and skills. Stroke is rarely a simple disease and often coexists with complex pathology and a diverse range of social, psychological and environmental factors. A specialist component of nursing in this situation may relate to the ability of the nurse to work with this complexity, drawing on a wider range of knowledge and expertise. In any case, it is apparent that stroke services provide considerable opportunities for both students and registered nurses to develop their knowledge and range of skills.

As in many aspects of UK health services, the development of new nursing roles, and opportunities for professional development, means that nurses are taking on activities traditionally performed by others, and are developing new roles to deliver new interventions and services. For example, considerable work has been undertaken in the development of interprofessional competences for the management of post-stroke dysphagia (Boaden et al. 2006). The nursing role in this is not uncontested, however. It would be churlish not to acknowledge the potential benefits these developments may bring to patients by reducing waiting times for swallowing assessments and increased patient safety at mealtimes due to enhanced skills in the nursing workforce. This may strengthen the contribution of nurses to service development in the short term, but in the long term does not ensure that the values and expertise that nurses bring to service development are safeguarded for the future.

The drive to increase the specialist nature of stroke nursing must therefore be balanced with the recognition of the importance of essential, generalist care for patients and families. Ultimately, this may define the perceived quality of the overall stroke service. To do this, we need to articulate the focus of nursing care rather than individual interventions, highlighting the broad issues for which nurses have a special affinity. These should reflect the theories that nurses espouse such as holistic family-centred care, partnership working and therapeutic communication. We need to ensure that these issues feature overtly in our consideration of the direct and indirect consequences of current and future role developments.

Developing acute stroke nursing

It has been clearly demonstrated that organising patient care within specialist stroke units provides clear and meaningful benefits for patients, including lower mortality and morbidity (Stroke Unit Trialists' Collaboration 2007). This evidence is now part of the underpinning recommendations for the delivery of UK stroke services in the *National Clinical Guidelines for Stroke* (Intercollegiate Stroke Working Party 2008a) and national stroke strategies (e.g. Department of Health 2007; Welsh Assembly Government 2006). Encouragingly, there has been a steady increase in the proportion of hospitals in England that have stroke units from 75% in 2001, to 84% in 2004, to 96% in 2008 (Intercollegiate Stroke Working Party 2008c).

To date there is limited evidence to indicate why or how stroke units are effective, which makes it difficult for effective implementation in a local context. There are, for example, no nationally accepted minimum standards for what constitutes a 'stroke unit', although there are classifications based on broad types of services. A pragmatic approach was adopted by the British Association of Stroke Physicians in 2005 (see http://www.basp.ac.uk/LinkClick.aspx ?fileticket=h6zszwmXQfk%3D&tabid=653&mid=1053&language=en-GB) in designation of three levels of stroke unit, differentiated by the availability of specialist staff and resources to deliver aspects of acute stroke care. A similar approach was taken in Australia (National Stroke Foundation 2007), producing a four-category classification. The Brain Attack coalition in the US, however, took a somewhat different approach in making consensus recommendations for constituents of a Comprehensive Stroke Center (Alberts et al. 2005). Ideally, however, the development or the redesignation of a stroke unit requires considerable planning and support, including amongst other things, specialist resources and training and development for staff. Conceptual clarity about what constitutes a stroke unit is therefore urgently required.

Based on a review of stroke unit trials (Langhorne & Pollock 2002), six features that characterise stroke units have been identified, as follows:

- Comprehensive assessment of medical problems, impairments and disabilities
- Active physiological management
- Early mobilisation and the avoidance of bed-rest
- Early setting of rehabilitation plans involving carers
- Early assessment and planning of discharge needs
- Skilled nursing care

The term 'skilled nursing care' is not further defined and there is little empirical research in the literature identifying exactly what nurses are skilled in. For example, nursing has often ascribed itself specialist status in skin care and the management of incontinence. However, the evidence to support these elements as exclusively or particularly nursing roles is somewhat limited.

Increasing numbers of admissions to stroke units, and increased proportions of hospital-stay spent within them, will inevitably increase the overall workload of stroke nursing. Further, there is little to indicate optimal nurse to patient ratios in relation to nurse-sensitive patient outcomes. In the absence of established evidence-based workload models for stroke unit nursing, the UK National Stroke Nursing Forum published a position statement on staffing, based on expert opinion and extrapolation from the wider literature on nursing staffing. This recommends one nurse to every two acute stroke patients in the first 36 hours, and a general staffing profile of 12.5 Whole Time Equivalent nurses for every 10 beds, excluding ward management and administration staff.

The political agenda shaping stroke service development

Successful service development depends on various factors, including the fit between health and social care strategy, and development plans being considered at a local level. There are many drivers for change, including a professional sense of obligation to improve the experience of service users. Ensuring a synergy of the priorities between professionals and those who develop and implement public policy and service commissioners is likely to maximise success. Whilst there are some differences between the policy contexts of the four UK countries, and between Western countries more broadly, core themes include:

- Maximising efficiency and effectiveness
- Encouraging integrated working across professional groups and organisations
- Building capacity in primary health care and community-based services, and
- More priority to the expectations and preferences of service users

Initiatives that access a wide variety of sources of support, and that make best use of available resources are most likely to succeed.

Stroke strategy

Stroke services in the United Kingdom are experiencing a period of unprecedented change, driven by a wide range of health policies and national reviews of stroke services. In England these include the National Service Frameworks for Older People and Long Term Conditions (Department of Health 2001, 2005a), the National Audit Office (2005) report *Reducing Brain Damage: Faster Access to Better Stroke Care*. These have culminated in the National Stroke Strategy launched in late 2007 (Department of Health 2007). Chapter 1 provides more detail of these. By providing an indication of how services should be organised and structured across the disease trajectory, the stroke strategy provides nurses with an opportunity to demonstrate how nursing expertise can support its delivery. Whilst the publication of national stroke strategies provides significant impetus and direction for service development, a range of other resources are available to facilitate service development. Although not exhaustive, the following sections provide a brief overview of the some of the most relevant resources.

Access to the evidence base

The National Stroke Strategy provides a synthesis of the evidence base for practice for use in the design of service models, focusing on their structure and organisation rather than content. The National Clinical Guidelines (Intercollegiate Stroke Working Party 2008a), however, provide a complete overview of the existing evidence base for stroke care, integrating syntheses of the evidence with best practice statements together with a service user perspective. Profession-specific summaries of the relevant evidence are available from professional organisations. For nursing, profession-specific guidelines are available from the National Stroke Nursing Forum (http://www.uclan.ac.uk/nsnf) and can be downloaded at http://www.rcplondon.ac.uk/pubs/contents/0bcf7680-7e4b-4cd1-a863-6080efde9a12.pdf. The opportunities and challenges for nursing focus on transformation of guideline recommendations into local practice protocols that reflect local capacity, and influencing the commissioning of research to plug gaps in the evidence base. For example, consider once more the recommendations for palliative care, which are underpinned by consensus and extrapolation from the cancer literature. The clinical contexts of stroke and cancer are obviously very different, particularly for the approximately one-third of patients who die within the first four weeks after stroke (Roberts & Goldacre 2003).

The development of stroke pathways

Stroke patients access a wide variety of support and services, from formal statutory health and social care providers to a range of community organisations and the voluntary sector. It may be unsurprising, then, that services can initially seem complex and impenetrable from the perspective of service users. The need for continuity in the provision of stroke services is well documented (e.g. Morris et al. 2007), and a variety of initiatives have been developed to promote smooth transitions between service providers and professionals through enhanced teamwork and communication. The development of stroke pathways at a local level provides a useful opportunity to identify transition points, and plan interventions that adequately prepare patients and family members for the transitions. These interventions are likely to include elements of patient and family support, and liaison between services; these have been incorporated into specialist nursing roles with promising results. For example, a clinical trial of specialist nursing outreach, which continued to support patients in the immediate period post transfer from hospital to home, demonstrated a positive benefit in subjective health status (Burton & Gibbon 2005).

Stroke-related competences

Much of the development in stroke care appears to be focused on the 'stroke pathway': what should happen and when, and who should have the competences to do it. For example, the UK organisation Skills for Health provides six competences for stroke care (http://www.skillsforhealth.org.uk/):

- Monitoring individuals diagnosed with stroke
- Responding to the needs of individuals with stroke or TIA
- Assessing individuals' risk of stroke and TIA
- Assessing individuals with suspected stroke or TIA
- Developing management plans for individuals with stroke or TIA
- Implementing interventions for individuals who have had a stroke or TIA

It is worth noting that these frameworks are broad, and provide an indication of general activities rather than specific interventions that should be undertaken. The demonstration of competency requires underpinning knowledge and skills, and access to the evidence base for practice. Any competency framework enables services to make practice explicit, bringing important benefits for the organisation of staff education, training and development. However, what these lack in any meaningful way is the importance of the organisational culture and context of care delivery. For example, how should stroke services be delivered to facilitate satisfaction, acceptability, participation in rehabilitation, adaptation and coping, and a sense of being cared for?

Stroke registers

The benefits of developing a comprehensive stroke register at organisational level are clearly understood, although there is some variation in their content. The collection of routine clinical data on patient and clinical characteristics, service factors and outcomes is particularly useful in monitoring the effectiveness of care, and planning future resource needs. The development of stroke registers also provides nursing with the opportunity to influence the routine collection of data, which can then subsequently be used to inform research questions. For example, stroke nurse consultants have been leading the collection of routine data on post-stroke urinary continence to identify variation in practice, and to explore relevant patient outcomes across different stroke services (French et al. 2007). Such information provides the opportunity to explore the patterns within data, generating research hypotheses for testing.

Stroke audit

Having evidence-based standards for practice in National Clinical Guidelines provides an opportunity to audit the degree to which services meet these standards. In England, Wales and Northern Ireland, the Intercollegiate Stroke Working Party have developed and led the biennial National Stroke Sentinel Audit. This initiative provides an overview of local performance, together with regional and national comparisons, which can be used to highlight priorities for local stroke service and practice development. A similar approach is being led in Australia through clinician representatives at the National Stroke Foundation.

Patient-led services

Internationally, changes in relationships between the public, patients and health care provider organisations are bringing about changes in service orientation. The publication of *Creating a Patient-led NHS* (Department of Health 2005b) intended to refocus the organisation and delivery of health services closer to the needs and aspirations of patients. In stroke, there are a wide range of sources of information about the experiences and expectations of patients. These include an extensive qualitative research literature (e.g. Murray et al. 2003) and internet-based sources (e.g. http://www.dipex.org). The importance of involving patients and carers in the development of stroke services was highlighted in the National Service Framework (Department of Health 2001), although no strategies were identified to demonstrate how this should be done, or what degree of involvement should be attempted. Whilst many attempts reported in the literature are merely consultative, it would appear that more active engagement of services users is possible in, for example, setting priorities for service development and supporting action planning; this is likely to require considerable preparatory work and external facilitation (Jones et al. 2008).

Stroke networks

Delivering the evidence base for stroke care will make considerable demands on services including the capacity and capability within the stroke service itself. Effective delivery will also have consequences for many other health and social care organisations, the voluntary and independent sectors, and other sources of support within community settings that are accessed by those affected by stroke (Department of Health 2007).

In some respects, these challenges have been addressed by providers of services for people with other diagnoses such as cancer and cardiac disease. It would seem sensible to use knowledge and experience from previous work in helping stroke services move forward. In England, stroke has now been incorporated into the cardiac network structure, which has demonstrated considerable success in service development through education, evidence dissemination, service redesign and modernisation. Cardiac networks should be working with local stroke services to identify workforce education and training needs, facilitating the implementation of evidence-based practice through dissemination and service development activities. Whether the success of the cardiac network model can be transferred to stroke will only become evident as networks begin to evaluate their impact on service delivery, and ultimately patient outcomes. The role of networks is also discussed in Chapter 1.

Nursing leadership

Clinical leadership is underpinned by the premise that transformational or facilitative styles of leadership in the workplace empower staff to deliver care of the highest quality (Bass 1990). Whilst the processes and mechanisms that link clinical leadership to patient outcomes are complex, the ability to influence and develop staff and build relationships with other disciplines appears to be crucial (Cunningham & Kitson 2000). Leadership is change and movement focused, and focuses on motivating and inspiring staff to realign their work around a shared strategic direction. It differs from the management role, which is primarily concerned with operational delivery through attention to planning and budgeting, staffing and problem-solving (Kotter 1990).

Most clinical leadership programmes in the UK are generic, and focus predominantly on the leadership skills of the individual participants. They usually include personal assessment and development, action learning, workshops on core leadership issues, mentorship, and a patient perspective through observation of care or patient narratives. However, there are a wide range of specific patient and clinical issues that need to be considered when relating these generic models of clinical leadership development to the context of stroke services. These include:

- The challenge of enabling an environment that promotes patient activation rather than the provision of passive care
- Multi-professional working within the context of modernising services
- Promoting patient motivation and managing negative emotional reaction
- Involving family members in an appropriate level of decision-making
- Dealing with chronic and complex health and social care needs across disciplines and service boundaries
- Managing specific stroke-related care needs such as communication, eating and drinking and the associated needs of dignity and respect

Meaningful consideration of these issues requires a specialist focus that draws on both generalist leadership skills and expert leadership skills developed within the context of stroke patient care.

The Department of Health has provided funds for a leadership programme for nurses and allied health professionals working in stroke services to address these issues. The programme was underpinned by an action learning approach, where participants were provided with a mix of peer support and challenge to take forward developments within their own service. Development priorities were identified through a synthesis of work-based learning activities designed to critically evaluate stroke policy, patient and carer priorities, teamworking, and personal leadership skills and resources to facilitate change.

Conclusion

Nurses have a responsibility for ensuring that the profession responds appropriately to new strategies and emerging evidence for stroke services. In many respects the UK political context of stroke care is one that is likely to be encouraging for some time to come. Consequently, some urgency is required in the development of stroke services to make best use of current opportunities. It is important to recognise that nursing also has a wealth of knowledge about patient care, and experience in the management of change, which will be vital to the success of national stroke strategies.

However, there is also a responsibility to ensure that the drive for evidence and strategy implementation reflects the core role domains and values of nursing. Development of stroke services without development and incorporation of nursing knowledge and practice will sell patients and health care professions short. However, an uncritical approach risks undermining aspects of nursing that are valued by patients and families, and limits the international development of the nursing contribution to stroke care. Development of stroke nursing is an important cornerstone of stroke service development, and this book is part of this process.

References

Alberts, MJ, Latchaw, RE, Selman, WR, Shephard, T, Hadley, MN et al., 2005, Recommendations for comprehensive stroke centers: a consensus statement from the Brain Attack Coalition, *Stroke*, vol. 36, no. 7, pp. 1597–1616.

Bass, BM, 1990, *Bass and Stoghill's Handbook on Leadership Theory, Research and Managerial Applications*, The Free Press, London.

Boaden, E., Davies, S., Storey, L., & Watkins, C, 2006, *Inter-professional Dysphagia Framework*, University of Central Lancashire, Preston.

Burton, CR, 2000, A description of the nursing role in stroke rehabilitation, *Journal of Advanced Nursing*, vol. 32, no. 1, pp. 174–181.

Burton, C, 2003, Therapeutic nursing in stroke rehabilitation: a systematic review, *Clinical Effectiveness in Nursing*, vol. 7, pp. 124–133.

Burton, C, & Gibbon, B, 2005, Expanding the role of the stroke nurse: a pragmatic clinical trial, *Journal of Advanced Nursing*, vol. 52, no. 6, pp. 640–650.

Burton, CR, Bennett, B, & Gibbon, B, 2009, Embedding nursing and therapy consultantship: the case of stroke consultants, *Journal of Clinical Nursing*, vol. 18, no. 2, pp. 246–254.

Cunningham, G, & Kitson, A, 2000, An evaluation of the RCN Clinical Leadership Development Programme: Part 2, *Nursing Standard*, vol. 15, no. 13–15, pp. 34–40.

Department of Health, 1999, *Nurse, Midwife and Health Visitor Consultants: Establishing Posts and Making Appointments (HSC 1999/217)*, The Stationery Office, London.

Department of Health, 2001, *The National Service Framework for Older People*, Department of Health, London.

Department of Health, 2005a, *The National Service Framework for Long Term Conditions*, Department of Health, London.

Department of Health, 2005b, *Creating a Patient-led NHS – Delivering the NHS Improvement Plan*, Department of Health, London.

Department of Health, 2007, *National Stroke Strategy*, Department of Health, London.

French, B., Burton, C., & Thomas, LH, 2007, *Incontinence After Stroke: Collaboration on Minimum Data Set Construction by a National Network of Nurse Consultants*, Nursing Communication in Multidisciplinary Practice: Proceedings of the 6th European Conference of Acendio, Oud Consultancy, Amsterdam.

Gibbon, B, 1999, An investigation of interprofessional collaboration in stroke rehabilitation team conferences, *Journal of Clinical Nursing*, vol. 8, no. 3, pp. 246–252.

Grimshaw, JM, Thomas, RE, Maclennan, G, Fraser, C, Ramsay, CR et al., 2004, Effectiveness and efficiency of guideline dissemination and implementation strategies, *Health Technology Assessment*, vol. 8, no. 6.

Henderson, VA, 1980, Preserving the essence of nursing in a technological age, *Journal of Advanced Nursing*, vol. 5, no. 3, pp. 245–260.

Intercollegiate Stroke Working Party, 2007, *National Sentinel Stroke Audit: Phase I (Organisational Audit) 2006: Phase II (Clinical audit) 2006*, Royal College of Physicians, London.

Intercollegiate Stroke Working Party, 2008a, *National Clinical Guidelines for Stroke*, 3rd edn, Royal College of Physicians, London.

Intercollegiate Stroke Working Party, 2008b, *National Sentinel Audit for Stoke 2008. National and Local Results for the Process of Stroke Care Audit 2008*, Royal College of Physicians, London.

Intercollegiate Stroke Working Party, 2008c, *National Sentinel Stroke Audit. Phase 1 Organisational audit 2008. Report for England, Wales and Northern Ireland*, Royal College of Physicians, London.

Jamtvedt, G, Young, JM, Kristoffersen, DT, O'Brien, MA, & Oxman, AD, 2006, *Audit and feedback: effects on professional practice and health care outcomes*, Cochrane Database, Issue 2, Art. No. CD000259.

Jones, SP, Auton, MF, Burton, CR, & Watkins, CL, 2008, Engaging service users in the development of stroke services: an action research study, *Journal of Clinical Nursing*, vol. 17, no. 10, pp. 1270–1279.

Kirkevold, M, 1992, Balancing values and norms in the nursing care of stroke patients, *Rehabilitation Nursing Research*, vol. 1, pp. 24–33.

Kirkevold, M, 1997, The role of nursing in the rehabilitation of acute stroke patients: toward a unified theoretical perspective, *Advances in Nursing Science*, vol. 19, no. 4, pp. 55–64.

Kotter, JP, 1990, *A force for change: How leadership differs from management*, Free Press, New York.

Langhorne, P, & Pollock, A, 2002, What are the components of effective stroke unit care? *Age and Ageing*, vol. 31, no. 5, pp. 365–371.

Manley, K, & McCormack, B, 2003, Practice development: purpose, methodology, facilitation and evaluation, *Nursing in Critical Care*, vol. 8, no. 1, pp. 22–29.

Morris, R, Payne, O, & Lambert, A, 2007, Patient, carer and staff experience of a hospital-based stroke service, *International Journal for Quality in Health Care*, vol. 19, no. 2, pp. 105–112.

Murray, J, Ashworth, R, Forster, A, & Young, J, 2003, Developing a primary care-based stroke service: a review of the qualitative literature, *British Journal of General Practice*, vol. 53, no. 487, pp. 137–142.

National Audit Office, 2005, *Reducing Brain Damage: Faster Access to Better Stroke Care*, The Stationery Office, London.

National Stroke Foundation, 2007, *National Stroke Audit Organisational Report: Acute Services*, National Stroke Foundation, Melbourne.

O'Connor, SE, 1993, Nursing and rehabilitation: the interventions of nurses in stroke patient care, *Journal of Clinical Nursing*, vol. 2, pp. 29–34.

Pennington, L, Roddam, H, Burton, C, Russell, I, Godfrey, C et al., 2005, Promoting research use in speech and language therapy: a cluster randomized controlled trial to compare the clinical effectiveness and costs of two training strategies, *Clinical Rehabilitation*, vol. 19, no. 4, pp. 387–397.

Roberts, SE, & Goldacre, MJ. 2003, Case fatality rates after admission to hospital with stroke: linked database study, *British Medical Journal*, vol. 326, no. 7382, pp. 193–194.

Rycroft-Malone, J, Seers, K, Titchen, A, Harvey, G, Kitson, A et al., 2004, What counts as evidence in evidence-based practice? *Journal of Advanced Nursing*, vol. 47, no. 1, pp. 81–90.

Stroke Unit Trialists' Collaboration, 2007, *Organised inpatient (stroke unit) care for stroke (Cochrane Review)*, Oxford, Issue 4, Art No: CD000197, Cochrane Database of Systematic Reviews.

Waters, KR, 1987, The role of nursing in rehabilitation care, *Science and Practice*, vol. 5, pp. 17–21.

Welsh Assembly Government, 2006, *National Service Framework for Older People in Wales*, Welsh Assembly Government, Cardiff.

Chapter 3

What is a stroke?

Anne W. Alexandrov

Key points

- Stroke is common and complex neurovascular disease, which makes it an important public health issue and a healthcare professional priority topic.
- Given the complexity of the disease, the variety of ways it can present, and the differences between treatment regimes for best outcomes of different types of stroke, it is essential that all clinical staff involved with stroke have a thorough understanding of its underpinning anatomy, physiology and disease processes.
- This chapter details neurological examinations and tools to support stroke assessment.

Stroke is fascinating, it's so complicated; you name it, a stroke patient can have problems with it. Stroke patients used to be, you know, needed a lot of care but we couldn't do much else. All that has changed. Now, we're learning so much more about it, and about the possibilities, and developing new treatments and ways to deliver these. It's an exciting place to work.

(Stroke specialist nurse, New South Wales)

Introduction

As the third most common cause of death and a leading cause of adult disability in most countries, stroke is an important neurovascular disease. This chapter provides an overview of the processes entailed in development of a stroke, the relevant normal neurological anatomy and physiology, and the neurovascular clinical examination used to identify stroke.

Stroke development processes

Stroke is broadly divided into two main categories: ischaemic infarction and intracerebral haemorrhage. Ischaemic stroke is by far the commonest, accounting for approximately 70% or more of stroke events (Adams et al. 2007). It is defined as a rapidly evolving syndrome of sudden onset, with a non-epileptic neurological deficit associated with a well-circumscribed volume of infarcted brain tissue within a discrete vascular territory. The original World Health Organisation definition of stroke differentiated ischaemic stroke from transient ischaemic attack (TIA) by the development of infarction, in terms of signs or symptoms enduring beyond 24 hours. However, as infarction may be clinically silent (that is, there may be no lasting signs or symptoms) in TIA, many practitioners favour a tissue-based definition consisting of a negative magnetic resonance imaging diffusion-weighted imaging sequence to definitively differentiate acute ischaemic stroke from TIA. Many clinicians prefer to talk in terms of acute stroke syndrome, rather than differentiate between TIA and stroke, and UK guidelines consider that using 'brain attack' to describe any neurovascular event, 'may be a clearer and less ambiguous term to use' (National Collaborating Centre for Chronic Conditions 2008).

When blood flow to an area is disrupted through occlusion of blood vessels, two major zones of injury develop: the core ischaemic zone and the 'ischaemic penumbra'. In the core zone, very low blood flow means oxygen and glucose supply is inadequate and stores are rapidly depleted. This results in the death of brain cells (neurons and supporting glial cells) within this area. Between this core area and the tissue that is normally perfused there lies a rim, or band, of mild to moderately ischaemic tissue, which may remain viable for some hours. In this 'ischaemic penumbra' blood is still able to flow through collateral arteries linking with branches of the occluded vessels. This is a time-limited process, and cells in the penumbra will die if reperfusion is not established within hours because collateral circulation is not adequate to meet cellular oxygen and glucose requirements in the long term.

Ischaemic stroke develops through a number of mechanisms and the TOAST classification is probably the most common method of categorisation. This system was developed for the Trial of Org 10172 (Danaparoid) in **Acute Stroke Treatment** – TOAST (Adams et al. 1993) and consists of the following subcategories of stroke mechanism for ischaemic stroke.

Large artery atherosclerosis

There is significant (greater than 50%) stenosis (or narrowing) of a major brain artery or cortical branch artery presumably due to atherosclerosis, with infarct size generally greater than 1.5 cm. Within this category mechanisms resulting in stroke include intracranial thrombosis as well as intra- and extracranial artery to artery embolisation, such as that occurring with rupture of a carotid plaque. Clinical findings of this type of ischaemic stroke include impairments following damage occurring in cortical, brainstem or cerebellar locations. Patients with this stroke mechanism often demonstrate evidence of widespread atherosclerotic disease, such as intermittent claudication, coronary artery disease, extracranial carotid stenosis and/or TIA occurring in the same vascular territory. For this categorisation, there should not be any indication of a cardioembolic mechanism (Adams et al. 1993). In the Stroke Data Bank of the US National Institute of Neurological Disorders and Stroke (NINDS), large artery atherosclerosis was responsible for about 6% of strokes, with another 4% categorised as tandem artery occlusions (Foulkes et al. 1988).

Cardioembolism

This mechanism produces a stroke as a result of emboli that arise from within the heart. At least one cardiac source must be identified to use this classification, and large artery atherosclerosis must be ruled out; that is, the categories of large artery atherosclerosis and cardioembolism are mutually exclusive (Adams et al. 1993). Conditions associated with cardioembolism are listed in Table 3.1. Patients with cardioembolic stroke may have evidence of multiple brain emboli over a period of time. About 14% of NINDS Stroke Data Bank patients were classified as having cardioembolic stroke (Foulkes et al. 1988).

Table 3.1 Conditions associated with cardioembolic stroke.

High-risk sources	Medium-risk sources
Mechanical prosthetic valves	Mitral valve prolapse
Mitral stenosis with atrial fibrillation	Mitral annulus calcification
Atrial fibrillation	Mitral stenosis without atrial fibrillation
Left atrial/atrial appendage thrombus	Left atrial turbulence
Sick sinus syndrome	Atrial septal aneurysm
Recent myocardial infarction (<4 weeks)	Patent foramen ovale
Left ventricular thrombus	Atrial flutter
Dilated cardiomyopathy	Lone atrial fibrillation
Akinetic left ventricular segment	Bioprosthetic cardiac valve
Atrial myxoma	Non-bacterial thrombotic endocarditis
Infective endocarditis	Congestive heart failure
	Hypokinetic left ventricular segment
	Myocardial infarction (>4 weeks, <6 months)

Small vessel occlusion

This type of stroke is commonly referred to as a lacunar stroke. Originally thought to be caused exclusively by lipohyalinosis (small vessel disease with deposits of eosinophilic cells within the vessel walls), small vessel occlusion secondary to atherosclerosis is now considered to be a common mechanism. Patients with lacunar stroke present with symptoms that include pure sensory or motor dysfunction, or combined sensory and/or motor findings. Such strokes usually occur in the subcortex and brainstem, and these patients often have long-standing hypertension, diabetes, hyperlipidaemia and/or are smokers (Adams et al. 1993). In the NINDS Stroke Data Bank, 19% of stroke patients were classified as having small vessel occlusions (Foulkes et al. 1988).

Stroke of other determined aetiology

This category includes unusual stroke mechanisms such as non-atherosclerotic vasculopathies, hypercoagulable states, haematological disorders, arterial dissections, venous thrombosis, cocaine or other illegal drug-associated cause, and unusual embolic sources (iatrogenic gas or small particles; neoplasms, parasites, fat). Stroke location and size varies depending on the associated cause, and cardiac embolism and large artery atherosclerotic lesions must be ruled out (Adams et al. 1993).

Stroke of undetermined aetiology

This classification of stroke mechanism, which is also called 'cryptogenic' stroke, is reserved for patients in whom no aetiological factor can be identified, patients with incomplete aetiological work-up, or patients with more than one contributing aetiological factor (Adams et al. 1993). Because determination of stroke mechanism can be challenging, not surprisingly, in the NINDS Stroke Data Bank, 28% of patients fell into this TOAST category (Foulkes et al. 1988). Patients with occult right-to-left intrathoracic vascular shunts may mistakenly be placed into this category when a thorough work-up is not performed. For example, patent foramen ovale (PFO) was identified in 50–56% of young stroke patients previously diagnosed with cryptogenic stroke (Cabanes et al. 1993; Lechat et al. 1989; Webster et al. 1988), resulting in recategorisation as cardioembolism.

Stroke due to haemorrhage

Haemorrhage typically constitutes less than 30% of stroke events (Broderick et al. 2007; Foulkes et al. 1988). Intraparenchymal haemorrhage (IPH, also referred to as intracerebral haemorrhage – ICH) associated with hypertensive emergency is the most frequently encountered form of haemorrhagic stroke.

Less commonly, IPH may result from amyloid angiopathy (most common in older persons) or rupture of an arteriovenous malformation or aneurysm. Sub-arachnoid haemorrhage resulting from rupture of an intracranial aneurysm is a less common, but important cause of haemorrhagic stroke, with the Asian population carrying the highest reported incidence of this worldwide (Johnston et al. 2002).

Risk factors for stroke

Stroke is a vascular disease carrying a similar set of risk factors to those recognised for cardiovascular disease. Risk factors can be classified as non-modifiable and modifiable (Goldstein et al. 2006). Non-modifiable stroke risk factors are characteristics which patients cannot change, including age, low birth weight, race-ethnicity and genetic factors. Modifiable risk factors can be broken into first and second tier factors. The first tier modifiable stroke risk factors in order of importance include hypertension, diabetes mellitus, cigarette smoking, atrial fibrillation and left ventricular dysfunction. Within this first tier, hypertension, diabetes and cigarette smoking contribute to about 50% of the total risk for stroke compared to other factors, making these the three most important areas for stroke prevention. Second tier risk factors include hyperlipidaemia, asymptomatic carotid stenosis, sickle cell disease, oestrogen replacement therapy, diet, obesity and body fat distribution, alcohol and/or drug abuse, sleep-disordered breathing, migraine and hypercoagulable states. Many second tier risk factors are associated with development of first tier risk factors; for example, obesity is a risk factor for both hypertension and diabetes. This indicates need for vigilant management of all contributing risk factors to prevent first-ever or secondary stroke. More on risk factor management can be found in Chapter 13.

Anatomy, physiology and related stroke clinical findings

The brain and spinal cord make up the central nervous system (CNS) and are among the most delicate organs of the body. Structural protection is provided to these structures because of their importance in the control of all human body systems. The skull forms a non-expanding, rigid bony vault that holds the brain, with one large opening at its base called the foramen magnum through which the brainstem projects and connects to the spinal cord (Standring 2004). Because the cranium cannot expand in size in adults, an increase in brain tissue (e.g. due to oedema), cerebrospinal fluid (CSF) or blood collection (e.g. haematoma) will result in compression of the brain, and an increase in intracranial pressure if treatment is not available quickly.

The meninges lie just beneath the skull and vertebral column, and consist of three layers, the dura mater, arachnoid mater and pia mater. The dura mater makes up the outermost layer of meninges; the term 'dura' in Latin means 'tough'. This layer supports the brain and spinal cord, holding nerves and blood vessels in place (Standring 2004; Waxman 2000). Within the double layers of the dura mater are venous sinuses that collect blood drained from intracranial and meningeal veins for return to the systemic venous circuit via the internal jugular veins (Standring 2004). Within the cranium four extensions of the dura mater provide direct support for brain structures and separate specific areas of the brain:

- The falx cerebri vertically divides the right and left hemispheres of the brain from the frontal to the occipital lobe.
- The tentorium cerebelli forms a tent-like extension between the occipital lobes and the cerebellum, separating the cerebrum from the brainstem and cerebellum. Brain structures located above the tentorium cerebelli are commonly called 'supratentorial', with those below the tentorium referred to as 'infratentorial', making up a region of the brain often called the posterior fossa.
- The falx cerebelli divides the two lobes of the cerebellum.
- The diaphragma sellae creates a roof-like covering for the sella turcica, which houses the pituitary gland (Standring 2004; Waxman 2000).

The arachnoid mater lies directly under the dura mater, with the area between these two meninges considered a 'potential space', containing a large number of unsupported small veins. These can tear during traumatic impact, resulting in development of a subdural haematoma (Standring 2004). The arachnoid is a delicate membrane with fine threads of elastic tissue called trabeculae connecting the arachnoid to the pia mater, creating a web-like structure called the subarachnoid space. Large arteries are carefully bound by trabeculae to the surface of the brain from the point at which they enter the skull (Standring 2004; Waxman 2000). Within the subarachnoid space, CSF freely circulates; rupture of an intracranial artery within the subarachnoid space causes blood and CSF to mix, and is referred to as subarachnoid haemorrhage. CSF is absorbed into arachnoid villi, membranous tufts that project into the superior sagittal and transverse venous sinuses and provide conduits into the venous system. Because the normal adult produces approximately 20 ml of CSF per hour, arachnoid villi reabsorption is largely driven by increased hydrostatic pressure within the subarachnoid space as CSF volume continuously builds. Should these delicate structures become obstructed with blood, as in subarachnoid haemorrhage, reabsorption may be significantly impacted resulting in an increase in CSF over time, commonly referred to as communicating hydrocephalus (Standring 2004).

The pia mater adheres directly to brain and spinal cord tissue, following all the folds and convolutions of the CNS surface. The pia is rich in small blood vessels that supply a large volume of arterial blood to the CNS. Within the lateral, third and fourth ventricles, tufts of pia mater form a portion of the choroid plexus, responsible for CSF production (Standring 2004; Waxman 2000).

Four CSF-filled canals lined with ependymal cells make up the ventricular system (see Figure 3.1). At the uppermost part of the system, two lateral ven-

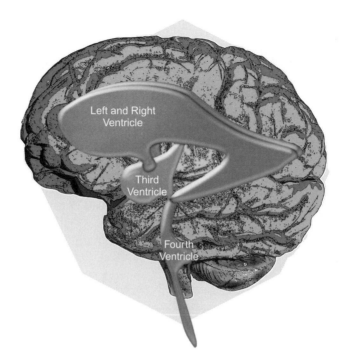

Figure 3.1 The ventricular system. Reproduced with permission of Stephen DiBiase Designs.

tricles extend from the frontal to the occipital lobes (Standring 2004; Waxman 2000). The right lateral ventricle is commonly the site for cannulation when CSF drainage by ventriculostomy or shunt, and/or intracranial pressure monitoring is required. The two lateral ventricles are connected by the foramen of Monro to the third ventricle, which lies directly above the midbrain of the brainstem. The aqueduct of Sylvius, or cerebral aqueduct, connects the third with the fourth ventricle, which is located between the brainstem and the cerebellum. Two openings at the base of the fourth ventricle, the foramina of Luschka and Magendie, open into the subarachnoid space (Standring 2004). Blockage of the CSF flow within the ventricular system, which may develop from a cerebellar infarct with oedema formation, is called a non-communicating hydrocephalus. Normal circulation of CSF is prevented, causing dilation of the ventricles from trapped CSF, and increased intracranial pressure (Waxman 2000).

The ventricular system and subarachnoid space are filled with CSF, which protects the CNS through a 'shock absorbing' mechanism during traumatic injury. While not well understood, it probably also plays a role in providing glucose to nourish neurons. CSF flows from the lateral ventricles, through the foramen of Monro into the third ventricle, through the cerebral aqueduct into the fourth ventricle, and out of the foramen of Magendie and the foramina of Luschka into the subarachnoid space of the brain and spinal cord; see Table 3.2 (Standring 2004; Waxman 2000).

Table 3.2 Composition of cerebrospinal fluid (CSF).

CSF Characteristics and components	Normal values
pH	7.35 to 7.45
Appearance	Clear and colourless
Specific gravity	1.007
Total volume	135 to 150 ml
Pressure:	
• Lumbar	70 to 200 cmH$_2$O
• Intraventricular	0 to 15 mmHg
Cell content:	
• White blood cells	0
• Red blood cells	0
• Lymphocytes	0–10
Glucose	50 to 75 mg/dl; typically 66% of blood glucose
Protein	5 to 25 mg/dl

Arterial circulation

The brain makes up only 2% of the body's weight but uses approximately 20% of resting cardiac output to maintain its vital functions. It requires approximately 750 ml of blood flow per minute, extracting up to 45% of arterial oxygen to meet normal metabolic needs (Alexandrov 2003; Standring 2004). There are no reserves of either oxygen or glucose in the brain, so disruption of arterial blood flow dramatically affects normal cellular function. Two pairs of arteries, the internal carotids and the vertebral arteries, provide blood to the brain; these pairs comprise the anterior and posterior circulations, and are connected at the base of the brain to form the circle of Willis (see Figure 3.2) (Alexandrov 2003; Standring 2004). Arterial distribution for the brain is illustrated in Figure 3.3.

The anterior circulation derives from the right and left internal carotid arteries and their branches. Originating as the common carotids, the left common carotid takes off from the arch of the aorta, and the right common carotid from the innominate artery. The common carotid splits at the level of the cricothyroid junction to form the external and internal carotid arteries, with the face, scalp and skull fed by branches of the external carotid artery. The internal carotid artery (ICA) enters the base of the skull through an opening in the petrous bone. The ICA gives off the right and left middle cerebral arteries (MCAs), the right and left anterior cerebral arteries (ACAs) that are connected by the anterior communicating artery (AcomA), and the two posterior communicating arteries – PcomAs (Alexandrov 2003). Eighty per cent of blood flow to the cerebral hemispheres is provided by the anterior circulation, includ-

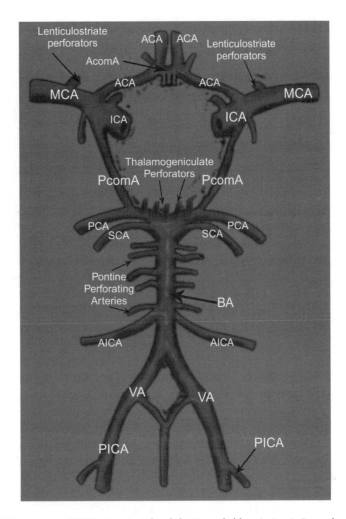

Figure 3.2 The circle of Willis (see text for definition of abbreviations). Reproduced with permission of Stephen DiBiase Designs.

ing to the frontal lobes, most of the parietal and temporal lobes and subcortical structures located above the brainstem (Alexandrov 2003; Mohr et al. 2004; Standring 2004). The ophthalmic artery (OA) is also derived from the ICA just before it divides into the ACA and MCA. The OA supplies blood to the optic nerve and eye; if the ICA is occluded, the OA may reverse its course to supplement the anterior circulation's arterial blood volume (Alexandrov 2003).

The posterior circulation is derived from the two vertebral arteries (VA), which originate from the subclavian arteries and travel posteriorly through small openings in the lateral spinous processes of the cervical spine. The VAs enter the skull through the foramen magnum; at the level of the pons, the VAs fuse to form the basilar artery (BA). Two important arterial branches are derived from the terminal portion of the VAs prior to their fusion into the BA, namely, the posterior inferior cerebellar arteries (PICAs). The BA gives rise to two major infratentorial branches, the anterior inferior cerebellar arteries

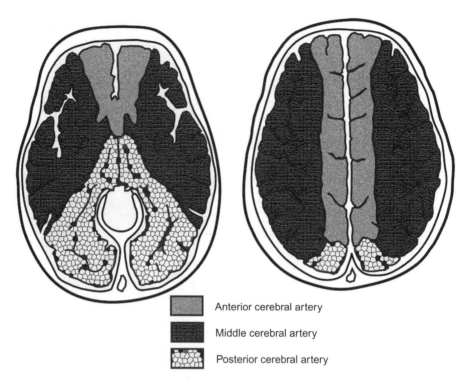

Figure 3.3 Arterial distribution for the brain. Reproduced with permission of Stephen DiBiase Designs.

(AICAs) and superior cerebellar arteries (SCAs); along with the PICAs, these arteries supply blood to the cerebellum. The distal BA gives off the two posterior cerebral arteries (PCAs) that supply the posterior regions of the cerebral cortex (Alexandrov 2003; Standring 2004).

The circle of Willis (Figure 3.2) is a unique vascular supply system made up of the major branches of the anterior and posterior circulation. Each side of the anterior circulation is connected by the AcomA which lies between the two ACAs; the posterior circulation is connected to the anterior circulation by the two PcomAs (Standring 2004). Approximately 50% of the population has a complete circle of Willis; atretic (small, non-functional or hypoplastic) segments are common, however, and are often found in the A1 branch of the ACAs, the P1 branch of the PCAs, and the posterior communicating arteries (Alexandrov 2003). When the circle of Willis is complete, it can support a degree of collateral blood flow if an artery is occluded, although sufficient arterial blood supply is not guaranteed.

Venous circulation

The brain's venous drainage occurs through venous sinuses, many housed in the dura mater. Brain capillaries drain blood into venules, which connect to cerebral veins and ultimately empty blood into venous sinuses. The sinuses empty blood into the internal jugular veins, which in turn empty into the superior vena cava. The brain's veins have relatively thinner walls than veins in the general circulation, lacking a muscular layer or valves (Standring 2004).

Cerebrum

The cerebrum comprises 80% of the brain's weight (Standring 2004) and is composed of right and left hemispheres separated by the longitudinal fissure and connected at the base by the corpus callosum. The cerebral cortex makes up the outer aspect, consisting of grey matter that constitutes neuronal cell bodies. White matter lies directly below the cerebral cortex in what is referred to as the subcortical region, consisting of the myelinated axons of the cortex's neurons, which communicate impulses from neuronal cell bodies to other areas of the CNS.

The cerebrum has four anatomical divisions: the frontal, parietal, temporal and occipital lobes. A fifth lobe is sometimes listed, called the rhinencephalon or limbic lobe, although others see this structure deep within the cerebrum as anatomically associated with the temporal lobe (Gloor 1997; Standring 2004). The cerebral cortex's primary functions include intellect, language, sensory and motor functions (Standring 2004). Cerebral cortical cell architecture was classified in 1909 by Brodmann, who identified more than 100 unique areas of specialised cortical function (Figure 3.4). The functions within Brodmann's classification that are commonly assessed by nurses are presented below within each section detailing the lobes of the cerebrum.

Frontal lobes

These lie beneath the frontal bone, are separated from the parietal lobe posteriorly by the central sulcus (fissure of Rolando), and from the temporal lobe inferiorly by the lateral fissure (Sylvian fissure). The frontal lobes' major functions include cognitive function (orientation, memory, insight, judgement, arithmetic and abstraction), expressive language (verbal and written), and voluntary motor function.

- *Cognition* is controlled in Brodmann's areas 9 to 12 (ACA territory), in the prefrontal cortex, located just behind the forehead (Mohr et al. 2004; Standring 2004); this region focuses on intellectual appraisal and response to environmental stimuli. Intellectual capacity is blended with socially learned and accepted emotional responses and practices; autonomic nervous system responses, such as tachycardia in relation to perceived threats, are also triggered in this brain area. Injury here may dramatically alter intellectual capacity and social responses to environmental stimuli, profoundly affecting quality of life.
- *Expressive language* is housed in Brodmann's area 44 (MCA territory), also called Broca's area. This region is located in the inferior frontal gyrus close

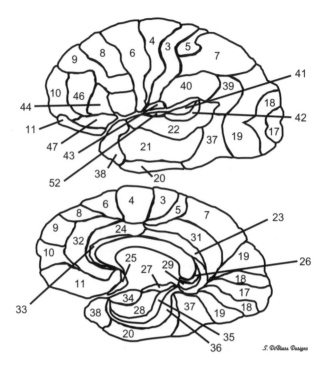

Figure 3.4 Brodmann areas of the cortex, numbered according to Brodmann's original plan; numbers missing in this series are 13–16 and 48–51. Brodmann's original plan does not specify these locations clearly. Reproduced with permission of Stephen DiBiase Designs.

to the motor strip's facial distribution. It is on the left side of the frontal lobe in most people, designating the left hemisphere as dominant in function, although occasionally it may be located in the right frontal hemisphere (Mohr et al. 2004; Standring 2004). Broca's area is responsible for formation of both verbal and written communication. Injury to this area of the brain results in disability ranging from word-finding difficulties to an expressive or non-fluent aphasia with significant compromise to verbal and written communication.

- *Voluntary (pyramidal) motor function* is controlled in Brodmann's area 4 (MCA territory), which is also called the motor strip. Because most voluntary motor tracts cross over to the opposite side as they descend through the brainstem, the right motor strip represents voluntary motor function for the left side of the body and vice versa (Mohr et al. 2004; Standring 2004). Figure 3.5 represents a graphic called the motor homunculus that is commonly used to depict the layout of motor function in area 4. The homunculus appears as an upside-down man; the foot of the homunculus is illustrated on the superior medial aspects of the frontal lobes, with the knees, hips, trunk and shoulders extending along the lateral surfaces, and the hands, thumb, head, face and tongue represented in a lateral inferior distribution extending to the Sylvian fissure. The larger the areas illustrated on the homunculus, the greater the amount of frontal cortex dedicated to the par-

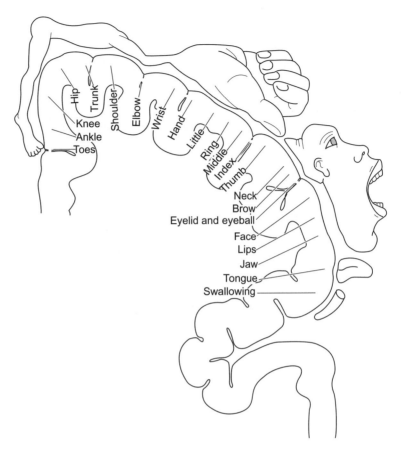

Figure 3.5 Motor homunculus. Reproduced from Patestas & Garter, *A Textbook of Neuroanatomy* 2nd Edition, copyright 2007 with permission of Blackwell Publishing.

ticular motor function (Standring 2004). For example, the hands require significantly more motor control than the trunk of the body and are therefore represented by a larger graphical distribution on the homunculus. When the motor strip is damaged by stroke or injury, motor function on the opposite side of the body is impaired. Table 3.3 summarises the clinical examination techniques used to assess frontal lobe function.

Parietal lobe

The parietal lobes are situated posterior to the frontal lobe on the opposite side of the central sulcus. Posteriorly, the parieto-occipital fissure separates the parietal lobe from the occipital lobe. The primary function of the parietal lobes is integration of sensory stimuli such as awareness of body parts and their positioning, recognition of the size, shape and texture of objects, and interpretation of touch, pressure and pain.

Similar to the frontal lobe's motor strip, the parietal lobe contains a sensory strip (Brodmann's areas 1, 2 and 3; MCA territory) that is also organised in

Table 3.3 Frontal lobe function examination techniques.

Brodmann's area	Arterial territory	Related clinical examination
9, 10, 11, 12	Anterior cerebral artery	Orientation to time, place and person Short- and long-term memory Cognitive insight Judgement, decision-making ability Abstract processes (e.g. spell a word backwards) and arithmetic (e.g. subtract 7 from 100, five times)
4	Middle cerebral artery	Grade motor function on a scale from 0 (absent) to 5 (normal): • 0/5 = No movement • 1/5 = Flicker of movement • 2/5 = Cannot overcome gravity • 3/5 = Cannot overcome resistance • 4/5 = Weak power • 5/5 = Normal power Arm pronator drift Deep and superficial tendon reflexes Speech articulation Facial expression testing (CN VII – motor component) Clench teeth (CN V – motor component mandibular branch) Dysphagia testing
44	Middle cerebral artery	Expressive language; word finding difficulties; fluency of language

the layout of a sensory homunculus, or upside-down man (Figures 3.5 and 3.6), representing those areas that receive and analyse sensory information from different areas of the body. These areas are concerned with both deep and internal sensations as well as cutaneous sensations such as touch, with sites of greater sensory need occupying larger areas on the sensory strip (Standring 2004). When injury occurs to this site, sensory loss or alteration on the opposite side of the body results.

Brodmann's areas 5 and 7 (MCA territory) are considered associative areas that further assess sensory stimuli to determine the precise purpose, relevance and importance of sensory data. This area is concerned with awareness of body parts, perceptual orientation in space, and recognition of environmental spatial relationships (Standring 2004). When injury occurs in these areas, perceptual neglect or inattention may occur (Mohr et al. 2004; Standring 2004).

Brodmann's area 22 (MCA territory) is also called Wernicke's area. Most commonly located on the left side of the cerebral cortex, it is concerned with reception of both written and verbal language. It is intricately connected to other parts of the brain concerned with auditory and visual functions, as well as cognitive appraisal, emotion and ultimately expressive language (Standring 2004). When this area is injured, disability ranging from minor receptive language dysfunction to receptive or fluent aphasia is likely. Those with receptive aphasia retain the ability to produce language, but its content is illogical, described as 'word salad'. When brain injury includes areas responsible for both expression (Broca's) and reception (Wernicke's) of language, a global

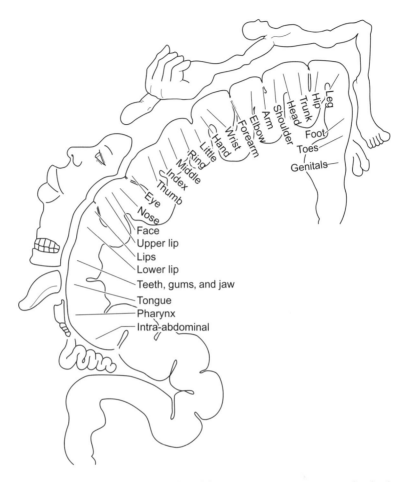

Figure 3.6 Sensory homunculus. Reproduced from Patestas & Garter, *A Textbook of Neuroanatomy* 2nd Edition, copyright 2007 with permission of Blackwell Publishing.

aphasia may result, significantly impacting quality of life through loss of most or all language ability. Table 3.4 summarises clinical examination techniques used to assess parietal lobe function.

Temporal lobe

The temporal lobe lies in a lateral position beneath the temporal bone and separated from the frontal and parietal lobes by the lateral fissure. The primary functions of the temporal lobe include hearing, speech, behaviour and memory (Standring 2004).

Brodmann's areas 41 and 42 (MCA territory) are the primary auditory areas that receive sound impulses and assist in determining both the source and the meaning of sound. Auditory loss may be the outcome of injury to these areas. The portion of the temporal lobe where the frontal, parietal and temporal lobes meet is an interpretive area for auditory, visual and somatic association

Table 3.4 Parietal lobe function examination techniques.

Brodmann's area	Arterial territory	Related clinical examination
1, 2, 3	Middle cerebral artery	Primary sensory testing: • Pin prick • Touch • Vibration • Position sense
5, 7	Middle cerebral artery	Complex sensory testing: • Stereognosia • Double simultaneous stimulation (visual and tactile) • Graphaesthesia
22	Middle cerebral artery	Receptive language

Table 3.5 Occipital lobe function examination techniques.

Brodmann's area	Arterial territory	Related clinical examination
17, 18, 19	Posterior cerebral artery	Visual field testing Visual acuity testing

responsible for integrating input into complex thought and memory. Seizures originating from this region may produce auditory, visual and sensory hallucinations. Clinical examination of temporal lobe function is primarily centred on auditory function; while loss of function may be associated with acute stroke, it is less common.

Occipital lobe

The most posterior lobes in the cerebrum are the occipital lobes which are concerned with interpretation of visual stimuli. Brodmann's area 17 (PCA territory) is the primary visual cortex, receiving impulses from the optic nerve (cranial nerve II). Impulses received here are referred to Brodmann's areas 18 and 19 (PCA territory), the visual associative areas responsible for interpretation and integration. Cortical blindness is likely following injury to the occipital lobes, where the ability to receive and interpret visual stimuli is lost, although the eye structures themselves remain intact (Mohr et al. 2004; Standring 2004). Clinical examination techniques pertinent to the occipital lobe are presented in Table 3.5.

Subcortical region

Fibre tracts from the cerebrum converge in the area of the brain known as the *internal capsule* as they progress toward the brainstem and spinal cord. This area's arterial supply is derived from small perforating arterial branches of the

MCA that originate at the proximal portion of each hemisphere's main arterial trunk. Afferent (sensory) stimuli destined for the cortex travel through the internal capsule from brainstem to thalamus to internal capsule to cerebral cortex. Efferent (motor) fibres leaving the cortex pass through the internal capsule en route to the brainstem and spinal cord (Standring 2004). With injuries to this area of the brain, pure sensory or motor, or a combined sensory and motor loss on the opposite side of the body may occur, with preservation of cortical function (Mohr et al. 2004). One exception to this rule is when discrete fibres from language centres are intercepted, resulting in presentation of aphasia in association with a subcortical lesion.

The *basal ganglia* comprise four pairs of nuclei (see below) that regulate involuntary (extrapyramidal) motor function and are located deep within the white matter of the cerebral hemispheres. The basal ganglia receive input from the cerebral cortex that stimulates basal ganglia output, which is then sent to the brainstem and thalamus for relay back to the frontal cortex. The basal ganglia integrate associated movements and postural adjustments with voluntary motor movement; they suppress skeletal muscle tone as needed to provide fluid, smooth motor function. Damage to the basal ganglia typically results in tremor or other involuntary movements, rigid non-fluid muscle tone, and slowness of movement without paralysis. The basal ganglia include:

- Corpus striatum (caudate nucleus, putamen and nucleus accumbens)
- Globus pallidus
- Substantia nigra
- Subthalamic nucleus

The *thalamus* is made up of two ovoid masses of grey matter that form the lateral walls of the third ventricle. These serve as a relay station and gatekeeper for both motor and sensory stimuli, preventing or enhancing transmission of impulses based on situational need. Sensory and/or motor dysfunction may occur with thalamic injury as normal impulse pathways are interrupted (Mohr et al. 2004).

Located below the thalamus is the *hypothalamus*, connected to the pituitary gland by the hypothalamic or pituitary stalk. The hypothalamus coordinates many neural systems associated with emotion, including the limbic system, to control bodily behavioural responses. It is the primary control centre for internal homeostasis, stimulating autonomic nervous system responses and endocrine system functions in relation to body needs. Through these mechanisms, the hypothalamus plays a significant role in temperature regulation, regulation of food and water intake, control of pituitary hormone release, and overall autonomic nervous system function (Standring 2004). Table 3.6 presents clinical examination techniques for the subcortical region.

Cerebellum

The cerebellum (Figure 3.7) is also called the 'hind brain'. It is separated from the cerebrum by the tentorium cerebelli, and accounts for one-fifth of the

Table 3.6 Subcortical function examination techniques.

Arterial territory	Related clinical examination
Middle cerebral artery	Grade motor function on a scale from 0 (absent) to 5 (normal): • 0/5 = No movement • 1/5 = Flicker of movement • 2/5 = Cannot overcome gravity • 3/5 = Cannot overcome resistance • 4/5 = Weak power • 5/5 = Normal power Arm pronator drift Deep tendon and superficial reflexes Speech articulation Facial expression testing (CN VII – motor component) Clench teeth (CN V – motor component mandibular branch)
Middle cerebral artery	Expressive language; word finding difficulties; fluency of language Receptive language
Middle cerebral artery	Primary sensory testing: • Pin prick • Touch • Vibration • Position sense

brain's overall size. It consists of two lateral hemispheres connected by the vermis. Similar to the cerebrum, it is composed of an outer layer of grey matter, or cortex, with a core of white matter tracts beneath (Standring 2004).

The cerebellum transmits impulses to descending motor pathways to integrate spatial orientation and equilibrium with posture and muscle tone, ensuring synchronised adjustments in movement that maintain overall balance and motor coordination. The cerebellum monitors and adjusts motor activity simultaneously with movement, enabling control of fine motor function. Cerebellar injury results in ataxia, which clinically presents as preservation of motor strength without control or coordination of motor function. The anterior inferior cerebellar artery (AICA) has very poor collateral blood supply, making this arterial territory highly susceptible to ischaemia. Typical presentation of an AICA territory stroke may include vertigo without hearing loss or tinnitus, and gaze-evoked nystagmus (Mohr et al. 2004). Cerebellar function examination techniques are presented in Table 3.7.

Brainstem

The brainstem is made up of three major divisions, the midbrain, pons and medulla oblongata. This area of the brain is packed with sensory and motor pathways that travel between the spinal cord and the brain, as well as centres that regulate vital mechanisms in the body.

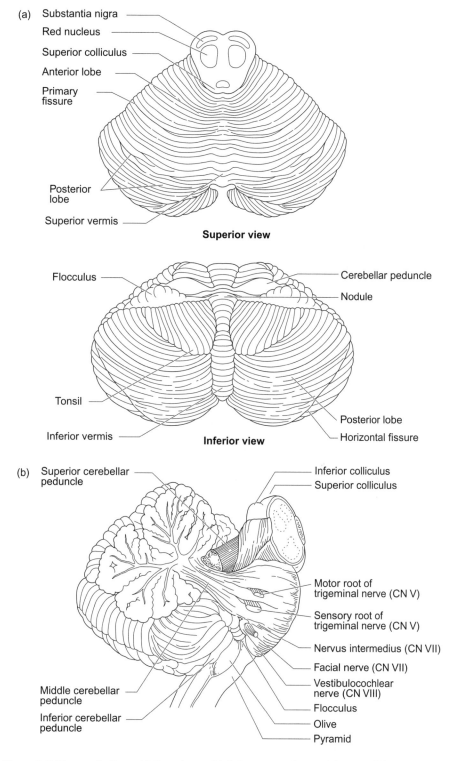

Figure 3.7 The cerebellum. (a) Superior and inferior views. (b) Lateral view of the cerebellum and medulla. Reproduced from Patestas & Garter, *A Textbook of Neuroanatomy* 2nd Edition, copyright 2007 with permission of Blackwell Publishing.

Table 3.7 Cerebellar function examination techniques.

Arterial territory	Related clinical examination
Superior cerebellar artery	Finger–nose–finger
Anterior inferior cerebellar artery	Romberg's balance testing
Posterior inferior cerebellar artery	Speech articulation
	Tandem gait testing
	Heel–shin testing
	Gaze-evoked nystagmus testing
	Dysphagia testing

Note: Cerebellar dysfunction commonly occurs alongside brainstem dysfunction.

The *midbrain* joins the brainstem to the diencephalon above it and the pons below it. Cranial nerves III and IV originate in the midbrain (Table 3.8) and the cerebral aqueduct is located in this area. Major functions of the midbrain include relay of stimuli to and from the brain through ascending sensory tracts and descending motor pathways (Standring 2004).

The *pons* is positioned directly above the medulla and also participates in the relay of information to and from the brain through sensory and motor pathways. The upper surface of the fourth ventricle is made up of the superior part of the pons. Two respiratory control centres are located in the pons; the apneustic centre controls the length of inspiration and expiration, while the pneumotaxic centre controls respiratory rate. Cranial nerves V (trigeminal), VI (abducens), VII (facial) and VIII (acoustic) are located in the pons (Table 3.8). The medial longitudinal fasciculus (MLF), an important fibre tract in the pons, connects cranial nerves III, IV and VI with the vestibular portion of the acoustic nerve and pontine paramedian reticular formation, also located in the pons. The MLF fosters coordinated and appropriate movements of the eyes in response to noise, motion, position and arousal; this is used by clinicians assessing the structural integrity of the brainstem by caloric testing (Mohr et al. 2004; Standring 2004).

The *medulla oblongata* is situated between the pons and the spinal cord. Voluntary motor fibres cross over (decussate) in the pyramids of the medulla, giving rise to the terminology pyramidal fibres, which is often used to describe voluntary motor function. This crossing over explains why stimuli from the right side of the brain control movement for the left side of the body and vice versa. The medulla oblongata houses the centres for control of involuntary functions such as swallowing, vomiting, hiccoughing, coughing, heart rate, arterial vasoconstriction, and respiration. The medullary respiratory centre works with both the apneustic and pneumotaxic centres in the pons to control respiratory function, and is responsible for the rhythm of respiration. Cranial nerves IX (glossopharyngeal), X (vagus), XI (spinal accessory) and XII (hypoglossal) are also located in the medulla oblongata; see Table 3.8 (Standring 2004).

The brainstem's *reticular formation* (RF) is located at the core of the brainstem and is active in modulating sensation, movement, consciousness, reflexive

Table 3.8 Cranial nerve anatomy, physiology and assessment.

Cranial nerve	Anatomy	Physiology	Assessment
I. Olfactory (sensory)	Cell body located in the nasal mucosa; axon passes through the ethmoid's cribriform plate, to olfactory bulbs, with temporal lobe interpretation of smell	Smell; participates in the stimulation of additional systems that are triggered by smell interpretation, including peristalsis, salivation and sexual stimulation	Rarely tested; with the eyes closed, the patient is presented with different familiar non-irritating odours. Commercial kits such as 'Sniffin' Sticks' may be used
II. Optic (sensory)	Retinal ganglionic cells converge in the optic disc, forming the optic nerve. Nerve fibres travel through the optic chiasm, the lateral geniculate body, and terminate in the occipital lobe	Vision, including visual acuity and peripheral vision	• Ophthalmoscope inspection of the optic fundi • Visual acuity: Often deferred in critical care; pocket-size Snellen cards may be used but are usually impractical • Visual fields: The 4 quadrants of vision are tested by confrontation in the cooperative patient, or by assessing blink to threat in the uncooperative patient • Visual neglect may be tested using double simultaneous stimulation (DSS) by having the patient identify simultaneous movement in both the examiner's right and left fingers. Note: Neglect is *not* visual loss, but inability to discriminate between two simultaneous stimuli
III. Oculomotor (motor)	Cell body located in the midbrain. Supplies motor fibres to the superior, inferior and medial recti, as well as the inferior oblique of the eye. Also supplies the levator muscle of the eyelid and gives off parasympathetic fibres to the ciliary muscles and iris	Extraocular movements; moves the eye in the following directions: superior rectus – elevation medial rectus – adduction (medially) inferior rectus – depression (downward) inferior oblique – extorsion (up and in) Raises eyelid and constricts the pupil.	• Assess for unilateral eyelid drooping (III) • Assess pupil size (range 1–6 mm) and symmetry. Note: 20% of people have anisocoria – a difference in pupil size of 0.5 mm. Anisocoria is normal if pupil light response is normal (III) • Assess pupil response to light: Direct response – the pupil of the eye directly receiving the light stimulus contracts; consensual response – the pupil of the eye not receiving the light stimulus contracts. Pupillary response is noted to be brisk, sluggish or non-reactive (III)
IV. Trochlear (motor)	Cell body located in the midbrain. Supplies motor fibres to the superior oblique muscle of the eye	Extraocular movements; moves the eye down and in (intorsion)	• Eye movement is coordinated through the internuclear pathway of the medial longitudinal fasciculus (MLF), and involves the integrated responses of the III, IV and VI cranial nerves, as well as input from the VIII nerve *(continued)*

Table 3.8 *Continued*

Cranial nerve	Anatomy	Physiology	Assessment
VI. Abducens (motor)	Cell body located in the pons. Supplies motor fibres to the lateral rectus muscle	Extraocular movements; moves the eye laterally (abduction)	• Eye movement is assessed to determine ability for the eyes to move in the 6 cardinal directions of movement; the conscious patient is asked to follow the examiner's finger movements with his/her eyes; the examiner moves his/her finger to trace the pattern of either an 'H' or an 'X' with a horizontal line through the middle; deviations in eye movement are noted. • In the unconscious patient, the oculocephalic reflex (doll's eyes) can be assessed once the cervical spine has been checked and neck can be safely manipulated; the patient's head is turned side to side with the eyes held open; normally, the eyes should move in the opposite direction of the head; eyes that remain in a fixed position indicate dysfunction of the midbrain/pontine region which houses the nuclei of cranial nerves III, IV and VI
V. Trigeminal (sensory and motor)	Cell body located in the pons; gives off 3 branches: ophthalmic (sensory), maxillary (sensory) and mandibular (sensory and motor)	Ophthalmic branch: Provides sensation to the cornea, ciliary body, iris, lacrimal gland, conjunctiva, nasal mucosa, forehead and nose Maxillary branch: Provides sensation to the skin of the cheek and nose, lower eyelid, upper jaw, teeth, mouth mucosa and maxillary sinuses Mandibular branch: Provides sensation to lower jaw, and motor function to muscles of mastication	• The ophthalmic branch is tested by eliciting a corneal reflex; in the unconscious patient, normally a blink should occur in response to gentle contact with the cornea by a cotton wisp • The maxillary branch is tested with dull/sharp discrimination using a pin • The mandibular branch is a mixed motor and sensory branch and may be tested by palpating muscles of the jaw during clenching of the teeth

Nerve			Testing
VII. Facial (sensory and motor)	Cell body located in the pons. Supplies sensory fibres to the anterior two-thirds of the tongue and soft palate. Supplies motor fibres to the muscles of the face	Taste and sensation for the anterior two-thirds of the tongue and soft palate. Serves as the primary motor nerve for facial expression	• Facial expression is tested by having the patient puff out the cheeks, smile/show teeth, tightly close the eyes, and lift the eyebrows. Asymmetry is noted • Taste is rarely tested
VIII. Acoustic (sensory)	Cell body located in the pons Cochlear sensory fibres originate in the ganglia of the cochlea, transmitting auditory sensation to the organ of Corti in the ear, pons and temporal lobe Vestibular sensory fibres originate in the semicircular canals of the ear and vestibular ganglion, terminating in the pons	Hearing Equilibrium	• Whispered word testing may be considered • In the unconscious patient, the oculovestibular reflex (ice water caloric testing) may be conducted to determine the integrity of the brainstem. The III, IV, VI and VIII nerves are stimulated through injection of iced water into the ear canal while keeping the head in a midline/neutral position with the eyes held open. Confirm that the tympanic membrane is intact prior to performing the procedure. The normal response is a conjugate nystagmus with deviation in the direction of the irrigated ear with a slow rhythmic quality. Absent eye movement or dysconjugate movement indicates brainstem injury. This procedure may produce nausea and vomiting in the conscious patient
IX. Glossopharyngeal (sensory and motor)	Cell body located in the medulla oblongata Sensory divisions transmit stimuli from the external ear, tympanic membrane, upper pharynx and posterior one-third of the tongue to the medulla Motor divisions supply voluntary control of the stylopharyngeus muscle and innervate the parotid gland	Stylopharyngeus muscle elevation for swallowing and speech Parotid gland secretion General sensory (pain, touch, temperature) function as specified	• The IX and X nerves are commonly tested together • Assess for symmetrical elevation of the palate, posterior pharynx and uvula • Palpate the larynx during swallowing, assessing for symmetrical laryngeal elevation • Have the patient repeat a word with a 'K' sound (e.g. Kitty Kat) and listen for complete/discrete pronunciation of the 'K' • Assess gag reflex

(continued)

Table 3.8 *Continued*

Cranial nerve	Anatomy	Physiology	Assessment
X. Vagus (sensory and motor)	The major parasympathetic nerve of the body, vagus is Latin for wandering; it originates in the medulla oblongata and travels as far as the splenic flexure of the colon. Motor components supply the pharynx, larynx, thoracic and abdominal viscera; sensory components transmit larynx, oesophagus, trachea, carotid bodies, and thoracic and abdominal viscera, as well as stretch and chemoreceptors from the aorta	Provides the majority of parasympathetic innervation to the regions specified. Effects include digestion, defecation, slowing of heart rate and reduction of contraction strength	
XI. Spinal accessory (motor)	Cell body located in the medulla oblongata with two roots: cranial and spinal. Cranial root innervates muscles of the larynx and pharynx; spinal root innervates trapezius and sternocleidomastoid muscles	Plays a role in swallowing and phonation. Innervates the muscles that turn the head and elevate the shoulders (shoulder shrug)	• Have the patient shrug his/her shoulders against resistance while the examiner pushes the shoulders downward • With resistance applied to one side of the face, have the patient turn his/her head against the resistance; repeat procedure with resistance applied to the opposite side of the face
XII. Hypoglossal (motor)	Cell body located in the medulla oblongata; sends off motor fibres to the tongue	Tongue movement.	• Have the patient push his/her tongue into a cheek while resistance is applied against the cheek; repeat the procedure with resistance applied to the other cheek. • Have the patient stick his/her tongue out and move it side to side • Have the patient repeat a word with an 'L' sound (e.g. lollypop, la-la-la) and listen for complete/discrete pronunciation of the 'L'

Table 3.9 Brainstem function examination techniques.

Arterial territory	Related clinical examination
Vertebral arteries Basilar artery Superior cerebellar artery Anterior inferior cerebellar artery Posterior inferior cerebellar artery	Cranial nerves III–XII (see Table 3.8) Dysphagia testing Level of consciousness: • Alert = awake • Lethargic = sleepy, dull, indifferent • Obtunded = deeply sleeping • Stuporous = arousable to noxious stimuli (localises or withdraws) • Comatose = unresponsive with absent or reflex response (decorticate, decerebrate, or spinal cord reflex arc) to noxious stimuli Voluntary motor function: • 0/5 = No movement • 1/5 = Flicker of movement • 2/5 = Cannot overcome gravity • 3/5 = Cannot overcome resistance • 4/5 = Weak power • 5/5 = Normal power Deep tendon and superficial reflexes Primary sensory function: • Pin prick • Touch • Vibration • Position sense Respiratory pattern, heart rate and blood pressure

Note: Cerebellar dysfunction commonly occurs alongside brainstem dysfunction.

behaviour and the activities of the cranial nerves arising from the brainstem (III–XII) (Standring 2004). Ascending RF is commonly called the reticular activating system (RAS), because it is responsible for increasing wakefulness, vigilance and responsiveness of cortical and thalamic neurons to sensory stimuli. Specifically, the RAS activates both the relay and diffuse projection nuclei of the thalamus to increase distribution of sensory stimuli throughout the cerebral cortex; additionally, the RAS activates the hypothalamus resulting in diffuse cortical and autonomic stimulation. Injury to the thalamic or hypothalamic RAS pathways may result in impaired consciousness (Bleck 1999). Table 3.9 presents the clinical examination pertinent to the brainstem.

Standardised instruments for acute neurological assessment

All assessments and supporting instruments require appropriate training in order to produce reliable assessment findings. A number of instruments have been constructed to support clinicians in conducting an acute neurological assessment, including:

- Glasgow Coma Scale – GCS (Teasdale & Jennett 1974)
- Intracerebral Haemorrhage Score – ICHS (Hemphill, III et al. 2001)
- Hunt and Hess Score – H-H (Johnston et al. 2002)

- National Institutes of Health Stroke Scale – NIHSS (Goldstein & Samsa 1997)

Glasgow Coma Scale (GCS)

The GCS is the most widely utilised neurological assessment instrument. It tests three categories of functioning to gauge level of consciousness (LOC): eye opening, best verbal response and best motor response (Table 3.10). Each category should be reported separately; the highest possible total score is 15, and the lowest is 3, with scores of 7 or less indicating significant LOC dysfunction. Commonly used across a wide variety of diagnoses, it is not a substitute for complete neurological assessment. Additionally, those using the GCS should bear in mind that it was developed to gauge severity in patients with traumatic brain injury (Teasdale & Jennett 1974), which explains its limited 'fit' with stroke presentation. Importantly, the GCS is insensitive to detection of focal neurological deficit and is based on recording the patient's best response; because of this, the tool will fail to capture deficits limited to one side of the body, or fluctuating signs. Scores of verbal response are confounded by endotracheal intubation. Although the GCS was validated for use in traumatic brain injury, it is currently also used as a measure of LOC in haemorrhagic stroke (Broderick et al. 2007).

Table 3.10 Glasgow Coma Scale (E + M + V) = 3–15.

	Activity	Score	Characteristics
Eye opening	None	1	Even to supra-orbital pressure
	To pain	2	Pain from sternum/limb/supra-orbital pressure
	To speech	3	Non-specific response, not necessarily to command
	Spontaneous	4	Eyes open, not necessarily aware
Motor response	None	1	To any pain; limbs remain flaccid
	Extension	2	Shoulder adducted and shoulder and forearm internally rotated
	Flexor response	3	Withdrawal response or assumption of hemiplegic posture
	Withdrawal	4	Arm withdraws to pain, shoulder abducts
	Localises pain	5	Arm attempts to remove supra-orbital/chest pressure
	Obeys commands	6	Follows simple commands
Verbal response	None	1	No verbalisation of any type
	Incomprehensible	2	Moans/groans, no speech
	Inappropriate	3	Intelligible, no sustained sentences
	Confused	4	Converses but confused, disoriented
	Oriented	5	Converses and oriented

Intracerebral Haemorrhage Score (ICHS)

The ICHS was developed to support acute trials in therapies for intraparenchymal haemorrhage (Broderick et al. 2007). The score consists of five components: GCS score, volume of the haemorrhage, presence of intraventricular haemorrhage, infratentorial location of the bleed, and patient age (Table 3.11). Scores of 3 have been associated with 70% mortality, while scores of 4 or more have been associated with 90–100% mortality rates.

Hunt and Hess Score (H-H)

The H-H Score is used to grade clinical severity of non-traumatic subarachnoid haemorrhage – SAH (Johnston et al. 2002). The score consists of five grades ranging from minimal (grade 1) to severe (grade 5) SAH clinical presentations (Table 3.12).

National Institutes of Health Stroke Scale (NIHSS)

The NIHSS was developed to support acute ischaemic stroke treatment trials and has demonstrated reliability when used with a range of appropriately

Table 3.11 Intracerebral Haemorrhage Score.

Component	Score
Glasgow Coma Scale score:	
GCS = 3–4	2
GCS = 5–12	1
GCS = 13–15	0
ICH volume (cm^3):	
ICH ≥30 ml	1
ICH <30 ml	0
Intraventricular component?	
Yes – intraventricular component present	1
No – no intraventricular haemorrhage	0
Infratentorial origin of ICH?	
Yes – Infratentorial in origin	1
No – not Infratentorial in origin	0
Age in years:	
Age ≥80 years	1
Age <80 years	0
Total score:	*0–6*

Table 3.12 Hunt and Hess Score.

Grade	Clinical features
1	Asymptomatic, mild headache, slight nuchal rigidity
2	Moderate to severe headache, nuchal rigidity No neurological deficit other than cranial nerve palsy
3	Drowsiness/confusion; mild focal neurological deficit
4	Stupor; moderate-severe hemiparesis
5	Coma; decerebrate posturing

trained clinicians (Goldstein & Samsa 1997). It is considered the only valid tool to assess stroke deficit severity (Adams et al. 2007). The NIHSS consists of a total of 14 categories that test LOC, extraocular movement, visual fields, facial expression, arm and leg motor function, cerebellar function, sensory function, language fluency, speech articulation and neglect or extinction (Table 3.13). Total possible score ranges from 0 (no neurological deficit) to 42 (severe neurological deficit). Each item within the scale must be scored unless it is deemed 'untestable'. While the NIHSS appears complex on first glance, experience with the instrument may result in rapid completion, taking as little as five to seven minutes. The NIHSS is mandated as an assessment supporting practice within Joint Commission on Accreditation of Healthcare Organization (JCAHO) Stroke Centers in the US, because it provides a common language with which to gauge stroke severity and improvement following treatment with intravenous thrombolysis and/or intra-arterial rescue therapies.

Other instruments to assess stroke-related impairment are also used; for example, tools such as the Scandinavian Stroke Scale can also provide an index of overall stroke impairment severity and the Barthel Index a broad measure of disability, through to targeted instruments such as the Action Research Arm Test, which provides a focused view of effects in one limb. In addition, a range of broader tools have been employed, such as the Medical Outcomes Study Short Form 36 (SF-36) and the Stroke-Specific Quality of Life tool, to examine effects of stroke within a whole-life context.

Conclusion

This chapter provides a brief overview of normal anatomy and physiology, disease processes associated with development of a stroke, and tools commonly used to gauge severity and detail of the physiological impact of the stroke on the individual. This comprises basic and fundamental knowledge essential for all clinicians involved with stroke patients, in order to understand the disease processes as a first step towards care and treatment of the person.

Table 3.13 National Institutes of Health Stroke Scale Score (http://www.ninds.nih.gov/disorders/stroke/strokescales.htm).

1a. Level of consciousness: The investigator must choose a response, even if a full evaluation is prevented by such obstacles as an endotracheal tube, language barrier, orotracheal trauma/bandages. A 3 is scored only if the patient makes no movement (other than reflexive posturing) in response to noxious stimulation

0 = Alert; keenly responsive
1 = Not alert, but arousable by minor stimulation to obey, answer, or respond
2 = Not alert, requires repeated stimulation to attend, or is obtunded and requires strong or painful stimulation to make movements (not stereotyped)
3 = Responds only with reflex motor or autonomic effects or totally unresponsive, flaccid, areflexic

1a: _____

1b. LOC questions: The patient is asked the month and his/her age. The answer must be correct - there is no partial credit for being close. Aphasic and stuporous patients who do not comprehend the questions will score 2. Patients unable to speak because of endotracheal intubation, orotracheal trauma, severe dysarthria from any cause, language barrier or any other problem not secondary to aphasia are given a 1. It is important that only the initial answer be graded and that the examiner not 'help' the patient with verbal or non-verbal cues

0 = Answers both questions correctly
1 = Answers one question correctly
2 = Answers neither question correctly

1b: _____

1c. LOC commands: The patient is asked to open and close the eyes and then to grip and release the non-paretic hand. Substitute another one step command if the hands cannot be used. Credit is given if an unequivocal attempt is made but not completed due to weakness. If the patient does not respond to command, the task should be demonstrated to them (pantomime) and score the result (i.e., follows none, one or two commands). Patients with trauma, amputation, or other physical impediments should be given suitable one-step commands. Only the first attempt is scored

0 = Performs both tasks correctly
1 = Performs one task correctly
2 = Performs neither task correctly

1c: _____

2. Best gaze: Only horizontal eye movements will be tested. Voluntary or reflexive (oculocephalic) eye movements will be scored but caloric testing is not done. If the patient has a conjugate deviation of the eyes that can be overcome by voluntary or reflexive activity, the score will be 1. If a patient has an isolated peripheral nerve paresis (CN III, IV or VI) score a 1. Gaze is testable in all aphasic patients. Patients with ocular trauma, bandages, pre-existing blindness or other disorder of visual acuity or fields should be tested with reflexive movements and a choice made by the investigator. Establishing eye contact and then moving about the patient from side to side will occasionally clarify the presence of a partial gaze palsy

0 = Normal
1 = Partial gaze palsy. This score is given when gaze is abnormal in one or both eyes, but where forced deviation or total gaze paresis are not present
2 = Forced deviation, or total gaze paresis not overcome by the oculocephalic maneuver

2: _____

(continued)

Table 3.13 *Continued*

3. Visual: Visual fields (upper and lower quadrants) are tested by confrontation, using finger counting or visual threat as appropriate. Patient must be encouraged, but if they look at the side of the moving fingers appropriately, this can be scored as normal. If there is unilateral blindness or enucleation, visual fields in the remaining eye are scored. Score 1 only if a clear-cut asymmetry, including quadrantanopia is found. If patient is blind from any cause score 3. Double simultaneous stimulation is performed at this point. If there is extinction patient receives a 1 and the results are used to answer question 11	0 = No visual loss 1 = Partial hemianopia 2 = Complete hemianopia 3 = Bilateral hemianopia (blind including cortical blindness)	3: _____
4. Facial palsy: Ask, or use pantomime to encourage the patient to show teeth or raise eyebrows and close eyes. Score symmetry of grimace in response to noxious stimuli in the poorly responsive or non-comprehending patient. If facial trauma/bandages, orotracheal tube, tape or other physical barrier obscures the face, these should be removed to the extent possible	0 = Normal symmetrical movement 1 = Minor paralysis (flattened nasolabial fold, asymmetry on smiling) 2 = Partial paralysis (total or near total paralysis of lower face) 3 = Complete paralysis of one or both sides (absence of facial movement in the upper and lower face)	4: _____
5 & 6. Motor arm and leg: The limb is placed in the appropriate position: extend the arms (palms down) 90 degrees (if sitting) or 45 degrees (if supine) and the leg 30 degrees (always tested supine). Drift is scored if the arm falls before 10 seconds or the leg before 5 seconds. The aphasic patient is encouraged using urgency in the voice and pantomime but not noxious stimulation. Each limb is tested in turn, beginning with the non-paretic arm. Only in the case of amputation or joint fusion at the shoulder or hip may the score be '9' and the examiner must clearly write the explanation for scoring as a '9'	0 = No drift, limb holds 90 (or 45) degrees for full 10 seconds 1 = Drift, Limb holds 90 (or 45) degrees, but drifts down before full 10 seconds; does not hit bed or other support 2 = Some effort against gravity, limb cannot get to or maintain (if cued) 90 (or 45) degrees, drifts down to bed, but has some effort against gravity 3 = No effort against gravity, limb falls 4 = No movement 9 = Amputation, joint fusion explain: _____	**5a.** **L Arm** _____ **5b.** **R Arm** _____ **6a.** **L Leg** _____ **6b.** **R Leg** _____
7. Limb ataxia: This item is aimed at finding evidence of a unilateral cerebellar lesion. Test with eyes open. In case of visual defect, insure testing is done in intact visual field. The finger–nose–finger and heel–shin tests are performed on both sides, and ataxia is scored only if present out of proportion to weakness. Ataxia is absent in the patient who cannot understand or is paralyzed. Only in the case of amputation or joint fusion may the item be scored '9', and the examiner must clearly write the explanation for not scoring. In case of blindness test by touching nose from extended arm position	0 = Absent 1 = Present in one limb 2 = Present in two limbs If present, is ataxia in Right arm 1 = Yes 2 = No 9 = amputation or joint fusion, explain _____ Left arm 1 = Yes 2 = No 9 = amputation or joint fusion, explain _____ Right leg 1 = Yes 2 = No 9 = amputation or joint fusion, explain _____ Left leg 1 = Yes 2 = No 9 = amputation or joint fusion, explain _____	7: _____

Table 3.13 *Continued*

8. Sensory: Sensation or grimace to pin prick when tested, or withdrawal from noxious stimulus in the obtunded or aphasic patient. Only sensory loss attributed to stroke is scored as abnormal and the examiner should test as many body areas [arms (not hands), legs, trunk, face] as needed to accurately check for hemisensory loss. A score of 2, 'severe or total,' should only be given when a severe or total loss of sensation can be clearly demonstrated. Stuporous and aphasic patients will therefore probably score 1 or 0. The patient with brain stem stroke who has bilateral loss of sensation is scored 2. If the patient does not respond and is quadriplegic score 2. Patients in a coma (item 1a = 3) are automatically given a 2 on this item

0 = Normal; no sensory loss
1 = Mild to moderate sensory loss; patient feels pinprick is less sharp or is dull on the affected side; or there is a loss of superficial pain with pinprick but patient is aware he/she is being touched
2 = Severe to total sensory loss; patient is not aware of being touched in the face, arm, and leg

8: _____

9. Best language: A great deal of information about comprehension will be obtained during the preceding sections of the examination. The patient is asked to describe what is happening in the attached picture, to name the items on the attached naming sheet, and to read from the attached list of sentences. Comprehension is judged from responses here as well as to all of the commands in the preceding general neurological exam. If visual loss interferes with the tests, ask the patient to identify objects placed in the hand, repeat, and produce speech. The intubated patient should be asked to write. The patient in coma (question 1a = 3) will arbitrarily score 3 on this item. The examiner must choose a score in the patient with stupor or limited cooperation but a score of 3 should be used only if the patient is mute and follows no one step commands
(The patient's language will be tested by having the patient identify standard groups of objects and by reading a series of sentences. Comprehension of language should be judged as the physician performs the entire neurologic examination. The physician should give the patient adequate time to identify the objects on the sheet of paper. Only the first response is measured. If the patient misidentifies the object and later corrects himself, the response is still considered abnormal. The physician should then give the patient a sheet of paper with the series of sentences. The examiner should ask the patient to read at least three sentences. The first attempt to read the sentence is measured. If the patient misreads the sentence and later corrects himself, the response is still considered abnormal. If the patient's visual loss precludes visual identification of objects or reading, the examiner should ask the patient to identify objects placed in his/her hand and the examiner should judge the patient's spontaneous speech and ability to repeat sentences. If the examiner judges these responses as normal, the score should be 0. If the patient is intubated or is unable to speak, the examiner should check the patient's writing)

0 = No aphasia, normal
1 = Mild to moderate aphasia; some obvious loss of fluency or facility of comprehension, without significant limitation on ideas expressed or form of expression. Reduction of speech and/or comprehension, however, makes conversation about provided material difficult or impossible. For example in conversation about provided materials examiner can identify picture or naming card from patient's response
2 = Severe aphasia; all communication is through fragmentary expression; great need for inference, questioning, and guessing by the listener. Range of information that can be exchanged is limited; listener carries burden of communication. Examiner cannot identify materials provided from patient response
3 = Mute, global aphasia; no usable speech or auditory comprehension

9: _____

(continued)

Table 3.13 *Continued*

10. Dysarthria: If patient is thought to be normal an adequate sample of speech must be obtained by asking patient to read or repeat words from the attached list. If the patient has severe aphasia, the clarity of articulation of spontaneous speech can be rated. Only if the patient is intubated or has other physical barrier to producing speech, may the item be scored '9', and the examiner must clearly write an explanation for not scoring. Do not tell the patient why he/she is being tested (The primary method of examination is to ask the patient to read and pronounce a standard list of words from a sheet of paper. If the patient is unable to read the words because of visual loss, the physician may say the word and ask the patient to repeat it. If the patient has severe aphasia, the clarity of articulation of spontaneous speech should be rated. If the patient is mute or comatose (item 9, Best Language = 3) or has an endotracheal tube, this item can be rated as 9 – untestable)	0 = Normal 1 = Mild to moderate; patient slurs at least some words and, at worst, can be understood with some difficulty 2 = Severe; patient's speech is so slurred as to be unintelligible in the absence of or out of proportion to any dysphasia, or is mute/anarthric 9 = Intubated or other physical barrier, explain_____	10: _____
11. Extinction and inattention (formerly neglect): Sufficient information to identify neglect may be obtained during the prior testing. If the patient has a severe visual loss preventing visual double simultaneous stimulation, and the cutaneous stimuli are normal, the score is normal. If the patient has aphasia but does appear to attend to both sides, the score is normal. The presence of visual spatial neglect or anosagnosia may also be taken as evidence of abnormality. Since the abnormality is scored only if present, the item is never untestable	0 = No abnormality 1 = Visual, tactile, auditory, spatial, or personal inattention or extinction to bilateral simultaneous stimulation in one of the sensory modalities 2 = Profound hemi-inattention or hemi-inattention to more than one modality. Does not recognize own hand or orients to only one side of space _____	11: _____

References

Adams, HP, Jr, Bendixen, BH, Kappelle, LJ, Biller, J, Love, BB et al., 1993, Classification of subtype of acute ischemic stroke – definitions for use in a multicenter clinical trial. TOAST. Trial of Org 10172 in Acute Stroke Treatment, *Stroke*, vol. 24, no. 1, pp. 35–41.

Adams, HP, Jr, del Zoppo G, Alberts, MJ, Bhatt, DL, Brass, L et al., 2007, Guidelines for the early management of adults with ischemic stroke: a guideline from the American Heart Association/American Stroke Association Stroke Council, Clinical Cardiology Council, Cardiovascular Radiology and Intervention Council, and the Atherosclerotic Peripheral Vascular Disease and Quality of Care Outcomes in Research Interdisciplinary Working Groups: the American Academy of Neurology affirms the value of this guideline as an educational tool for neurologists, *Stroke*, vol. 38, no. 5, pp. 1655–1711.

Alexandrov, AV, 2003, *Cerebrovascular Ultrasound in Stroke Prevention and Treatment*, Blackwell-Futura, Armonk, New York.

Bleck, TP, 1999, Levels of consciousness and attention, in *Textbook of Clinical Neurology*, C Goetz & E Pappert, eds., Saunders, Philadelphia.

Broderick, J, Connolly, S, Feldmann, E, Hanley, D, Kase, C et al., 2007, Guidelines for the management of spontaneous intracerebral hemorrhage in adults: 2007 update: a guideline from the American Heart Association/American Stroke Association Stroke Council, High Blood Pressure Research Council, and the Quality of Care and Outcomes in Research Interdisciplinary Working Group, *Stroke*, vol. 38, no. 6, pp. 2001–2023.

Cabanes, L, Mas, JL, Cohen, A, Amarenco, P, Cabanes, PA et al., 1993, Atrial septal aneurysm and patent foramen ovale as risk factors for cryptogenic stroke in patients less than 55 years of age. A study using transesophageal echocardiography, *Stroke*, vol. 24, no. 12, pp. 1865–1873.

Foulkes, MA, Wolf, PA, Price, TR, Mohr, JP, & Hier, DB, 1988, The Stroke Data Bank: design, methods, and baseline characteristics, *Stroke*, vol. 19, no. 5, pp. 547–554.

Gloor, P, 1997, *The Temporal Lobe and Limbic System*, Oxford University Press, New York.

Goldstein, LB, & Samsa, GP, 1997, Reliability of the National Institutes of Health Stroke Scale – extension to non-neurologists in the context of a clinical trial, *Stroke*, vol. 28, no. 2, pp. 307–310.

Goldstein, LB, Adams, R, Alberts, MJ, Appel, LJ, Brass, LM et al., 2006, Primary prevention of ischemic stroke: a guideline from the American Heart Association/ American Stroke Association Stroke Council: cosponsored by the Atherosclerotic Peripheral Vascular Disease Interdisciplinary Working Group; Cardiovascular Nursing Council; Clinical Cardiology Council; Nutrition, Physical Activity, and Metabolism Council; and the Quality of Care and Outcomes Research Interdisciplinary Working Group: the American Academy of Neurology affirms the value of this guideline, *Stroke*, vol. 37, no. 6, pp. 1583–1633.

Hemphill, JC, III, Bonovich, DC, Besmertis, L, Manley, GT, & Johnston, SC, 2001, The ICH score: a simple, reliable grading scale for intracerebral hemorrhage, *Stroke*, vol. 32, no. 4, pp. 891–897.

Johnston, SC, Higashida, RT, Barrow, DL, Caplan, LR, Dion, JE et al., 2002, Recommendations for the endovascular treatment of intracranial aneurysms: a statement for healthcare professionals from the Committee on Cerebrovascular Imaging of the American Heart Association Council on Cardiovascular Radiology, *Stroke*, vol. 33, no. 10, pp. 2536–2544.

Lechat, P, Lascault, G, Mas, JL, Loron, P, Klimczac, K et al., 1989, Prevalence of patent foramen ovale in young patients with ischemic cerebral complications, *Archives des maladies du coeur et des vaisseaux*, vol. 82, no. 6, pp. 847–852.

Mohr, JP, Choi, DW, Grotta, JS, & Wolf, PA, 2004, *Stroke: Pathophysiology, Diagnosis, and Management*, 3rd edn, Churchill Livingstone, New York.

National Collaborating Centre for Chronic Conditions, 2008, *Stroke – National Clinical Guideline for Diagnosis and Initial Management of Acute Stroke and Transient Ischaemic Attack (TIA)*, Royal College of Physicians, London.

Standring, S, 2004, *Gray's Anatomy: The Anatomical Basis for Clinical Practice*, 39th edn, Elsevier Churchill Livingstone, London.

Teasdale, G, & Jennett, B, 1974, Assessment of coma and impaired consciousness. A practical scale, *Lancet*, vol. 2, no. 7872, pp. 81–84.

Waxman, SG, 2000, *Correlative Neuroanatomy*, Lange, New York.

Webster, MW, Chancellor, AM, Smith, HJ, Swift, DL, Sharpe, DN et al., 1988, Patent foramen ovale in young stroke patients, *Lancet*, vol. 2, no. 8601, pp. 11–12.

Chapter 4

Acute stroke nursing management

Anne W. Alexandrov

Key points

- Historically, stroke care comprised supportive care only; those days are past.
- Timely initiation of appropriate interventions can make the difference between life and death, independence and dependency – 'Time is brain'.
- Hyperacute and acute stroke care entails identification of stroke aetiology, and proactive management to achieve haemodynamic stability, thrombolysis, arrest or evacuation of haemorrhage.
- Ongoing priorities include prevention of complications and initiation of rehabilitation programmes.
- Education of patients and families, and preparation for hospital discharge and life after stroke are also priorities.
- This chapter contains protocols and criteria to support service delivery.

Current roles of nurses working with stroke patients are multifaceted, diverse and expanding; many are specialist skills. Key attributes include promoting cohesion, facilitating interagency communication and cross-boundary service developments. Essential care-giving skills and relationship-centred care must not be devalued as this is what attracts many people. Stroke nursing is gaining recognition but needs to be pro-active in driving service developments, developing roles in specialist areas of acute, rehabilitation and community care; crossing boundaries between hospital and community and bridging gaps in existing services. At the same time, nurses must remain patient-focused and involve service users at all stages of development.

(Stroke nurse focus groups: summary of preliminary analysis;
Perry et al. 2004)

Introduction

Recent decades have seen a radical shift in attitudes towards management of stroke. Stroke has always been seen as an end result of chronic disease, but now it is also recognised as an acute disease event in which swift and appropriate treatment can effect major benefits in terms of patient outcomes. This chapter provides an overview of priority-driven acute stroke care, with discussion of the evidence supporting diagnostic and treatment processes, and stroke service configuration to deliver this. Mechanisms supporting ongoing quality improvement will be highlighted as well as guidelines supporting governmental and accreditation requirements aimed at achieving improved acute stroke outcomes.

Priorities in acute stroke management

Management of acute stroke patients is organised around several priorities aimed at ensuring optimal patient outcomes. A first priority is stabilisation and ensuring the safety of the patient. In ischaemic stroke, this proceeds in tandem with provision of reperfusion therapies aimed at recanalisation of obstructed arterial vessels thereby restoring brain perfusion and minimising disability. Following reperfusion therapy, or in patients who lack an indication for reperfusion therapy (e.g. transient ischaemic attack (TIA) or patient arrival to the hospital beyond the therapeutic time window and services available), the next priority is determination of pathogenic mechanism (explained in Chapter 3). This is achieved by provision of a comprehensive work-up to determine probable cause of ischaemic stroke or TIA and will inform appropriate secondary prevention.

In haemorrhagic stroke, immediate foci include two almost simultaneous priorities:

- Determination of haemorrhage mechanism (e.g. hypertensive intraparenchymal haemorrhage, anticoagulation-related haemorrhage, aneurysmal subarachnoid haemorrhage, vascular malformation haemorrhage, or traumatic haemorrhage mimicking acute stroke)
- Prevention of haemorrhagic expansion to limit neurological disability

In the case of lesions amenable to surgical or endovascular treatment, the focus of care should immediately shift to provision of definitive methods for haemorrhage control. However, in the case of large haemorrhages, with devastating neurological deficit, the focus should shift to palliative care.

For both ischaemic and haemorrhagic stroke, provision of secondary prevention measures, along with therapies that prevent complications associated with neurological disability, and evaluation for the most appropriate type and level of rehabilitation services are also early priorities during acute hospitalisation. The duration of acute stage hospitalisation varies internationally as well as locally, and is associated with severity of neurological deficit, development of complications, and the structure of health service provision, including payment mechanisms.

Hyperacute stroke management

Pre-hospital and emergency evaluation

While systems and personnel requirements vary throughout the world, most countries offer some system of emergency response, stabilisation and transport of patients to hospitals for definitive diagnosis and treatment. Accurate recognition of stroke is prerequisite for early initiation of treatment and use of valid and reliable pre-hospital stroke scales have been shown to improve accuracy (Table 4.1) (Adams et al. 2007; Kidwell et al. 2000; Kothari et al. 1999). Use of pre-hospital standardised protocols (Table 4.2) further benefits pre-hospital care by outlining care priorities, limiting the time spent on-scene, and expediting the rapid direct transport of suspected stroke patients to hospitals capable of delivering acute stroke treatment (Morris et al. 2000; Porteous et al. 1999; Rossnagel et al. 2004; Rymer & Thrutchley 2005; Silliman et al. 2003; Suyama & Crocco 2002). Collectively, these scales and protocols increase the number of stroke patients eligible for reperfusion therapies.

Within the Emergency Department (ED), interdisciplinary staff must be alert to the recognition of acute stroke patients because, for various reasons, including knowledge deficits amongst the population, a significant number of acute stroke patients arrive by private transport instead of ambulance (Morris et al. 2000; Schroeder et al. 2000; Schwamm et al. 2005; Williams et al. 2000; Wojner-Alexandrov et al. 2005). Use of simple scales such as the Face Arm Speech Test (Harbison et al. 2003) or the ROSIER Scale (Recognition of Stroke in the Emergency Room (Nor et al. 2004); Table 4.1) in the triage area of the ED may result in rapid identification of patients with possible stroke or TIA (Kothari et al. 1999). Emergency triage of an acute stroke or TIA patient using the Emergency Severity Index (ESI) typically locates the patient in category 2 (Figure 4.1), although concurrent airway, breathing and/or haemodynamic instability will trigger triage to category 1 (Tanabe et al. 2004, 2005). All suspected stroke, and TIA patients with or without current neurological deficit, should be rapidly identified in the triage area. Evidence from studies of patients with TIA and minor strokes indicates that very early intervention (within 24 hours) can avert stroke recurrence (National Collaborating Centre for Chronic Conditions 2008) although whether it requires hospitalisation to achieve this has not been demonstrated. Internationally, stroke guidelines recommend that patients with suspected TIA should be managed in services that allow rapid assessment and treatment to be undertaken within 24–48 hours of symptom onset (National Collaborating Centre for Chronic Conditions 2008; National Stroke Foundation 2008). All patients suspected of stroke should be admitted for diagnosis, and if indicated, reperfusion therapy.

Establishment of the time of stroke symptom onset, or the time the patient was last seen symptom free, is a high priority for triage personnel. To expedite emergency management of suspected stroke patients, many EDs have implemented standing orders that empower nurses to institute care prior to assessment by an emergency physician. Along with assessment and management of

Table 4.1 Valid and reliable stroke scales.

Stroke scale	Scale elements

Los Angeles Prehospital Stroke Scale (LAPSS)	Last time patient known to be symptom free: Date _____ Time _____
	Screening criteria:
	Age ≥45 years: Yes Unknown No
	No history of seizures or epilepsy: Yes Unknown No
	Symptoms present ≤24 hours: Yes Unknown No
	Not previously bedridden or wheelchair bound: Yes Unknown No
	
	If all above elements are 'unknown' or 'yes':
	
	Blood glucose 60 to 400 mg/dl: Yes No
	
	Examination:
	Facial smile grimace: Normal Right droop Left droop
	Grip: Normal Right weak Left weak
	                                     No right grip No left grip
	Arm strength: Normal Right drift Left drift
	                                     Right falls Left falls
	
	Based on examination, patient has unilateral weakness: Yes No
	
	If items are yes or unknown, meets criteria for stroke

Cincinnati Prehospital Stroke Scale (CPSS Scale)	Facial droop: Normal – both sides of face move equally Abnormal – one side of face does not move as well as the other Arm drift: Normal – both arms move the same or both arms do not move at all Abnormal – one arm either does not move or drifts down compared to the other Speech: Normal – says correct words with no slurring Abnormal – slurs words, says the wrong words, or is unable to speak Time: Onset time of stroke symptoms: _____ Transport FAST to Stroke Center Hospital
Recognition of Stroke in the Emergency Room (ROSIER)	**GCS** E= M= V= **BP=** ***BM=** ***If BM <3.5 mmol/L treat urgently and reassess once blood glucose normal** Has there been loss of consciousness or syncope? Y(–1) N(0) Has there been seizure activity? Y(–1) N(0) Is there a NEW ACUTE onset (or on awakening from sleep) I. Asymmetric facial weakness Y(+1) N(0) II. Asymmetric arm weakness Y(+1) N(0) III. Asymmetric leg weakness Y(+1) N(0) IV. Speech disturbance Y(+1) N(0) V. Visual field defect Y(+1) N(0) *Total Score (–2 to +5)= Provisional diagnosis Stroke [ ] Non-stroke [ ] (specify) *Stroke is unlikely but not completely excluded if total scores are ≤0. BM = blood glucose; BP = blood pressure (mmHg); GCS = Glasgow Coma Scale; E = eye; M = motor; V = verbal component.

Note: These scales have been validated within the pre-hospital environment in US stroke patients. Other valid and reliable pre-hospital stroke scales may be available in different countries worldwide.

Table 4.2 American Stroke Association guidelines for pre-hospital management of suspected acute ischaemic stroke (Adams et al. 2007).

Category	Components
Components of the medical history recommended for collection in the pre-hospital setting	• Symptom onset time • Recent medical problems: stroke; myocardial infarction; trauma; surgery; bleeding • Co-morbid diseases: hypertension; diabetes mellitus • Medications: anticoagulants; insulin; antihypertensives
Recommended pre-hospital management	• Manage airway, breathing and circulation • Monitor cardiac rhythm • Obtain intravenous access • Supplemental oxygen • Assess blood glucose • Nil orally • Notify receiving Emergency Department of on route status • Rapidly transfer to the nearest 'stroke capable' Emergency Department; spend minimal time on scene
Practices NOT recommended in the pre-hospital environment	• Do *NOT* use dextrose-containing intravenous fluids unless there is evidence of hypoglycaemia • Do *NOT* lower blood pressure • Do *NOT* administer excessive intravenous fluid

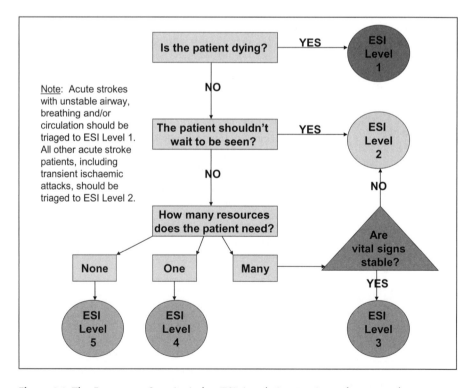

Figure 4.1 The Emergency Severity Index (ESI) in relation to triage of acute stroke.

airway, breathing and circulation, coupled with a brief primary neurological disability assessment, these independent nursing measures most commonly include:

- Calling a 'Code Stroke' alert in the hospital, so that the Stroke Team is mobilised to the ED, if this has not been automatically triggered by ambulance call to the ED
- Administering 100% oxygen by non-rebreather mask, only where appropriate
- Establishing two 0.9% (normal) saline intravenous lines
- Ordering and drawing initial blood samples, e.g. for complete blood count, blood chemistry and glucose, coagulation profile, cardiac enzymes
- Ordering an immediate non-contrast computed tomography (CT) scan of the head
- Completing a 12-lead electrocardiogram
- Ordering an upright portable chest X-ray if indicated by airway or oxygenation assessment findings
- Completing the National Institutes of Health Stroke Scale (NIHSS; see Table 3.13, Chapter 3)
- Ordering and collecting a drug screen panel, if indicated
- In the case of patients with significant neurological disability (e.g. with decreased level of consciousness), insertion of a urinary catheter

The Brain Attack Coalition (BAC) Guidelines (Alberts et al. 2000, 2005) identify the need for physician evaluation of an acute stroke patient within 10 minutes of arrival to the ED, completion of a non-contrast CT within 25 minutes of hospital arrival and CT diagnostic interpretation within 45 minutes of hospital arrival. These guidelines are closely adhered to in the most experienced stroke centres throughout the world, in keeping with the philosophy that, 'time is brain'. The BAC Guidelines were designed to facilitate timely administration of reperfusion therapies in appropriate candidates, and stipulate that if treating with tissue plasminogen activator (tPA), the thrombolytic bolus dose should be administered within 60 minutes of arrival to the hospital. However, completion of a thorough work-up for tPA treatment candidacy may be sufficiently completed in less than 60 minutes by experienced Stroke Teams. Where patients arrive at the hospital in less than 60 minutes of the current standard time window for treatment with intravenous tPA, rapid, expert response is paramount to achieve optimal stroke outcomes. Many departments have instituted an Emergency Stroke Care Quality Scorecard based on the BAC Guidelines (Figure 4.2) to drive and support ongoing improvement of ED systems and processes.

Once essential assessments have been conducted, the patient stabilised and a quick primary neurological disability assessment performed, rapid progress to non-contrast CT is paramount (Adams et al. 2007). Non-contrast CT is highly sensitive for the presence of blood, allowing practitioners to identify haemorrhage and so exclude reperfusion therapies from the treatment plan (Adams et al. 2007; Alberts et al. 2000; Grotta et al. 1999; Kidwell et al. 2004; Patel et al. 2001). In the case of hyperacute ischaemic stroke (symptoms

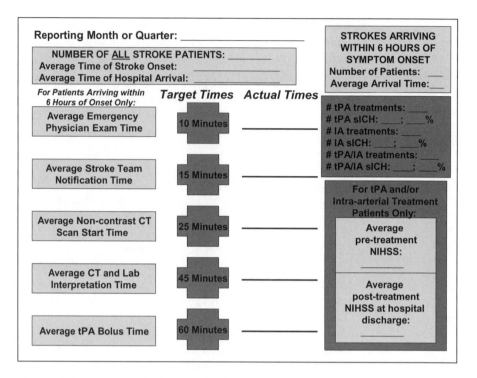

Figure 4.2 Emergency Stroke Care Quality Scorecard.

occurring six to eight hours prior to hospital arrival), the non-contrast CT should be normal or contain only early infarct signs such as sulcal effacement, blurring of the grey and white matter interface or a hyperdense artery sign. When this is the case, care progresses to rapid completion of neurological examination by means of a valid tool, such as the NIHSS (Dewey et al. 1999; Dominguez et al. 2006; Goldstein & Samsa 1997; Josephson et al. 2006; Kasner 2006; Lyden et al. 1994, 1999, 2005). Of paramount importance is whether impairment patterns follow neurovascular territory in the brain, which assists with localisation of the arterial occlusion.

Use of additional neuroimaging technologies to image vessel occlusion is unnecessary to make a tPA treatment decision within current standard protocols, but for the future may help refine decision-making for patients who present outside the current 4.5-hour time window for intravenous tPA administration yet have good potential for reperfusion. Additional neuroimaging technologies may also complement the diagnostic work-up; CT angiography (CTA) and transcranial Doppler (TCD) may be completed quite rapidly and may increase clinicians' confidence in the diagnosis of ischaemic stroke, although small vessel occlusions may be missed using these technologies (Adams et al. 2007). Magnetic resonance imaging (MRI) is usually impractical within the first 4.5 hours of symptom onset except in advanced stroke centres where rapid MRI protocols have been established with no more than 20-minute scanning times (Adams et al. 2007). In the case of haemorrhagic stroke, additional neuroimaging with CTA and/or catheter angiography should be considered for intraparenchymal haemorrhages occurring outside a territory suggestive of a hypertensive mechanism, to exclude an aneurysmal or arteriovenous malformation mechanism (Adams et al. 2007).

Delivery of reperfusion therapies in acute ischaemic stroke

Once ischaemic stroke has been diagnosed, the patient should be positioned with the head of the bed flat. Flat, zero-degree positioning has been shown to increase blood flow by 20% through the residual arterial lumen affected by stroke (Wojner-Alexander et al. 2005); additionally, early (under 48 hours) development of increased intracranial pressure (ICP) is unlikely, making this position an important first step in enhancing perfusion within penumbral territory. Ischaemic stroke patients arriving within 4.5 hours of symptom onset who meet current criteria for tPA treatment should be rapidly thrombolysed with intravenous tPA (IV-tPA) (Adams et al. 2007; Alberts et al. 2000, 2005). In most US hospitals, administration of IV-tPA does not require written consent because patients with acute stroke are at significant risk for severe neurological disability, warranting emergency medical treatment with all available approved therapies. The position in the UK is that IV-tPA is a recognised and licensed treatment so explanation and verbal agreement only is required or a medical 'best interests' decision if the patient is unable to participate in decision-making. Good practice denotes providing information to the patient and relatives as appropriate. The US approach of waiving of written consent for IV-tPA treatment in ischaemic stroke mirrors that applied, for example, for major traumatic injury requiring emergency surgery, or acute myocardial infarction warranting emergency reperfusion. Additionally, because neurological disability may preclude a stroke patient's ability to sign their own written consent, waiting to obtain consent from the legally designated family member may prevent administration of IV-tPA in a timely manner, thereby worsening subsequent neurological disability.

Numerous studies have demonstrated the safety and benefit of IV-tPA for the treatment of acute ischaemic stroke (Albers et al. 2000; Hacke et al. 1998, 2004; Hill & Buchan 2005; Steiner et al. 1998; The National Institute of Neurological Disorders and Stroke rt-PA Stroke Study Group 1995; Wahlgren et al. 2007). A potentially serious adverse event of IV-tPA is symptomatic intracerebral haemorrhage (sICH), defined as an increase of four or more points on the NIHSS associated with a post-treatment finding of haemorrhage on non-contrast CT (Adams et al. 2007). However, in the hands of well-trained, experienced Stroke Teams, sICH is a relatively rare event. Stroke Teams with high IV-tPA treatment rates typically have sICH rates lower than the 6.4% sICH rate observed in the NIH National Institutes of Neurological Disorders and Stroke (NINDS) tPA trial that led to national drug approval in the US in 1996; this suggests that experience with IV-tPA administration is associated with reduced treatment complications.

It is also important to consider the risk of sICH in relation to the risk of significant neurological disability. For example, using the data from the NINDS tPA trial (1995), about 6 out of 100 patients treated with IV-tPA may be at risk for development of an sICH; applying the data from the phase IV European 'Safe Implementation of Thrombolysis in Stroke Monitoring Study' – SITS-MOST (Wahlgren et al. 2007), about 2 out of 100 patients treated with IV-tPA may be at risk to develop an sICH. Additionally, in the NINDS tPA Trial (1995), 39% of patients receiving IV-tPA compared to only 26% of placebo patients achieved a modified Rankin Score (mRS) of 0–1 by three months, and these patients had a 30% greater chance of sustaining either minimal or no neurological disability at three months compared to placebo patients. Interestingly, SITS-MOST data also demonstrated that 39% of subjects receiving tPA had attained an mRS of 0–1 by three months (Wahlgren et al. 2007), providing significant validation of both the safety and benefit of IV-tPA in the treatment of acute ischaemic stroke patients.

Clearly, the odds of significant neurological improvement with reduction of devastating neurological disability outweigh the risks associated with IV-tPA treatment. In fact, where resistance to the use of IV-tPA for ischaemic stroke remains, it is likely due to the challenge of updating emergency systems that have slow approaches to stroke care, practitioners that may be unwilling to take on the practice of emergency stroke management, and/or health systems with significant financial constraints that are unwilling to support the cost of swift diagnostic imaging, emergency medical and nursing management, and the cost of IV-tPA. However, it is important to recognise that hyperacute stroke practice today equates to 'stat' (immediate) emergency management, and is likely to continue down this path for years to come as researchers explore other methods aimed at enhancing or restoring brain perfusion to ward off neurological disability.

Adherence to an evidence-based protocol for administration of IV-tPA is closely tied to patient outcome. While optimal, weighing ischaemic stroke patients in the ED is rarely undertaken, and was not undertaken in any of the IV-tPA trials. Instead, patients or family are asked to provide approximate weight data, or in the absence of this information, weight is estimated by the Stroke Team. Dosage of IV-tPA is then calculated using the formula:

$$0.9 \text{ mg of tPA per 1 kg of patient weight}$$

The total dose of tPA should never exceed 90 mg, so when the calculated dose exceeds this level, it is dropped back to the 90 mg limit. Once the total dose has been calculated, 10% of the total is given as an intravenous bolus over 1 minute; the remaining 90% of the dose is then infused over the next 60 minutes.

Safety measures that are advocated to ensure that the exact amount of tPA ordered is given include the following:

- Double check and verify among Stroke Team members the estimated patient weight used in the calculation of total tPA dose.
- Double check the total dose calculation.

- Withdraw and discard from the tPA vial the amount of drug that exceeds the total dose. (Clinical example: Each vial of tPA contains a total of 100 mg/100 ml fluid once reconstituted. If the total dose to be given is 68 mg, the Stroke Team nurse should withdraw and discard 32 ml of the reconstituted tPA, leaving only the 68 ml in the vial for infusion.)
- Withdraw with a 10 ml syringe a 10% bolus dose. (Clinical example: If the total dose to be given is 68 mg, the 10% bolus dose amounts to 6.8 mg or 6.8 ml.)
- Administer the bolus dose over one minute via the intravenous line that will be dedicated to the tPA infusion.
- Attach the intravenous tubing to the tPA bottle, or other administration device, e.g. syringe driver, and clear the line of air; ensure that no tPA is wasted while clearing the air from the line.
- Attach the tPA infusion to an infusion pump (or prepare the syringe driver) and set for 60 minutes to deliver the drug remaining in the vial.
- Ensure that once the infusion is complete, all tPA remaining in the tubing reaches the patient before the infusion is discontinued.
- Once discontinued, flush the intravenous line with 3–5 ml normal saline.

Prior to administration of the bolus, as well as throughout the tPA infusion and post-infusion 24-hour period, it is paramount that blood pressure is precisely and accurately measured and controlled to maintain the parameters noted in Table 4.3 (Adams et al. 2007). Inability to appropriately control blood pressure is the most common reason associated with sICH in IV-tPA-treated patients; all deviations from specified blood pressure parameters must be immediately acted upon with intravenous antihypertensive agents to ensure patient safety. Pharmaceutical agents that allow for rapid, precise, non-aggressive blood pressure reduction are best, because dropping the blood pressure too low will result in decreased blood flow through the residual arterial lumen which may worsen perfusion within the ischaemic penumbra (Adams et al. 2007; Castillo et al. 2004; Johnston & Mayer 2003).

Use of non-invasive oscillometric automatic blood pressure (NIBP) cuffs had originally been thought to be dangerous in IV-tPA treated patients because of intense mechanical compression of the arm that might facilitate bruising. However, no study has been undertaken to investigate this, and these devices are regularly used in many facilities without deleterious effects. It cannot be concluded that NIBPs are entirely safe, but neither is there any indication at present that they are unsafe; future investigations by nurses may assist in quantifying safety concerns with these devices during and after treatment with IV-tPA.

Elevated glucose levels should also be identified early in the hyperacute phase due to their association with poor neurological outcome; when present, elevated glucose should be treated with short-acting insulin prior to treatment with tPA to achieve a value ranging from 80 to 110 mg/dl (Adams et al. 2007; Baird et al. 2002; Gray et al. 2004; Scott et al. 1999; Williams et al. 2002). Consensus management in the UK aims to maintain blood glucose levels in the range of 4–9 mmol/l in the first 24–48 hours post-stroke, and consider starting a glucose-potassium infusion at 10 mmol/l.

Table 4.3 Control of blood pressure in intravenous tPA treated patients.

Phase of management	Blood pressure control guidelines
Preparing for tPA administration	*If blood pressure is >185 mmHg systolic or >110 mmHg diastolic, administer:* • Labetalol 10 to 20 mg IV over 1 to 2 minutes, may repeat once; or • Nitropaste 1 to 2 inches; or • Nicardipine infusion, 5 mg/hour; titrate up by 0.25 mg/hour at 5- to 15-minute intervals, maximum dose 15 mg/hour *If blood pressure remains >185 mmHg systolic or >110 mmHg diastolic, do NOT give tPA bolus*
During and after tPA treatment	• Monitor blood pressure every 15 minutes during treatment • Immediately post-treatment, vital signs frequency for the next 24 hours should be: every 15 minutes for 2 hours; every 30 minutes for 6 hours; every hour for 16 hours • Maintain systolic blood pressure <180 mmHg and diastolic blood pressure <105 mmHg *If blood pressure >180 mmHg and diastolic blood pressure >105 mmHg, administer:* • Labetalol 10 mg IV over 1 to 2 minutes; may repeat every 10–20 minutes to a total of 300 mg (consider labetalol infusion if repeated injections are necessary) or • Nicardipine infusion, 5 mg/hour; titrate up by 0.25 mg/hour at 5- to 15-minute intervals, maximum dose 15 mg/hour or • Sodium nitroprusside if unable to control blood pressure with nicardipine

Note: Adapted from the American Stroke Association 2007 Guidelines (Adams et al. 2007).

Additionally, the presence of fever in acute stroke patients is also associated with poor outcome and these patients should be rapidly returned to normothermic levels using routine measures such as paracetamol or cooling blankets (Adams et al. 2007; Azzimondi et al. 1995; Castillo et al. 1998; Ginsberg & Busto 1998; Hajat et al. 2000; Reith et al. 1996; Wang et al. 2000; Zaremba 2004).

Other nursing priorities during and after delivery of IV-tPA include close monitoring for neurological change using an objective quantifiable tool such as the NIHSS to alert clinicians to improvement or deterioration warranting repeat of a 'stat' non-contrast CT to rule out sICH. Sudden onset of neurological deterioration in the first 24 hours from treatment with IV-tPA is associated with either sICH or arterial reocclusion, which may occur in up to 22% of patients (Alexandrov et al. 2004). By closely assessing patients for neurological change, reocclusion can be immediately identified and, in some cases, acted upon by means of intra-arterial rescue (Adams et al. 2007). Lastly, nurses and other interdisciplinary providers involved in the care of patients treated with IV-tPA must remember that once the drug has been administered, no invasive procedures may be performed for the next 24 hours unless there is a life-threatening need AND only when the invasive procedure is being performed in a compressible or surgically controlled manner.

For ischaemic stroke patients with arterial occlusions evident on neuroimaging that may be treated within eight hours of symptom onset, use of intra-arterial rescue procedures are options that are enthusiastically being adopted in many countries throughout the world. Options include intra-arterial tPa, clot extraction using devices such as the MERCI™ retriever or Penumbra™, angioplasty, and/or intra- and extracranial stent placement (Adams et al. 2007); often these treatment strategies are combined to ensure both clot clearance and vessel patency. Further research is required to quantify risks and benefits.

Arterial access is typically achieved through canalisation of the femoral artery. Serial angiograms are taken to diagnose the problem, strategise the treatment approach, and once treatment is complete, to evaluate the outcome. Patients undergoing intra-arterial treatment may require intubation and sedation depending on the procedure undertaken and the preference of the clinicians. Once the procedure is concluded, patients are often transported directly to MRI so that final infarct size can be determined. Nursing care of patients undergoing intra-arterial rescue procedures includes: airway management; weaning and extubation; close monitoring and control of blood pressure before, during and after the procedure; management of intra-procedural sedation; assessment of the groin arterial puncture site and/or maintenance of arterial sheaths when left in place; and ongoing neurological monitoring using a quantifiable tool such as the NIHSS to determine change from baseline scores.

Hyperacute treatment of haemorrhagic stroke

Once non-contrast CT evidence of haemorrhage has been obtained, the patient should be positioned with the head of the bed at 30 degrees because of the potential for development of increased ICP secondary to intracranial haemorrhage. Medical treatment of haemorrhagic stroke is closely associated with haemorrhage subtype, namely intraparenchymal haemorrhages (hypertensive, coagulopathic or amyloid origins), aneurysmal subarachnoid haemorrhage (SAH) or arteriovenous malformation (AVM) related haemorrhage.

Intraparenchymal haemorrhage (IPH) is the most common form of haemorrhagic stroke, producing bleeding into the brain tissues. In the case of hypertensive IPH, the most vulnerable areas of the brain include the basal ganglia, thalami and occasionally the pons (Broderick et al. 2007). Coagulopathic IPH may occur in a variety of locations depending on whether concurrent head trauma is a factor, and on the presence of amyloid angiopathy and/or significant concurrent hypertension (Broderick et al. 2007; Flibotte et al. 2004). In the case of pure amyloid-related IPH, the most common location is on the convexities of the grey matter of the brain, and this type of IPH is more common with elevated age and/or genetic predisposition. Unfortunately, IPH continues to challenge stroke practitioners in that surgical treatment has yet to be shown to be more effective than conservative non-surgical approaches, and no drug

---

Box 4.1 Guidelines for control of blood pressure in haemorrhagic stroke.

- IF systolic blood pressure is >200 mmHg or mean arterial pressure is >150 mmHg:CONSIDER aggressively lowering blood pressure with continuous intravenous infusion agents; reassess blood pressure every 5 minutes
- IF systolic blood pressure is >180 mmHg or mean arterial pressure is >130 mmHg
  AND if there is evidence of elevated intracranial pressure (ICP):
  CONSIDER monitoring ICP and administering intermittent (e.g. labetalol) or continuous agents (e.g. nicardipine) to maintain cerebral perfusion pressure >60–80 mmHg
- IF systolic blood pressure is >180 mmHg or mean arterial pressure is >130 mmHg
  AND there is no evidence of increased ICP:
  CONSIDER modest reduction of blood pressure (e.g. 160/90 mmHg or mean arterial pressure of 110 mmHg) using either intermittent or continuous intravenous medications; re-examine the patient every 15 minutes to determine tolerance of lower blood pressure parameters

Note: Adapted from the American Stroke Association 2007 Guidelines (Adams et al. 2007).

---

therapy to date has yet to achieve a difference in the three-month outcome of this disease (Broderick et al. 2007). Considerations in the medical management of IPH include: close monitoring and control of blood pressure, rapid or early detection of coagulopathies and reversal of these conditions when present, identification of non-communicating hydrocephalus resulting from ventricular clot obstruction, ongoing neurological assessment, and in some cases institution of palliative care (Broderick et al. 2007).

Blood pressure limits set by expert consensus and medications for control of blood pressure in haemorrhagic stroke can be seen in Box 4.1. It remains unknown at this time whether hypertension occurs in response to haemorrhage expansion with increased ICP in haemorrhagic stroke, or whether prolonged elevation of blood pressure is responsible for haemorrhagic expansion in IPH. The two processes are clearly related, with the risk for haemorrhage expansion and clinical deterioration ranging from 14% to 38% within the first 24 hours of the initial bleed (Broderick et al. 2007; Brott et al. 1997; Fujii et al. 1998; Kazui et al. 1996). It is theoretically feasible that elevated blood pressure may exacerbate haemorrhage expansion and so current research is focusing on whether aggressive, early blood pressure reduction is associated with less expansion and better outcomes in IPH. Until the results of this work are known, the exact blood pressure parameters that are associated with improved stroke outcomes in IPH remain unverified by science. Additionally, Box 4.1 highlights the need for careful patient assessment in relation to blood pressure parameters: strategies for management of blood pressure differ in the presence of elevated ICP, because higher mean arterial pressures may be necessary to ensure achievement of optimal cerebral perfusion pressures (CPP).

Early identification of a concurrent coagulopathy is paramount to determining the need for additional treatment to support or augment the clotting cascade (Broderick et al. 2007; Flibotte et al. 2004). Coagulopathies may occur in patients treated with anticoagulants, as well as diseases such as chronic alcoholism (Alexandrov et al. 2007b; Broderick et al. 2007). Warfarin-related coagulopathies have been associated with significant ongoing expansion of IPH, and should be rapidly targeted for reversal. Traditional management of coagulopathies includes administration of vitamin K (phytonadione 10 mg intravenously delivered over 10 minutes), infusion of fresh frozen plasma, and/or cryoprecipitate (Broderick et al. 2007). This traditional treatment regimen can be challenging to administer without deleterious effects, because the overall volume of fluid administered is significant, and patients with underlying left ventricular dysfunction are at great risk for developing heart failure.

Factor VIIa (80 µg/kg given intravenously) has been shown to significantly reduce haemorrhage expansion in all-cause IPH while not demonstrating a significant difference in three-month outcome (Broderick et al. 2007; Mayer et al. 2005); whether factor VIIa may be a suitable choice for more rapid, low fluid volume control of purely coagulopathic IPH remains to be seen (Freeman et al. 2004), but it may be a reasonable theoretical choice in the early management of this disease. Prothrombin complex concentrate (PCC) consists of vitamin K dependent factors (II, VII, IX and X) and it may also be a reasonable choice for prevention of haemorrhage expansion (Broderick et al. 2007; Lankiewicz et al. 2006); however, PCC safety and dose for this use has not yet been established by clinical trials. It is also important to note that PCC factor concentrations may vary by batches and manufacturers, and it may not be readily available in many hospitals. Should factor VIIa or PCC be selected for treatment, cautious screening of patients for concurrent arterial and/or venous occlusive disease is paramount to the safe administration of these substances, since both will increase blood clotting systemically and therefore may exacerbate vessel occlusion sequelae, for example myocardial infarction, deep vein thrombosis, peripheral limb ischaemia (Broderick et al. 2007).

Serial non-contrast CT is important in IPH to document stability or expansion of haemorrhage, especially when significant clinical change is identified. In the case of subcortical or pontine IPH, extension into or obstruction of the ventricular system may occur, making insertion of ventriculostomy for drainage of cerebrospinal fluid necessary in many cases (Broderick et al. 2007). Ongoing research is investigating the efficacy of instillation of small amounts of tPA into intraventricular catheters to facilitate ventricular blood clot dissolution and drainage, once the haemorrhage size has stabilised (Naff et al. 2004); this treatment may hold promise in reducing the duration of ventricular drainage and the need for long-term shunting. Once inserted, ventricular drains should be levelled and zero balanced to the foramen of Monro, and ICP should be monitored closely, with the system open to drainage and the head of the patient's bed elevated to 30 degrees. Standard measures for treatment of increased ICP should be employed as indicated. Neurological status should be closely observed since haemorrhage enlargement is associated with poor clinical outcome and death.

The validity of using the NIHSS as a quantitative tool to capture neurological disability in haemorrhagic stroke has not yet been studied but this tool may be suitable since it does provide more complete neurological assessment data than the Glasgow Coma Scale (GCS) alone. Use of the GCS is also considered to be acceptable in IPH, but alone this instrument does not capture key elements of the neurological examination other than the 'best response' of factors most closely aligned with consciousness. The Intracerebral Haemorrhage Score

(ICHS) should also be calculated (Table 3.11, Chapter 3) because it provides a useful estimate of outcome from this devastating disease (Hemphill et al. 2001). In cases of large IPH with coma, the Stroke Team must cautiously decide whether heroic measures are in the patient's best interest, and consider consulting with family members about pursuing palliative care.

In the case of haemorrhages located in places deemed unusual for the forms of IPH discussed above, and/or the presence of SAH on non-contrast CT, imaging priorities shift to include angiographic capabilities (e.g. CTA or digital subtraction angiography (DSA)) to identify brain aneurysm or AVM (Broderick et al. 2007). Definitive treatment of arterial anomalies using endovascular catheter-based (e.g. detachable coils) or surgical procedures is an early consideration to reduce the risk for rebleeding.

Acute stroke management

General management priorities

Once the hyperacute phase of stroke management is complete, priorities shift to:

- Identifying aetiological stroke mechanisms
- Developing individualised secondary stroke prevention measures aimed at addressing these factors
- Prevention of complications
- Evaluation of rehabilitation needs
- Patient and family preparation for discharge from acute care services

Blood pressure control continues during the acute phase of hospitalisation for stroke, but goals may vary when haemodynamic factors suggest the need for higher pressures (e.g. persisting extracranial or intracranial vessel occlusions). By 24 hours, oral antihypertensive agents or those that may be given through enteral feeding tubes are added to the regimen and patients are progressively weaned from intravenous antihypertensive agents. Multiple agents are often required to achieve adequate blood pressure control and should be added slowly and adjusted to achieve the therapeutic effect over the course of hospitalisation (Adams et al. 2007; Broderick et al. 2007; Chobanian et al. 2003). Antihypertensive drugs should be selected based on consideration of numerous factors such as underlying renal function, history of myocardial infarction, left ventricular dysfunction, baseline cardiac rhythm, and even genetic factors (clinical trials data suggest that people of black ethnic origin may respond better to use of calcium channel blockers, as compared to angiotensin-converting enzyme inhibitors or angiotensin receptor blockers, due to their lower rates of renin-based hypertension (ALLHAT 2002)).

Blood glucose levels should continue to be closely monitored and controlled in patients with diabetes. The target range for blood glucose is 80–110 mg/dl (4–9 mmol/l), and practitioners should strive to maintain glucose in this range using insulin or oral agents as indicated by baseline values and response to treatment. Temperature should also be monitored as hyperthermia has been associated with poor neurological outcome and may also indicate an underlying infectious process requiring management (Adams et al. 2007; Broderick et al. 2007).

Swallow integrity must be assessed in all stroke patients with the patient kept 'nil orally' (NPO) until the ability to safely manage oral intake has been adequately assessed (Adams et al. 2007; Alberts et al. 2000). Chapter 5 provides a detailed overview of the measures used to screen and definitively diagnose swallow dysfunction in stroke patients alongside recommendations for nutritional support and rehabilitation. The risk of aspiration is high in patients with dysphagia and/or strokes that are associated with a decrease in level of consciousness (LOC). Vigilant nursing assessment of airway patency, breathing pattern, breath sounds and gas exchange is important in the prevention and early detection of aspiration. Although the head of the bed should be kept at zero degrees during the first 12–24 hours following ischaemic stroke to optimise lesion haemodynamics, in patients with decreased LOC and/or an inability to deal with secretions, side-lying positioning should be maintained instead of supine, to reduce aspiration risk. In cases where the patient was found on the floor and unconscious, aspiration may have occurred prior to hospitalisation and this should be noted in their record.

The prevalence of sleep apnoea in stroke patients ranges from 30% to 70% (Culebras 2005; Martinez-Garcia et al. 2005). It remains unclear how often sleep apnoea in stroke patients is of central, obstructive or mixed aetiologies, and while all patients suspected of this disorder should receive formal sleep studies, the early identification and management of sleep-associated disordered breathing should be promptly undertaken by stroke practitioners. The 'reversed Robin Hood syndrome' (RRHS) details the intravascular 'steal' of blood from neurovascular territories associated with stroke, which need optimal perfusion, to normal vascular territories during apnoeic episodes (Alexandrov et al. 2007a).

The pathophysiology supporting RRHS suggests that vasomotor reactivity in response to elevated carbon dioxide levels is lost in the arterial region of the stroke due to ischaemia, which depletes cellular adenosine triphosphate (ATP) stores; however, vasomotor reactivity is maintained in normally perfused areas of the brain. During apnoeic episodes with elevated arterial carbon dioxide levels, normal vasculature in the brain vasodilates, thereby 'stealing' arterial blood flow away from ischaemic regions that are unable to dilate in response to carbon dioxide levels. Quantifiable clinical worsening has been noted in response to RRHS due to increased penumbral ischaemia (Alexandrov et al. 2007a). Use of non-invasive modes of ventilation with continuous positive airway pressure (CPAP) has been shown to improve and maintain steady arterial flow through neurovascular territories in patients with sleep apnoea, while improving and maintaining clinical outcome (Martinez-Garcia et al. 2005). Nurses working with stroke patients will increasingly need to become expert in non-invasive ventilation with its growing use to combat sleep-disordered breathing problems such as apnoea.

Prolonged immobility contributes to the risk of: venous thromboembolism (VTE); pneumonia with reduced systemic perfusion; skin breakdown; physical deconditioning; and lethargy with mental confusion (Adams et al. 2007; Alberts et al. 2000; Bernhardt et al. 2008). These topics are covered in detail in Chapters 5, 7, 8, 9 and 11, and it is important to emphasise that once the hyperacute stage has ended (and there are no medical contraindications), patients should be moved to a mobilisation protocol that includes: moving out of bed to a chair; range of motion; and progressive ambulation. Patients should also be thoroughly assessed for their rehabilitation needs by members of the interdisciplinary Stroke Team (Adams et al. 2007; Alberts et al. 2000).

Development of VTE is a significant concern following stroke that is associated with prolonged immobility (Adams et al. 2007; Alberts et al. 2000; Broderick et al. 2007; Fraser et al. 2002; Gregory & Kuhlemeier 2003); institution of prophylactic measures to prevent VTE is the standard of care throughout most of the world. Methods of VTE prevention include anticoagulation, which carries the best supporting evidence in ischaemic stroke. Sequential compression devices (SCD) are currently being investigated; thigh-length compression stockings have been demonstrated as ineffective (The CLOTS Trial Collaboration 2009). In many instances, these preventative strategies are combined (e.g. anticoagulation combined with use of SCD) to provide optimal VTE prophylaxis (Adams et al. 2007; Alberts et al. 2000; Boeer et al. 1991; Broderick et al. 2007; Lacut et al. 2005). This is one part of a major international trial (the CLOTS trial: http://www.dcn.ed.ac.uk/clots/), an earlier component of which demonstrated that compression stockings alone are ineffective (The CLOTS Trial Collaboration 2009). The safety of using anticoagulation for VTE prophylaxis in IPH has not been established by large randomised clinical trials, although many experts assert that once the haemorrhage has stabilised, at approximately 72 hours from stroke onset, anticoagulation is probably safe and should be considered given its superiority to other prophylactic measures (Boeer et al. 1991; Broderick et al. 2007).

The routine insertion of urinary catheters in acute stroke patients should be discouraged, and instead patients should be individually assessed for the need for these devices. Chapter 6 provides detailed information related to continence, but within the context of this chapter, it is important to emphasise that urinary catheters should be considered when close tracking of intake and output takes precedence (e.g. concurrent congestive heart failure, myocardial stunning, use of triple H therapy – hypertension, hypervolaemia, haemodilution) and/or when urinary retention is a concern, but not routinely as a convenience to the nursing staff. Urine samples taken on admission should screen for bacterial contamination, and the need for culture and sensitivity testing may follow based on initial results. When patients are admitted with urinary tract infection (UTI), this should be clearly documented to exclude a diagnosis of hospital-acquired UTI.

Patients who smoke should be counselled to further reduce the risk of another stroke event and/or cardiac disease (Adams et al. 2007; Alberts et al. 2000). It is essential that family and significant others be involved in this process, because smoking cessation is often a 'family affair' that requires all those close to the patient to quit smoking as well, to ensure long-term sustainability. Use of nicotine patches or varenicline (Chantix/Champix) may complement a smoking cessation plan; Chapter 13 has details of this.

From hospital admission through till the point of hospital discharge, patients and their family members should also receive ongoing education about stroke that covers:

- Ischaemic and haemorrhagic stroke disease processes
- Stroke warning signs
- Rapid access to a hospital delivering hyperacute stroke care and use of emergency medical transport systems
- Risk factors for stroke and their modification
- Treatment for stroke
- Recovery from stroke
- Prevention of complications associated with stroke
- Hospital discharge planning (Adams et al. 2007; Alberts et al. 2000)

Specific management of ischaemic stroke

Box 4.2 presents components of a post IV-tPA protocol that outlines routine care. Special attention should be paid to arterial blood pressure control in tPA-treated patients due to the increased risk for sICH with elevated blood pressure post-tPA treatment (Adams et al. 2007). Use of protocols and care pathways for nursing and medical care may result in better adherence to blood pressure goals after treatment with IV-tPA and improve patient outcomes.

In patients with large infarctions affecting the cerebral hemispheres, and in particular in young patients lacking room within the cranial vault associated with atrophic age-related changes, hemicraniectomy may be considered as a life-saving technique when intracranial mass effects with the risk for herniation are a concern (Vahedi et al. 2007). Craniectomy may also be employed to treat cerebellar infarctions that risk compromise of brainstem structures due to oedema and obstructive hydrocephalus. Cautious patient selection and early

---

Box 4.2 Intravenous t-PA post-treatment order set.

- Activity – bed rest for 24 hours with head of bed at 0 degrees; turn side to side to protect airway as needed
- Vital signs: blood pressure and pulse every 15 minutes for the first 2 hours after completion of tPA drip, then every 30 minutes for 6 hours, then hourly for 16 hours
- Continuous cardiac monitoring; repeat aberrant cardiac rhythms and run ECG strip to document
- Record National Institutes of Health Stroke Scale (NIHSS) hourly for 24 hours; increase frequency of score if deterioration occurs in clinical examination
- Order stat non-contrast CT scan and notify Stroke Team stat for any deterioration in clinical examination
- Notify Stroke Team stat for any signs of oropharyngeal oedema
- Notify Stroke Team stat for any signs of excessive extracranial haemorrhage; apply pressure to external bleeding sites if necessary
- Hold all antithrombotic medications (antiplatelet and anticoagulation medications) for at least 24 hours
- Avoid all arterial or intravenous blood draws and intravenous line starts for 24 hours unless critically warranted by patient's condition and in a compressible site
- Do not insert Foley catheter and/or nasogastric/nasoenteric tube for 24 hours
- Nil orally
- Manage blood pressure according to parameters and methods listed in Table 4.3

Table 4.4 The CHADS-2 Score (Gage et al. 2001).

Component	Score
Congestive heart failure	1
Hypertension	1
Age ≥75 years	1
Diabetes mellitus	1
History of stroke or transient ischaemic attack	2
Recommendations based on CHADS-2 Score:	
CHADS-2 = 0: stroke risk low (1.0%/year)	Aspirin 75–325 mg/day
CHADS-2 = 1: stroke risk low/moderate (1.5%/year)	Warfarin (INR 2–3) or aspirin (as above)
CHADS-2 = 2: stroke risk moderate (2.5%/year)	Warfarin (INR 2–3)
CHADS-2 = 3: stroke risk high (5.0%/year)	Warfarin (INR 2–3)
CHADS-2 = 4 or higher: stroke risk very high (>7.0%/year)	Warfarin (INR 2–3)

timing for hemicraniectomy are important. Post-procedural serial assessments using the NIHSS are important after hemicraniectomy and should be accompanied by non-contrast CT to determine response to therapy. Bone removed during the procedure may be either stored in a Bone Bank or sewn into a pouch made in the patient's abdomen; the bone is replaced at around three months from the time of the brain infarction, and until that time, helmet precautions should be implemented.

Antiplatelet agents and statins are commonly used in the treatment and secondary prevention of ischaemic stroke, and further detail of this is given in Chapter 13.

The benefit of anticoagulation in atrial fibrillation to prevent stroke is well established and discussed in Chapter 13. The CHADS-2 score (Table 4.4) may provide one method to gauge risk of stroke in patients with atrial fibrillation to determine best medical treatment (Gage et al. 2001). When anticoagulation is selected, in the US it is typically withheld for the first three days from the time of stroke onset because of the risk of haemorrhagic transformation of the infarction. Intravenous heparin is started and then the patient is bridged to oral warfarin (Adams et al. 2007). The target international normalised ratio (INR) for patients with atrial fibrillation is an INR of 2–3, compared to patients with prosthetic heart valves who aim to achieve an INR of 2.5–3.5. Heparin is usually discontinued once the INR reaches 1.8 (usually by day three) and patients who are otherwise eligible for discharge may be released when this level is achieved if they can return to have their INR checked within two to three days after discharge.

Specific management of haemorrhagic stroke

In the case of SAH, secondary ischaemic stroke associated with refractory vasospasm is common, and medical strategies such as use of triple 'H' therapy (hypertension, hypervolaemia and haemodilution) are commonly employed, along with intra-arterial angioplasty, although definitive differences in clinical outcome have yet to be observed with these techniques (Zwienenberg-Lee et al. 2008). Nimodipine therapy is now widely acknowledged to have no direct effect on reduction of vasospasm, but probably increases the tolerance of ischaemia within brain tissues subjected to vasospasm. Use of dihydropyridine class calcium channel blockers such as nicardipine has recently emerged as a new strategy to combat vasospasm. Either by direct surgical implantation after open surgical flushing of the basal cisterns (Barth et al. 2007), or by intra-arterial infusion during direct intracranial arterial canalisation, dihydropyridines hold promise in their ability to prevent and treat vasospasm, while also providing likely neuroprotective effects through elevation of tissue thresholds to ischaemic insult.

There has been wide documentation about how SAH is associated with stunning of the myocardium (Lee et al. 2006; Samuels 2007), which further challenges use of hypertension and hypervolaemic management, placing patients at risk for development of heart failure due to significant left ventricular afterload and elevated preload. Judicious use of volume and pressure-driven therapies is paramount. Lastly, development of non-communicating hydrocephalus is common in SAH requiring management by ventriculostomy and often long-term shunt placement. Because early surgical or endovascular treatment is now the standard of care for aneurysmal SAH, development of increased ICP in patients with SAH is most commonly associated with either hydrocephalus that has not been properly identified and treated by ventriculostomy, or ischaemic infarction that develops secondary to refractory vasospasm.

Conclusion

Acute stroke management today is supported by aggressive front-line therapies that have moved the setting of care to Emergency Departments, Acute Stroke Units and Catheterisation Labs, away from a paradigm that was focused on supportive care only. Hyperacute stroke science requires an inquisitive interest and determination to reverse neurological dysfunction; nurses practising in this area must embrace this challenge and join this exciting expedition toward improvement of stroke outcomes.

References

Adams, HP, Jr, del Zoppo G, Alberts, MJ, Bhatt, DL, Brass, L et al., 2007, Guidelines for the early management of adults with ischemic stroke: a guideline from the American Heart Association/American Stroke Association Stroke Council, Clinical Cardiology Council, Cardiovascular Radiology and Intervention Council, and the Atherosclerotic Peripheral Vascular Disease and Quality of Care Outcomes in Research Interdisciplinary Working Groups: the American Academy of Neurology affirms the value of this guideline as an educational tool for neurologists, *Stroke*, vol. 38, no. 5, pp. 1655–1711.

Albers, GW, Bates, VE, Clark, WM, Bell, R, Verro, P et al., 2000, Intravenous tissue-type plasminogen activator for treatment of acute stroke: the Standard Treatment with Alteplase to Reverse Stroke (STARS) study, *Journal of the American Medical Association*, vol. 283, no. 9, pp. 1145–1150.

Alberts, MJ, Hademenos, G, Latchaw, RE, Jagoda, A, Marler, JR et al., 2000, Recommendations for the establishment of primary stroke centers. Brain Attack Coalition, *Journal of the American Medical Association*, vol. 283, no. 23, pp. 3102–3109.

Alberts, MJ, Latchaw, RE, Selman, WR, Shephard, T, Hadley, MN et al., 2005, Recommendations for comprehensive stroke centers: a consensus statement from the Brain Attack Coalition, *Stroke*, vol. 36, no. 7, pp. 1597–1616.

Alexandrov, AV, Molina, CA, Grotta, JC, Garami, Z, Ford, SR et al., 2004, Ultrasound-enhanced systemic thrombolysis for acute ischemic stroke, *New England Journal of Medicine*, vol. 351, no. 21, pp. 2170–2178.

Alexandrov, AV, Sharma, VK, Lao, AY, Tsivgoulis, G, Malkoff, MD et al., 2007a, Reversed Robin Hood syndrome in acute ischemic stroke patients, *Stroke*, vol. 38, no. 11, pp. 3045–3048.

Alexandrov, AW, Lao, AY, & Frey, JL, 2007b, Stroke in southwest native Americans, *International Journal of Stroke*, vol. 2, no. 1, p. 62.

ALLHAT, 2002, Major outcomes in high-risk hypertensive patients randomized to angiotensin-converting enzyme inhibitor or calcium channel blocker vs diuretic: The Antihypertensive and Lipid-Lowering Treatment to Prevent Heart Attack Trial (ALLHAT), *Journal of the American Medical Association*, vol. 288, no. 23, pp. 2981–2997.

Azzimondi, G, Bassein, L, Nonino, F, Fiorani, L, Vignatelli, L et al., 1995, Fever in acute stroke worsens prognosis: A prospective study, *Stroke*, vol. 26, no. 11, pp. 2040–2043.

Baird, TA, Parsons, MW, Barber, PA, Butcher, KS, Desmond, PM et al., 2002, The influence of diabetes mellitus and hyperglycaemia on stroke incidence and outcome, *Journal of Clinical Neuroscience*, vol. 9, no. 6, pp. 618–626.

Barth, M, Capelle, HH, Weidauer, S, Weiss, C, Munch, E et al., 2007, Effect of nicardipine prolonged-release implants on cerebral vasospasm and clinical outcome after severe aneurysmal subarachnoid hemorrhage: a prospective, randomized, double-blind phase IIa study, *Stroke*, vol. 38, no. 2, pp. 330–336.

Bernhardt, J, Dewey, H, Thrift, A, Collier, J, & Donnan, G, 2008, A very early rehabilitation trial for stroke (AVERT): phase II safety and feasibility, *Stroke*, vol. 39, no. 2, pp. 390–396.

Boeer, A, Voth, E, Henze, T, & Prange, HW, 1991, Early heparin therapy in patients with spontaneous intracerebral haemorrhage, *Journal of Neurology, Neurosurgery and Psychiatry*, vol. 54, no. 5, pp. 466–467.

Broderick, J, Connolly, S, Feldmann, E, Hanley, D, Kase, C et al., 2007, Guidelines for the management of spontaneous intracerebral hemorrhage in adults: 2007 update: a guideline from the American Heart Association/American Stroke Association Stroke Council, High Blood Pressure Research Council, and the Quality of Care and Outcomes in Research Interdisciplinary Working Group, *Stroke*, vol. 38, no. 6, pp. 2001–2023.

Brott, T, Broderick, J, Kothari, R, Barsan, W, Tomsick, T et al., 1997, Early hemorrhage growth in patients with intracerebral hemorrhage, *Stroke*, vol. 28, no. 1, pp. 1–5.

Castillo, J, Davalos, A, Marrugat, J, & Noya, M, 1998, Timing for fever-related brain damage in acute ischemic stroke, *Stroke*, vol. 29, no. 12, pp. 2455–2460.

Castillo, J, Leira, R, Garcia, MM, Serena, J, Blanco, M et al., 2004, Blood pressure decrease during the acute phase of ischemic stroke is associated with brain injury and poor stroke outcome, *Stroke*, vol. 35, no. 2, pp. 520–526.

Chobanian, AV, Bakris, GL, Black, HR, Cushman, WC, Green, LA et al., 2003, The Seventh Report of the Joint National Committee on Prevention, Detection, Evaluation, and Treatment of High Blood Pressure: the JNC 7 report, *Journal of the American Medical Association*, vol. 289, no. 19, pp. 2560–2572.

Culebras, A, 2005, Sleep apnea and stroke, *Reviews in Neurologic Disease*, vol. 2, no. 1, pp. 13–19.

Dewey, HM, Donnan, GA, Freeman, EJ, Sharples, CM, Macdonell, RA et al., 1999, Interrater reliability of the National Institutes of Health Stroke Scale: rating by neurologists and nurses in a community-based stroke incidence study, *Cerebrovascular Diseases*, vol. 9, no. 6, pp. 323–327.

Dominguez, R, Vila, JF, Augustovski, F, Irazola, V, Castillo, PR et al., 2006, Spanish cross-cultural adaptation and validation of the National Institutes of Health Stroke Scale, *Mayo Clinic Proceedings*, vol. 81, no. 4, pp. 476–480.

Flibotte, JJ, Hagan, N, O'Donnell, J, Greenberg, SM, & Rosand, J, 2004, Warfarin, hematoma expansion, and outcome of intracerebral hemorrhage, *Neurology*, vol. 63, no. 6, pp. 1059–1064.

Fraser, DG, Moody, AR, Morgan, PS, Martel, AL, & Davidson, I, 2002, Diagnosis of lower-limb deep venous thrombosis: a prospective blinded study of magnetic resonance direct thrombus imaging, *Annals of Internal Medicine*, vol. 136, no. 2, pp. 89–98.

Freeman, WD, Brott, TG, Barrett, KM, Castillo, PR, Deen, HG, Jr et al., 2004, Recombinant factor VIIa for rapid reversal of warfarin anticoagulation in acute intracranial hemorrhage, *Mayo Clinic Proceedings*, vol. 79, no. 12, pp. 1495–1500.

Fujii, Y, Takeuchi, S, Sasaki, O, Minakawa, T, & Tanaka, R, 1998, Multivariate analysis of predictors of hematoma enlargement in spontaneous intracerebral hemorrhage, *Stroke*, vol. 29, no. 6, pp. 1160–1166.

Gage, BF, Waterman, AD, Shannon, W, Boechler, M, Rich, MW et al., 2001, Validation of clinical classification schemes for predicting stroke: results from the National Registry of Atrial Fibrillation, *Journal of the American Medical Association*, vol. 285, no. 22, pp. 2864–2870.

Ginsberg, MD, & Busto, R, 1998, Combating hyperthermia in acute stroke: a significant clinical concern, *Stroke*, vol. 29, no. 2, pp. 529–534.

Goldstein, LB, & Samsa, GP, 1997, Reliability of the National Institutes of Health Stroke Scale – Extension to non-neurologists in the context of a clinical trial, *Stroke*, vol. 28, no. 2, pp. 307–310.

Gray, CS, Hildreth, AJ, Alberti, GK, & O'Connell, JE, 2004, Poststroke hyperglycemia: natural history and immediate management, *Stroke*, vol. 35, no. 1, pp. 122–126.

Gregory, PC, & Kuhlemeier, KV, 2003, Prevalence of venous thromboembolism in acute hemorrhagic and thromboembolic stroke, *American Journal of Physical Medicine and Rehabilitation*, vol. 82, no. 5, pp. 364–369.

Grotta, JC, Chiu, D, Lu, M, Patel, S, Levine, SR et al., 1999, Agreement and variability in the interpretation of early CT changes in stroke patients qualifying for intravenous rtPA therapy, *Stroke*, vol. 30, no. 8, pp. 1528–1533.

Hacke, W, Kaste, M, Fieschi, C, von Kummer R, Davalos, A et al., 1998, Randomised double-blind placebo-controlled trial of thrombolytic therapy with intravenous alteplase in acute ischaemic stroke (ECASS II) – Second European-Australasian Acute Stroke Study Investigators, *Lancet*, vol. 352, no. 9136, pp. 1245–1251.

Hacke, W, Donnan, G, Fieschi, C, Kaste, M, von Kummer R et al., 2004, Association of outcome with early stroke treatment: pooled analysis of ATLANTIS, ECASS, and NINDS rt-PA stroke trials, *Lancet*, vol. 363, no. 9411, pp. 768–774.

Hajat, C, Hajat, S, & Sharma, P, 2000, Effects of poststroke pyrexia on stroke outcome: a meta-analysis of studies in patients, *Stroke*, vol. 31, no. 2, pp. 410–414.

Harbison, J, Hossain, O, Jenkinson, D, Davis, J, Louw, SJ et al., 2003, Diagnostic accuracy of stroke referrals from primary care, emergency room physicians, and ambulance staff using the Face Arm Speech Test, *Stroke*, vol. 34, no. 1, pp. 71–76.

Hemphill, JC, III, Bonovich, DC, Besmertis, L, Manley, GT, & Johnston, SC, 2001, The ICH score: a simple, reliable grading scale for intracerebral hemorrhage, *Stroke*, vol. 32, no. 4, pp. 891–897.

Hill, MD, & Buchan, AM, 2005, Thrombolysis for acute ischemic stroke: results of the Canadian Alteplase for Stroke Effectiveness Study, *Canadian Medical Association Journal*, vol. 172, no. 10, pp. 1307–1312.

Johnston, KC, & Mayer, SA, 2003, Blood pressure reduction in ischemic stroke: a two-edged sword? *Neurology*, vol. 61, no. 8, pp. 1030–1031.

Josephson, SA, Hills, NK, & Johnston, SC, 2006, NIH Stroke Scale reliability in ratings from a large sample of clinicians, *Cerebrovascular Diseases*, vol. 22, no. 5–6, pp. 389–395.

Kasner, SE, 2006, Clinical interpretation and use of stroke scales, *Lancet Neurology*, vol. 5, no. 7, pp. 603–612.

Kazui, S, Naritomi, H, Yamamoto, H, Sawada, T, & Yamaguchi, T, 1996, Enlargement of spontaneous intracerebral hemorrhage: incidence and time course, *Stroke*, vol. 27, no. 10, pp. 1783–1787.

Kidwell, CS, Starkman, S, Eckstein, M, Weems, K, & Saver, JL, 2000, Identifying stroke in the field – prospective validation of the Los Angeles prehospital stroke screen (LAPSS), *Stroke*, vol. 31, no. 1, pp. 71–76.

Kidwell, CS, Chalela, JA, Saver, JL, Starkman, S, Hill, MD et al., 2004, Comparison of MRI and CT for detection of acute intracerebral hemorrhage, *Journal of the American Medical Association*, vol. 292, no. 15, pp. 1823–1830.

Kothari, RU, Pancioli, A, Liu, T, Brott, T, & Broderick, J, 1999, Cincinnati Prehospital Stroke Scale: reproducibility and validity, *Annals of Emergency Medicine*, vol. 33, no. 4, pp. 373–378.

Lacut, K, Bressollette, L, Le Gal G, Etienne, E, De Tinteniac, TA et al., 2005, Prevention of venous thrombosis in patients with acute intracerebral hemorrhage, *Neurology*, vol. 65, no. 6, pp. 865–869.

Lankiewicz, MW, Hays, J, Friedman, KD, Tinkoff, G, & Blatt, PM, 2006, Urgent reversal of warfarin with prothrombin complex concentrate, *Journal of Thrombosis and Haemostasis*, vol. 4, no. 5, pp. 967–970.

Lee, VH, Oh, JK, Mulvagh, SL, & Wijdicks, EF, 2006, Mechanisms in neurogenic stress cardiomyopathy after aneurysmal subarachnoid hemorrhage, *Neurocritical Care*, vol. 5, no. 3, pp. 243–249.

Lyden, P, Brott, T, Tilley, B, Welch, KM, Mascha, EJ et al., 1994, Improved reliability of the NIH Stroke Scale using video training. NINDS TPA Stroke Study Group, *Stroke*, vol. 25, no. 11, pp. 2220–2226.

Lyden, P, Lu, M, Jackson, C, Marler, J, Kothari, R et al., 1999, Underlying structure of the National Institutes of Health Stroke Scale: results of a factor analysis – NINDS tPA Stroke Trial Investigators, *Stroke*, vol. 30, no. 11, pp. 2347–2354.

Lyden, P, Raman, R, Liu, L, Grotta, J, Broderick, J et al., 2005, NIHSS training and certification using a new digital video disk is reliable, *Stroke*, vol. 36, no. 11, pp. 2446–2449.

Martinez-Garcia, MA, Galiano-Blancart, R, Roman-Sanchez, P, Soler-Cataluna, JJ, Cabero-Salt, L et al., 2005, Continuous positive airway pressure treatment in sleep apnea prevents new vascular events after ischemic stroke, *Chest*, vol. 128, no. 4, pp. 2123–2129.

Mayer, SA, Brun, NC, Begtrup, K, Broderick, J, Davis, S et al., 2005, Recombinant activated factor VII for acute intracerebral hemorrhage, *New England Journal of Medicine*, vol. 352, no. 8, pp. 777–785.

Morris, DL, Rosamond, W, Madden, K, Schultz, C, & Hamilton, S, 2000, Prehospital and emergency department delays after acute stroke: the Genentech Stroke Presentation Survey, *Stroke*, vol. 31, no. 11, pp. 2585–2590.

Naff, NJ, Hanley, DF, Keyl, PM, Tuhrim, S, Kraut, M et al., 2004, Intraventricular thrombolysis speeds blood clot resolution: results of a pilot, prospective, randomized, double-blind, controlled trial, *Neurosurgery*, vol. 54, no. 3, pp. 577–583.

National Collaborating Centre for Chronic Conditions, 2008, *Stroke: National Clinical Guideline for Diagnosis and Initial Management of Acute Stroke and Transient Ischaemic Attack (TIA)*, London.

National Stroke Foundation, 2008, *Clinical Guidelines for Stroke and TIA Management: A guide for general practice*, National Stroke Foundation, Melbourne.

Nor, AM, McAllister, C, Louw, SJ, Dyker, AG, Davis, M et al., 2004, Agreement between ambulance paramedic- and physician-recorded neurological signs with Face Arm Speech Test (FAST) in acute stroke patients, *Stroke*, vol. 35, no. 6, pp. 1355–1359.

Patel, SC, Levine, SR, Tilley, BC, Grotta, JC, Lu, M et al., 2001, Lack of clinical significance of early ischemic changes on computed tomography in acute stroke, *Journal of the American Medical Association*, vol. 286, no. 22, pp. 2830–2838.

Perry, L, Brooks, W, Hamilton, S, Ayers, T, Bennett, B et al., 2004, Exploring nurses' perspectives of stroke care. *Nursing Standard*, vol. 19, no.12, pp. 33–38.

Porteous, GH, Corry, MD, & Smith, WS, 1999, Emergency medical services dispatcher identification of stroke and transient ischemic attack, *Prehospital Emergency Care*, vol. 3, no. 3, pp. 211–216.

Reith, J, Jorgensen, HS, Pedersen, PM, Nakayama, H, Raaschou, HO et al., 1996, Body temperature in acute stroke: relation to stroke severity, infarct size, mortality, and outcome, *Lancet*, vol. 347, no. 8999, pp. 422–425.

Rossnagel, K, Jungehulsing, GJ, Nolte, CH, Muller-Nordhorn, J, Roll, S et al., 2004, Out-of-hospital delays in patients with acute stroke, *Annals of Emergency Medicine*, vol. 44, no. 5, pp. 476–483.

Rymer, MM, & Thrutchley, DE, 2005, Organizing regional networks to increase acute stroke intervention, *Neurologic Research*, vol. 27 Suppl 1, pp. S9–16.

Samuels, MA, 2007, The brain–heart connection, *Circulation*, vol. 116, no. 1, pp. 77–84.

Schroeder, EB, Rosamond, WD, Morris, DL, Evenson, KR, & Hinn, AR, 2000, Determinants of use of emergency medical services in a population with stroke symptoms: the Second Delay in Accessing Stroke Healthcare (DASH II) Study, *Stroke*, vol. 31, no. 11, pp. 2591–2596.

Schwamm, LH, Pancioli, A, Acker, JE, III, Goldstein, LB, Zorowitz, RD et al., 2005, Recommendations for the establishment of stroke systems of care: recommendations from the American Stroke Association's Task Force on the Development of Stroke Systems, *Stroke*, vol. 36, no. 3, pp. 690–703.

Scott, JF, Robinson, GM, French, JM, O'Connell, JE, Alberti, KG et al., 1999, Prevalence of admission hyperglycaemia across clinical subtypes of acute stroke, *Lancet*, vol. 353, no. 9150, pp. 376–377.

Silliman, SL, Quinn, B, Huggett, V, & Merino, JG, 2003, Use of a field-to-stroke center helicopter transport program to extend thrombolytic therapy to rural residents, *Stroke*, vol. 34, no. 3, pp. 729–733.

Steiner, T, Bluhmki, E, Kaste, M, Toni, D, Trouillas, P et al., 1998, The ECASS 3-hour cohort. Secondary analysis of ECASS data by time stratification – ECASS Study Group. European Cooperative Acute Stroke Study, *Cerebrovascular Diseases*, vol. 8, no. 4, pp. 198–203.

Suyama, J, & Crocco, T, 2002, Prehospital care of the stroke patient, *Emergency Medicine Clinics of North America*, vol. 20, no. 3, pp. 537–552.

Tanabe, P, Gimbel, R, Yarnold, PR, Kyriacou, DN, & Adams, JG, 2004, Reliability and validity of scores on The Emergency Severity Index version 3, *Academic Emergency Medicine*, vol. 11, no. 1, pp. 59–65.

Tanabe, P, Travers, D, Gilboy, N, Rosenau, A, Sierzega, G et al., 2005, Refining Emergency Severity Index triage criteria, *Academic Emergency Medicine*, vol. 12, no. 6, pp. 497–501.

The CLOTS Trials Collaboration, 2009, Effectiveness of thigh-length graduated compression stockings to reduce the risk of deep vein thrombosis after stroke (CLOTS trial 1): a multicentre, randomised controlled trial. *The Lancet*, vol 373, pp. 1958–1965.

The National Institute of Neurological Disorders and Stroke rt-PA Stroke Study Group, 1995, Tissue plasminogen activator for acute ischaemic stroke, *New England Journal of Medicine*, vol. 333, no. 24, pp. 1581–1587.

Vahedi, K, Hofmeijer, J, Juettler, E, Vicaut, E, George, B et al., 2007, Early decompressive surgery in malignant infarction of the middle cerebral artery: a pooled analysis of three randomised controlled trials, *Lancet Neurology*, vol. 6, no. 3, pp. 215–222.

Wahlgren, N, Ahmed, N, Davalos, A, Ford, GA, Grond, M et al., 2007, Thrombolysis with alteplase for acute ischaemic stroke in the Safe Implementation of Thrombolysis in Stroke-Monitoring Study (SITS-MOST): an observational study, *Lancet*, vol. 369, no. 9558, pp. 275–282.

Wang, Y, Lim, LL, Levi, C, Heller, RF, & Fisher, J, 2000, Influence of admission body temperature on stroke mortality, *Stroke*, vol. 31, no. 2, pp. 404–409.

Williams, JE, Rosamond, WD, & Morris, DL, 2000, Stroke symptom attribution and time to emergency department arrival: the delay in accessing stroke healthcare study, *Academic Emergency Medicine*, vol. 7, no. 1, pp. 93–96.

Williams, LS, Rotich, J, Qi, R, Fineberg, N, Espay, A et al., 2002, Effects of admission hyperglycemia on mortality and costs in acute ischemic stroke, *Neurology*, vol. 59, no. 1, pp. 67–71.

Wojner-Alexander, AW, Garami, Z, Chernyshev, OY, & Alexandrov, AV, 2005, Heads down: flat positioning improves blood flow velocity in acute ischemic stroke, *Neurology*, vol. 64, no. 8, pp. 1354–1357.

Wojner-Alexandrov, AW, Alexandrov, AV, Rodriguez, D, Persse, D, & Grotta, JC, 2005, Houston paramedic and emergency stroke treatment and outcomes study (HoPSTO), *Stroke*, vol. 36, no. 7, pp. 1512–1518.

Zaremba, J, 2004, Hyperthermia in ischemic stroke, *Medical Science Monitor*, vol. 10, no. 6, pp. RA148–RA153.

Zwienenberg-Lee, M, Hartman, J, Rudisill, N, Madden, LK, Smith, K et al., 2008, Effect of prophylactic transluminal balloon angioplasty on cerebral vasospasm and outcome in patients with Fisher grade III subarachnoid hemorrhage: results of a phase II multicenter, randomized, clinical trial, *Stroke*, vol. 39, no. 6, pp. 1759–1765.

Chapter 5

Nutritional aspects of stroke care

Lin Perry and Elizabeth Boaden

> Key points
>
> - Good nutrition is essential for recovery and rehabilitation; malnourished patients fare worse, stay in hospital longer, experience more complications and are more likely to die.
> - Eating is a source of pleasure and an intrinsic part of social lives.
> - Dysphagia affects between one-third and one-half of all stroke patients. Early recognition and management is becoming widely recognised and addressed within routine care.
> - Impairments that affect eating are dealt with in therapy programmes, but not those related to eating activities.
> - Recovery can be maximised through holistic assessment and with therapy focusing on the ability to eat and what is consumed.

I   *Since you mention food, is this a good point to ask how you are managing to eat, and what you're eating?*

S1   *Oh Diana will answer that.*

S2   *We haven't used the PEG for a while because gradually over the weeks he's been eating a lot better, ordinary food, within reason. We're very fond of stewed apples –*

S1   *Egg and bacon, macaroni cheese – all sorts of things.*

S2   *Egg and chips, chicken livers, he's very fond of.*

I   *This doesn't sound very much like puree! Or even soft!*

S2   *No he doesn't have puree now. We've given that up.*

S1   *Given that up completely!*

S2   *He eats pretty well ordinary food.*

S1   *I had pork steak –*

S2 *Pork chop.*
S1 *Pork chop! And pizza – I had pizza for my tea the other day! But I'm enjoying my food now.*

(I: Interviewer; S1: 72 years old, male stroke survivor;
S2: survivor's wife; 6 months post-stroke, London, UK)

Introduction

This chapter discusses food, nutrition and malnutrition following stroke, whereas nutrition as a risk factor and as a factor that may decrease the likelihood of stroke recurrence is discussed in Chapter 13. Nutritional status is central to health and disease. Malnutrition is due to not eating or absorbing enough essential components, such as vitamins, minerals, energy or protein. Over-nutrition is reflected in excessive, unbalanced or disproportionate intake, for example too much carbohydrate or fats without adequate vitamins or minerals (Keller 1993). Key characteristics of malnutrition have been identified as: poor appetite, not eating enough, muscle wasting and weight loss in the context of general health deterioration (Chen et al. 2001). However, measurements of these and related features during acute illness are difficult, because the signs, symptoms and effects of malnutrition are confounded by the features of the disease. Studies attempting to disentangle these factors and make between-study comparisons are hampered by the range of different criteria for malnutrition used (Reilly 1996). Nonetheless, nutritional screening and assessment are critical first steps towards ensuring adequate dietary intake. Because malnutrition has been linked with increased risk of death or dependency post-stroke, nutritional screening and assessment, as well as implementation of an action plan to overcome problems are essential components of stroke care (Davalos et al. 1996; Davis et al. 2004; Finestone et al. 1996; FOOD Trial Collaboration 2003). Furthermore, because food and eating are fundamental parts of our social lives and contribute to well-being, they have a substantial influence on quality of life after stroke (Perry & McLaren 2004).

Do stroke patients experience nutritional problems pre-stroke?

Nutrition and malnutrition

Eating enough to meet bodily requirements for energy, protein, fats and other nutrients to maintain health and activity is vital but food and eating are also intricately linked with psychosocial well-being and community life (Lupton 1996). People can often cope with eating poorly in the short term, especially if they were previously well-nourished. However, if this poor eating continues, especially if this is in addition to illness or disease, then outcomes are generally poor.

Older people tend to have a greater risk of malnutrition when they become ill due to the pre-existing physiological and social changes that are associated with normal ageing (Gariballa & Sinclair 1998). With stroke incidence increasing with age, a substantial proportion of stroke patients are affected by age-related nutritional changes. These include:

- Alterations in the gastrointestinal system: fewer taste buds; loss of teeth (with or without getting dentures); reduced gastric acid secretion and decreased gastrointestinal peristalsis
- Altered awareness of hunger, enjoyment in eating, and satiety – sense of fullness (Duffy et al. 1995)
- Social factors: those bereaved or living alone may be less motivated to cook or eat well
- Practical issues such as dependence on others for shopping or meals may limit choices
- Psychological factors, such as depression, may affect appetite and eating habits

Any or all of these factors may contribute to reduced dietary intake both of quality and quantity. Studies of community-living older people have revealed insufficient energy intake in almost 25% of women, and 22–29% of men (Finch et al. 1998), whilst dietary deficiencies across Europe were found in 24% of men and 47% of women (de Groot et al. 1999). High levels of nutritional risk and dietary inadequacies have been found in residential care settings, and in almost 10% of selected general practice patients (Edington et al. 1996; Vir & Love 1979). It is likely that some, perhaps many, stroke patients are under-nourished before their first stroke.

For those who have already experienced a stroke, the situation is compounded by effects of the stroke. In a cohort of stroke patients six months post-stroke 66% had some degree of disablement that affected eating (Perry & McLaren 2003a). Earlier studies had found 51% not cooking, 40–55% not shopping, 23% incapable of making a hot drink, 7–21% in receipt of mobile meals services and 39% dependent for eating (Ebrahim et al. 1987; Wilkinson et al. 1997).

Nutritional status on admission to hospital

Nutritional screening and assessment undertaken with stroke patients on admission to hospital have shown substantial nutritional problems in many people, which pre-dated the stroke. Comparison between studies is difficult because of the lack of an agreed clinical 'gold standard' assessment for 'nutritional risk' or malnutrition. However, there is general agreement that no single criterion is adequate and a combination of assessments is preferred. In the UK, the Malnutrition Universal Screening Tool (http://www.bapen.org.uk/pdfs/must/must_full.pdf) is becoming adopted as the screening tool of choice (http://www.bapen.org.uk/ofnsh/OrganizationOfNutritionalSupportWithinHospitals.pdf); however, to date this has not been studied with stroke patients. Table 5.1 shows assessments and findings from stroke patients. Further explanations of approaches to measuring nutrition (anthropometric, biochemical, clinical

Table 5.1 Timing, assessments and nutritional status identified of stroke patients.

Source	Timing	Assessments	Numbers (%) malnourished/ 'at risk'
Axelsson et al. (1989)	Within 4 days of admission	2 or more under reference limits: weight TSF MAMC albumin, prealbumin, transferrin	16 (16)
Unosson et al. (1994)	Within 48 hr of admission	1 abnormal value in each category Anthropometric: weight index/ MAC/TSF Blood tests: albumin/transthyretin/ alpha$_1$-antitrypsin Skin tests: delayed hypersensitivity with 3 antigens	4 (8)
Davalos et al. (1996)	At 7 days from admission	Albumin <35 g/l or TSF or MAMC <10th centile	17 (16)
Choi-Kwon et al. (1998)	Within 1 week of admission	1 biochemical + 2 anthropometric measurements: <80% reference values of lean body mass or TSF at 3 sites BMI <20 kg/m^2 lymphocytes <1500/mm^3 haemoglobin <12 g/dl albumin <35 g/l	30 (34)
Gariballa et al. (1998)	Within 48 hr of admission	TSF <5th centile MAC <5th centile BMI <20 kg/m^2 albumin <35 g/l	46 (23) 4 (2) 62 (31) 38 (19)
Westergren et al. (2001)	After admission to rehab (median 6 days post admission)	Modified SGA	20 (12) 32 (20) 'at risk'
Davis et al. (2004)	Within 24 hr of stroke	SGA	30 (16)
FOOD Trial (2003)	Within 7 days	Clinician judgement	279 (9)
Nip (2007)	Within 2 weeks of admission	MNA	7 (7) 66 (66) 'at risk'

TSF, Triceps skinfold; MAMC, mid-arm muscle circumference; MAC, mid-arm circumference; SGA, Subjective Global Assessment; MNA Mini Nutritional Assessment.

judgement) are discussed later in this chapter. Altogether these studies identified 7–34% but most frequently around 16% of patients as malnourished and up to 66% 'at risk' within the early days of hospital admission. Many patients show nutritional deterioration in hospital, in part at least due to effects of their stroke, or the effects of post-stroke care.

How does stroke affect dietary intake?

Effects of acute illness

Strokes, particularly ischaemic events, are now recognised as acute brain injury, in which an inflammatory component contributes to the pathological process (see Chapter 3). Acute injury is associated with a metabolic response, originally described as two phases, of ebb and flow. The ebb phase lasts around 24 hours, the latter lasts much longer and involves increased nutritional requirements. More recently this has been described as an initial period of acute stress and a longer-term anabolic (rebuilding) phase (Broom 1993). However, studies of acute stroke patients have not conclusively shown what this means in terms of dietary requirements. Whilst for some stroke patients, basal (resting) metabolic rates (BMRs) were increased (Chalela et al. 2004; Touho et al. 1990) for others no significant difference was seen in BMR. In these studies, BMR was predicted by the Harris Benedict equation (what would be expected for someone of that age, weight and height) and was compared with actual energy expenditure in stroke patients up to 90 days after admission (Esper et al. 2006; Finestone et al. 2003; Weekes & Elia 1992).

Despite lack of clear evidence of increased BMR, the energy 'cost' associated with physical activity may be affected by stroke-related disablement. On the one hand, activity-related energy expenditure may be less than estimated if disabilities restrict the type and duration of daily activities. Alternatively, the energy 'cost' of physical activity may be higher because of muscle inefficiency; stroke patients have to work relatively harder to complete the actions. In a small study of 13 middle-aged stroke patients and 13 age- and sex-matched controls, Platts et al (2006) measured oxygen uptake and reported significantly greater energy cost for stroke patients to walk a much shorter distance compared to controls. Studies comparing various energy predictive equations have yet to establish the best method to fine-tune calculation of energy requirements for individual stroke patients.

Stroke-related eating disabilities

Stroke produces a wide range of deficits that can affect ability to eat and so increase risk of malnutrition. These include inability to maintain head control and upright posture; loss of upper limb motor control and sensation; problems chewing and swallowing; and communication, visual, perceptual and attention deficits. Table 5.2 shows eating disabilities demonstrated by a cohort of patients

Table 5.2 Eating disabilities of a cohort of acute stroke admissions to a South London hospital, March 1998 to December 1999 (Perry 2002).

Eating disabilities* at hospital**	3–5 days after admission to hospital	Number	Percentage
Posture control	No functional impairment (0)*	325	56
	Mild impairment (1)	130	22
	Moderate impairment (2)	89	15
	Severe impairment (3)	43	7
**Median (25, 75 centile) scores		0 (0, 1)	
Arm movement	No functional impairment (0)	159	27
	Mild impairment (1)	209	35
	Moderate (2)	86	15
	Severe (3)	133	23
**Median (25, 75 centile) scores		1 (0, 2)	
Lip closure	No functional impairment (0)	449	76
	Partial impairment (1)	109	19
	Severe impairment (2)	29	5
**Median (25, 75 centile) scores		0 (0, 0)	
Chewing	No functional impairment (0)	369	63
	Partial impairment (1)	172	29
	Severe impairment (2)	46	8
**Median (25, 75 centile) scores		0 (0, 1)	
Swallowing	No functional impairment (0)	341	58
	Partial – can't tolerate 1 of 3 textures (1)	66	11
	Severe – can't tolerate 2 of 3 textures (2)	64	11
	Aspiration/high risk; nil orally (3)	116	20
**Median (25, 75 centile) scores		0 (0, 2)	
Communication	No functional impairment (0)	276	47
	Partial impairment (1)	149	25
	Severe impairment (2)	162	28
**Median (25, 75 centile) scores		1 (0, 2)	
Attention and praxis	No functional impairment (0)	417	71
	Partial impairment (1)	130	22
	Severe impairment (2)	39	7
**Median (25, 75 centile) scores		0 (0, 1)	
Visual field/ perceptual loss/ neglect	No functional impairment (0)	428	73
	Partial impairment (1)	132	23
	Severe impairment (2)	25	4
**Median (25, 75 centile) scores		0 (0, 1)	

n = 670 stroke patients, of whom 587 (586 for attention and praxis; 585 for visual fields) were able to be assessed using the
*Eating Disabilities Assessment Scale (McLaren & Dickerson 2000).
**Scale point scores.

admitted to a London hospital with acute stroke (Perry 2002), and Case example 5.1 shows what this meant for one of these patients. As well as physical problems, depression, which is common after stroke, may also influence dietary intake.

As a result of eating-related disabilities, many stroke patients need help to eat. Of the above cohort of 670 stroke patients, in the early days after admis-

---

Case example 5.1 Evelyn's problems in relation to eating.

Evelyn is an 82-year-old admitted to hospital with an ischaemic stroke. She is not tall, but is a large woman, and had a right hip replacement following a bad fall the year before. She lives next door to her daughter, Jenny. On admission she has a dense left hemiplegia, left visual inattention, and she answers questions appropriately, although attention is required to understand her. Dysphagia is identified, and she is placed nil orally with intravenous hydration commenced. However, her chewing and swallow function is not the only eating related problem: she is not able to keep herself upright (the safest position for eating); her left hand has minimal movement, and all activities are one-handed; she neglects part of her left spatial field, and needs prompting with a plate of food; her speech makes communicating hunger, thirst and food preferences an effort. She has a history of depression and says she feels a burden to her family.

---

sion, less than half (46.5%) ate independently, 4% were judged to require supervision, 26% needed assistance, 12.5% were fed and 11% were tube fed (Perry 2002). Similarly, Westergren et al. (2001) reported that 52.5% stroke patients needed help to eat on admission to rehabilitation.

Reliance upon assistance to eat increases the risk of inadequate intake and development of complications (Kayser-Jones & Schell 1997; Siebens et al. 1986; Unosson et al. 1994). Even minor difficulties in people who eat independently may result in inadequate dietary intake (Aquilani et al. 1999). Patients can be distressed by eating in public if their functional limitations mean that the way they eat does not match cultural expectations of well-mannered behaviour; as a result they may limit or curtail what they eat, and refuse to eat in company. This affects not just the stroke survivor, but carer, families and wider social networks (Jacobsson et al. 2000; Perry & McLaren 2003a; Sidenvall et al. 1996).

Chewing and dysphagia

Dysphagia is defined as 'eating and drinking disorders which may occur in the oral, pharyngeal and oesophageal stages of deglutition' (Royal College of Speech and Language Therapy 2006). Dysphagia is important because it can cause aspiration pneumonia, malnutrition, dehydration, weight loss and airway obstruction. Dysphagia can result in reduced stamina, increased complications, increased likelihood of pressure sores, less physical recovery, reduced wound healing and increased risk of anxiety or depression, infections and ultimately death (Kuhlemeier et al. 1989; Logemann 1998; Sala et al. 1998). Fear of choking can also result in anxiety and a self-imposed restriction on what is eaten.

Observational studies suggest that in the first 24 hours post-stroke, between 30 and 40% of conscious and assessable individuals have dysphagia. However, higher numbers have been reported at risk of aspiration in the acute phases of stroke, from 67% when screened during the first 72 hours, to 43% within seven days (Perry & Love 2001). Other studies have reported a recovery rate of 73% within seven days, with 11–19% reported with long-term (more than six months post-stroke) swallowing difficulties (Perry & McLaren 2003a; Smithard

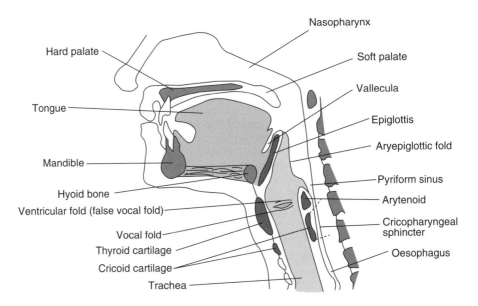

Figure 5.1 Lateral view of the anatomy of the head and neck.

et al. 1996). This is not a static condition, however, and deterioration as well as recovery is seen. This means it is important to train carers as well as hospital staff to identify when swallowing difficulties arise or relapse, and to ensure they know how, and are able to manage these difficulties appropriately (Boaden et al. 2006).

Figure 5.1 outlines the anatomy of head and neck, showing the main structures involved in swallowing, which requires coordination of six cranial nerves and 26 pairs of muscles. Swallowing needs muscle function to ensure stability, neuromuscular coordination, sensory and gastrointestinal function, normal heart and breathing control, as well as the autonomic nervous system to deliver overall coordination (Royal College of Speech and Language Therapy 2006). Any or all of these can be disrupted by stroke at any or every stage of the swallowing process.

The oral stage of swallowing

Absent or loose teeth or dentures significantly hinder chewing; they limit sensory feedback from nerves in teeth and temporo-mandibular (jaw) joints that control individual muscle movements that are needed to chew and adapt chewing to changes in food type. Problems with teeth and dentures are common amongst elderly people, and are often dealt with by people opting for softer diets, often with consequently reduced nutritional quality (Wayler & Chauncey 1983).

Inability to create good lip seal results in failure to generate the negative pressure in the mouth which is necessary to move food backwards through the oropharynx, as well as to prevent forward leakage of saliva, food and drinks. Poor tongue control, from damage affecting the hypoglossal nerve (cranial nerve (CN) XII), may result in failure to lift the back portion of the tongue, which prevents food and drink spilling into the pharynx pre-swallow whilst chewing. Sideways tongue movements, essential for chewing, may be limited; this can mean the tongue has difficulty controlling the food bolus, as well as problems stopping it leaking forwards and sideways. The tongue can also have problems with the rolling movement (sequential elevation) which is needed to move the food bolus back into the pharynx. Damage to the facial nerve (CN VII) in stroke patients causes loss of taste and sensation, and this loss of sensation can affect timing and movement at the upper oesophageal sphincter.

Reduced saliva production may result in teeth demineralisation, loss of mucosal protection and changes in the pH balance in the mouth. There may be difficulty forming and moving a food bolus, and subsequent digestion and gastric microbial control may be affected. Over one-third of acute stroke patients had mouths colonised with aerobic Gram-negative bacilli, which, if aspirated could cause chest infection (Millns et al. 2003). Further, facial paresis means cheek muscles do not have the normal increased muscle tension when chewing; this can allow food debris to lodge both sides of the gums, where aerobic bacteria can multiply, with increased risks of chest infection following aspiration.

The pharyngeal stage
Incoordination, unilateral or bilateral paresis of the soft palate (CN IX, X, XII) will allow nasal reflux. Pharyngeal paresis (from damage to CN IX) results in a decrease in muscle contraction in the base of tongue and constrictor muscles, and delayed bolus movement across the back of the pharynx. The consequence of this can be food residues in the valleculae and pyriform sinus, which can be inhaled post-swallow (Figure 5.2).

Delayed or absent superior and anterior hyoid movement with limited movement of the thyroid and cricoid cartilages causes incoordination of the cricopharyngeal opening, increasing the risk of aspiration. The cricopharyngeal sphincter opens in response to sensory information from the oral cavity, usually within 0.10 seconds of airway closure (Hiiemae & Palmer 1999). Three mechanisms protect the airway: the true and the false vocal folds coming together, and closure of the epiglottis to meet the arytenoids. This process works in reverse order to eject any material which penetrates the airway, normally assisted by expiration pre- and post-swallow. Abnormal inspiratory breathing patterns observed in stroke patients post-swallow may serve to suck pharyngeal residue into the airway (Selley et al. 1989).

The oesophageal stage
Oesophageal distension triggers coordinated waves of contraction by striated, and then smooth, oesophageal muscle fibres. With ageing, the oesophagus

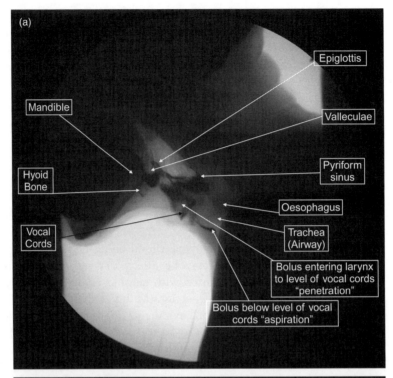

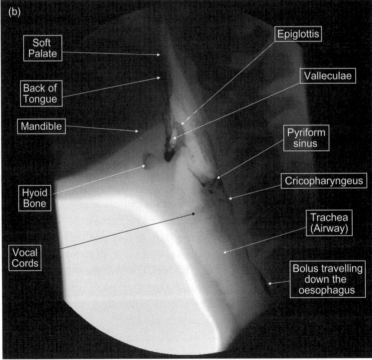

Figure 5.2 X-ray image, lateral view of the pharynx. Comparison of pre-swallow and post-swallow aspiration of bolus into trachea with residue in the valleculae and pyriform sinus. Anonymised X-ray images reproduced with permission of Chorley and South Ribble District General Hospital.

increasingly consists of smooth muscle, which explains the tendency for hiatus hernia and consequent increased risk of aspiration of refluxed material in older people, with development of aspiration pneumonitis (Marik 2001).

Posture and head control

Any disturbance of posture and sitting balance poses challenges for eating. The safest eating position is upright, with support as appropriate. Early assessments found almost 46% with postural instability (Table 5.1; McLaren & Dickerson 2000). Refer to Chapter 7 for more detail of posture and positioning.

Upper limb impairment

In the early weeks following stroke the main motor impairments around the shoulder and upper limb are: weakness, lack of active range of movement, reduced selective movement and dexterity (see Chapter 7). Broad measures of upper limb function and limb ataxia within 48 hours of admission have been reported to affect 79% and 35% patients (Brott et al. 1989). Observations of a selected group of patients eating at up to 14 days post-stroke revealed 57% unable to manipulate cutlery and/or transfer food from plate to mouth; arm movement impairment predicted reduced energy and protein intake (Jacobsson et al. 2000; McLaren & Dickerson 2000).

Problems with cognition and communication

Stroke causes a variety of communication problems, for example of expression, with dysphasia, dyspraxia and dysarthria; problems understanding the emotional tone of speech and lack of verbal comprehension, all ranging from subtle deficit to incomprehension (see Chapter 8). Reported incidence varies widely, from 18% to 74% of patients (Kalra et al. 1993; Taub et al. 1994). At 48 hours after admission communication deficits were found in 43%, with 59% dysarthric (Brott et al. 1989). The data reported relied predominantly upon subjective judgement, which perhaps has contributed to widely varying findings.

Inability to communicate food preferences and requirements was identified in 48% of patients taking oral diet at 8–10 days post-stroke and has been shown to be one of the factors that differentiates those with low dietary protein – less than 20% of reference nutrient intakes (McLaren & Dickerson 2000).

Visual and perceptual deficits

A wide range of visual, perceptual and attention deficits have been reported following stroke, including visual field deficits (hemianopias) and differing forms of apraxia, agnosia and neglect (inattention). Reported incidence varies widely, probably due to differing methods of assessment with varying sensitivity, differing patient populations and timing of assessment after stroke onset. At 48 hours after admission visual and/or sensory inattention was found in

38% of patients, and hemianopia in 46% (Brott et al. 1989). Detection of meal components features in tests for visuo-spatial neglect (Stone et al. 1991). Apraxia may directly affect ability to eat (Foundas et al. 1995), and as both neglect and apraxia negatively influence rehabilitation of activities of daily living, they may indirectly influence eating and nutritional status (Hochstenbach & Mulder 1999; Kalra et al. 1997).

Smell and taste

Smell and taste both contribute to the sensation of taste; complaints of altered 'taste' commonly arise from problems with smell. Taste disturbance has been reported in stroke patients with symptoms ranging from increased thresholds, reduced intensity of taste, loss of pleasant associations and conversion of some neutral to unpleasant sensations, development of smell and taste intolerance, food aversion and marked weight loss (Finsterer et al. 2004; Heckmann et al. 2005; Kim & Choi 2002; Pritchard et al. 1999). Case studies have reported taste disturbance in patients with lesions at a variety of locations, including pontine, midbrain, thalamic, internal capsule and insular haemorrhage and infarction, and unilateral cortical infarction (Finsterer et al. 2004; Heckmann et al. 2005; Kim & Choi 2002; Pritchard et al. 1999). In one consecutive cohort of people admitted with stroke 31 of 102 patients (30.5%) had reduced taste, most of whom had frontal lobe lesions. Of those with abnormal taste, 6 of 21 (28.6%) also experienced impaired smell; of those with normal taste, 4 of 33 (12.1%) had loss of ability to smell (Heckmann et al. 2005).

Oral hygiene

As discussed above, stroke patients may have difficulty clearing food from their mouths and may 'pocket' residues. If not removed after every meal, this may harbour bacterial growth, leading to bad breath and a bad taste in the mouth which may deter eating. Further this may pose additional risks of developing aspiration pneumonia if this material enters the lungs (Yoneyama et al. 2002).

Psychosocial effects

Mood disorder and appetite

Post-stroke depression is common both in acute stages and for some years afterwards. It has been found that 31–33% of patients were depressed at three weeks, with 25–31% affected during the first three months (Wade et al. 1987). Links have been demonstrated between nutrition and mood state, and a vicious cycle may become established as what people eat may affect mood, and depressed mood may be linked with altered food intake. Complex interrelationships are suggested. The most significant study of the effects of dietary intake in relation to mood entailed a 24-week period of semi-starvation for 32 young healthy male volunteers. A sustained intake of around 1470 kcal/day resulted in progressively increased tiredness, irritability, apathy, moodiness, depression and apprehension; and decreased ambition, concentration, self-discipline, and loss of mental alertness and drive to activity (Brozek 1985). Depressed mood post-stroke has been consistently linked with poorer outcomes, for example ability to carry out activities of daily living, social function, and mortality (Gillen et al. 2001).

Altered appetite and weight changes have been identified as core symptoms of depression although the relationship has remained unclear in stroke patients. Work with eating disordered and weight cycling participants has suggested that alterations to fatty acid intake, as a consequence of dietary restriction or manipulation, may be key contributors to mood disturbance (Bruinsma & Taren 2000; Chen et al. 1997). This may be relevant to stroke patients who experience sustained poor dietary intakes.

In exploring the relationship between mood state and nutritional status in hospitalised stroke patients, researchers failed to demonstrate a direct association between nutritional status and mood state, when assessed using Mini-Nutritional Assessment and the General Health Questionnaire, respectively. However, nutritional scores were significantly related to those for appetite, hunger, taste and smell, which in turn were linked to mood scores (Nip 2007). Comparing dietary intakes of those identified as depressed with those who were not depressed, the former consistently consumed less energy and protein. During the first two weeks of admission, depressed participants consumed mean (SD) 1227 (711) kcal energy and 46.7 (20) g protein per day compared to 1440 (677) kcal energy and 56 (20.2) g protein in those not depressed; this pattern was sustained, with depressed participants eating 299 kcal and 16.8 g less per day than those not depressed in the week before discharge (Nip 2007). This effect continued, with links between appetite, mood state and dietary intake still evident at six months post-stroke (Perry & McLaren 2004).

Altered body image may also have an effect on mood state, and hence dietary intake. The effects of stroke, such as uncontrolled drooling and facial palsy, have an obvious potential to affect the way people feel about themselves. However, even relatively subtle signs or symptoms (e.g. loss of sensation or tactile recognition in an upper limb, leading to reduced manual dexterity and clumsy eating) can have negative effects.

Impact of dietary provision and hospital meals

Dietary provision in hospital may influence what patients eat because they are directly dependent on what catering services provide and indirectly affected through the eating environment. Numerous results have flagged the deficiencies of both (e.g. Age Concern 2006). A recent focus on hospital food in the UK has resulted in national standards (Department of Health 2004), and the Better Hospital Food programme (http://195.92.246.148/nhsestates/better_hospital_food/bhf_content/protected_mealtimes/overview.asp) focused on recipes, snack-provision and the mealtime environment on wards. Nonetheless, it is salutary to note that whilst many patients are wholly dependent upon hospital meals, 31% of one cohort of stroke patients opted to consume additional food items, 17% consumed drinks not provided by the hospital; and 5% were prescribed supplements, with these supplementary items meeting an estimated 25–40% of daily energy and protein requirements (Nip 2007).

A requirement for modified consistency diets may also have psychosocial effects, singling the individual out as requiring 'special' food. This may bring attention to the person as different, cause embarrassment, and have a socially isolating effect. Even within the family, it may be perceived as burdensome, by the patient as well as family members.

Altogether, stroke patients are known to experience pre-existing malnutrition that may be compounded by metabolic consequences of acute illness; physical, psychological, social and emotional effects pose barriers to eating and adequate dietary intake. Whilst an integrated programme of eating rehabilitation focused on dysphagia amongst chronic stroke survivors has been described (Jacobsson et al. 1997), components are more often addressed separately, and may not be explicitly linked to eating.

How can stroke patients be helped to maintain adequate dietary intake?

Nutritional support is essentially a multidisciplinary activity; many professional and lay personnel contribute to ensuring adequate and acceptable dietary provision and intake for stroke patients. Professional roles tend to vary across locations; hence, this section focuses on what can and should be done, rather than who might do this.

Screening and assessment

Screening is the process used to identify those with established malnutrition or evidence of nutritional risk; once identified, these individuals can undergo dietetic assessment to identify the nature, source and extent of their problems. Nutritional screening is part of routine initial assessment, undertaken as soon as the patient's condition allows, ideally within the first 24 hours of admission or first contact. No single measurement is adequate and many composite screening tools have been developed. However, many have not demonstrated validity (ability to differentiate those with nutritional problems from those without) and all have limitations especially when used with acutely ill patients. Clinical examination is an important component but whilst malnutrition produces a range of clinical signs these tend to be subtle and non-specific until malnutrition is advanced. Reliance upon clinical signs for nutritional screening may not be effective; use of screening tools with demonstrated validity and reliability is recommended (National Institute for Health and Clinical Excellence (2006), for example the Malnutrition Universal Screening Tool.

Weight is commonly used. It is a component of many screening tools, and may be compared to percentile weight tables, ideal weight tables, previous or usual weight. Sequential weights can be recorded to track progress and response to nutrition support. However, weight has limitations as a nutritional index, particularly for stroke patients. Perry (2002) noted that only 48% of stroke patients were weighed at any point during admission, only rising to 56.5% following a nutritional support project. Equipment may not be available to weigh immobile patients; shifting fluid balance, differing scales, clothing and times of day for weighing may mean that changes do not reflect nutritional state. Weighing scales in institutions are often minimally maintained and calibrated, and may not be accurate. Weight measurement cannot differentiate muscle from fat and does not take account of overall bodily size unless height is used to calculate body mass index (BMI). The commonest BMI equation is Quetelet's Index: weight (kg) divided by height (m^2). A cut-off value of $18.5\,kg/m^2$ is often regarded as suggestive of malnutrition, or less than $20\,kg/m^2$ if accompanied by recent weight loss. However, this is the subject of considerable debate and in older people criteria may be higher (e.g. less than $23\,kg/m^2$ (Beck & Ovesen 1998)). Height may be difficult to measure in hospital patients, and may be misleading in older people. Knee height, ulnar length and demi-span may be measured instead and different calculations or tables applied (Perry & McLaren 2003b). The approaches taken to nutritional screening for Evelyn are shown in Case example 5.2.

Other anthropometric measures, such as arm circumference and skinfold measurements, are seldom used in acute clinical practice but may be useful in longer-term monitoring; biochemical tests are affected by acute illness and unreliable as nutritional indicators. Albumin has a long half-life and is a particularly poor nutritional index although, reflecting severity of illness, it may indicate prognosis. Recent dietary intake can be a useful pointer towards nutritional status. In 2006 the National Institute for Health and Clinical Excellence (NICE) issued a clinical guideline to help UK health care staff identify patients who are malnourished or at risk of malnutrition (National Institute for Health and Clinical Excellence 2006) and similar recommendations were issued from the Council of Europe (http://www.bapen.org.uk/res_council.html).

Many stroke patients experience nutritional deterioration during the course of treatment and rehabilitation; monitoring is therefore important, encompassing such aspects as nutritional intake, weight, gastrointestinal function and general clinical condition (National Institute for Health and Clinical Excellence 2006). As a minimum, weekly weighing has been advocated, with additional

---

Case example 5.2 Nutritional risk screening for Evelyn.

Evelyn is initially not easy to transfer, with left hemiplegia and a fairly recent right hip replacement. However, using hoist scales she is weighed as 70 kg, and her knee height measured at 47.5 cm, producing a height of 152 cm and a BMI of 30 (MUST score = 0). Asked whether her weight had changed recently, she denies this, but her notes for her hip replacement record her weight as 76 kg. She has therefore lost almost 8% of her body weight within the past six months (MUST score = 1). Evelyn was eating normally (according to both her and Jenny) up to the point of admission, but as she has severe dysphagia, not taking anything orally, and it can be predicted this will take some days at least to resolve, she scores 2 for acute disease effect, giving her a total score of 3. This is in the 'high-risk' category, despite her borderline obesity. Further, discussion with Jenny indicates that Evelyn has been on and off 'diets' all her life, and has a tendency to snack.

activities such as keeping food record charts recommended according to individual nutritional status.

Timing of initiation of nutritional support

There is no clear evidence to identify a 'safe' maximum period of starvation or nutritional depletion, and individual circumstances, degree of nutritional risk and actual dietary intake guide individual decisions. However, the clear association between malnutrition and increased mortality in stroke patients should be borne in mind, and the significant reduction in complications seen with fewer numbers of days spent with nil orally (Perry & McLaren 2003a). A major multinational trial, the FOOD Trial (Dennis et al. 2005a), reported early tube feeding 'associated with an absolute reduction in risk of death of 5·8% (95% confidence intervals (CI): −0.8 to 12.5, p = 0·09) and a reduction in death or poor outcome of 1.2% (95% CI: −4.2 to 6.6, p = 0.7)', recommending that 'dysphagic stroke patients should be offered enteral tube feeding via a nasogastric tube within the first few days of admission'.

Ethical dilemmas may be posed in relation to decision-making around initiation of tube feeding for severely impaired, acutely unwell stroke patients. Difficulties arise from not knowing the prognosis, not knowing values and preferences, and not being able to elicit them. Families may or may not be able to indicate the patient's perspective, and may have different views themselves (see Case example 5.3). Provision of nourishment is a fundamental and very emotive topic (Lupton 1996); excellent communication between and amongst families and health care professionals is essential. UK guidance flags artificial nutrition support as a medical intervention, decisions concerning which need

---

Case example 5.3 Difficult decisions for Margaret.

Margaret is 92 years old, had a leg amputated in a road traffic accident some years before, is living with her daughter Frances, son-in-law Martin and young adult grandchildren. On admission she has a dense hemiplegia, is incontinent, and her speech is only intelligible with effort. She is also has severe dysphagia, and is placed nil orally with subcutaneous hydration. Her swallow function is reassessed daily but by five days shows no sign of improvement. Repeat attempts by different clinicians to place a nasogastric tube over the next days fail. Margaret tells the nurses that she is too tired to do anything, and switches between saying she wants to eat and get better, to saying she can't cope anymore and just wants to die. Frances is desperate for her to make progress and come home; Martin is very anxious about whether Frances will cope with her mother who is more dependent than before the stroke. Gastroscopy shows a large sliding hiatus hernia and a gastrostomy is successfully placed after a longer than usual procedure. Recovery is slow and complicated by poor tolerance of feeding and leakage from the gastrostomy insertion site. Margaret remains low in spirit and does not engage with therapy, saying she is too tired. Despite weeks in hospital there is little change in Margaret. There are intermittent problems with the tube feeding, and her dysphagia and functional abilities show little improvement. Margaret is hoisted out of bed but otherwise remains bed-bound. Eventually, admission to nursing home care is arranged, once Frances finally agrees that return home is unrealistic.

to consider likely benefit, risks and harms. Where there is real concern that such an intervention may be futile, it is clearly important that this is discussed and understood by all concerned (Lennard-Jones 1998). The UK Mental Capacity Act of 2005 (http://www.opsi.gov.uk/ACTS/acts2005/ukpga_20050009_en_1) provides guidance on establishing whether and to what extent someone can contribute to decisions about their care, and when Lasting Power of Attorney can be used or a deputy appointed.

Managing eating disabilities

As eating-related disabilities are experienced across the spectrum from acute to long-term care, management strategies may need to span similar time frames.

Chewing difficulties

The risk of stroke is increased in people with both significant periodontal disease and no natural teeth (Elter et al. 2003). With increasing age the mouth changes shape and dentures no longer fit the gums, compounding difficulties in mastication. Dentures are only one-sixth as effective as teeth when chewing (Marks & Rainbow 2003), and although digestion has been shown to be independent of chewing, edentulous patients consumed less calcium, protein, niacin and vitamin C compared to individuals with intact dentition (Farrell 1956; Krall et al. 1998; Sheiham et al. 2001).

Poor jaw closure requires facilitated jaw support (manual assistance); if the tongue cannot move the bolus across the midline onto the teeth, the food bolus needs to be placed on the non-damaged side of the tongue in the short term, and tongue lateralisation exercises are needed in the long term. External pressure to the cheek in patients with unilateral facial weakness increases the negative intraoral pressure required for swallowing, prevents food falling between teeth and cheek, and assists the tongue to form food into a cohesive bolus. It may also help to avoid food of mixed textures that are difficult to chew, and to serve several smaller meals to allow the person to rest between meals.

Restorative and compensatory strategies for dysphagia management

Restorative (direct) therapy aims to change dysfunctional swallowing physiology (Table 5.3). Research evidence is currently limited in this area; clinical experience and some preliminary work suggests enhancing pre-swallow sensory input by prior rubbing or applying pressure to tongue or fauces, or the use of carbonated, cold, sour or electrical stimuli may lower the threshold for initiation of oropharyngeal motor activity and reduce delay in oral responses (Bulow et al. 2003; Power et al. 2006). Where the swallow is weak with poor laryngeal elevation, Mendelssohn's manoeuvre entails deliberately prolonging laryngeal elevation during mid-swallow, aiming to increase the proportion of bolus going into the oesophagus and decrease pharyngeal residues. The patient is taught to

Table 5.3 Compensatory strategies and restorative therapies for dysphagia.

Stage of swallow	Swallow disorder	Compensatory strategy	Restorative/rehabilitative exercises/therapy
Oral preparatory	Poor lip seal	Supported lip and jaw closure	Lip exercises
Oral preparatory	Poor cheek tone	Intraoral prosthesis, cheek hold technique (apply pressure to weak side), tilt head towards unaffected side	Cheek tone exercises
Oral preparatory	Poor sensation in oral cavity	Increase bolus taste, volume, density, temperature, carbonated drinks	Sensory awareness programme
Oral preparatory	Poor tongue movement	Modify consistency of bolus, pace rate of bolus presentation, avoid mixed consistencies, remove residue from oral cavity post swallow	Tongue lateralisation exercises
Oral preparatory	Poor chewing/jaw closure	Jaw support, diet modification	Chewing exercises
Oral transit	Poor tongue movement/oral transit	Head back posture	
Pharyngeal	Delayed swallow	Adapted cutlery and crockery to assist in self feeding, chin tuck posture, increase bolus taste, volume, density, temperature, fizzy drinks	Thermal stimulation, proprioceptive neuromuscular facilitation (PNF) to the fauceal arches
Pharyngeal	Reduced base of tongue movement	Chin tuck, clearing swallows, effortful swallow, decrease bolus size, increase bolus consistency	Tongue hold technique, gargle and yawn exercises, supersupraglottic swallow
Pharyngeal	Unilateral pharyngeal paresis	Head rotation to damaged side, head tilt to unaffected side, back or side lying, clearing swallows, liquid wash down	
Pharyngeal	Unilateral tongue and pharyngeal paresis	Head tilt to unaffected side, clearing swallows	
Pharyngeal	Reduced laryngeal closure	Chin tuck, head rotation to damaged side, supraglottic swallow, supersupraglottic swallow, alter bolus consistency	Supraglottic swallow, supersupraglottic swallow, breath hold manoeuvre, push–pull voicing
Pharyngeal	Reduced laryngeal elevation	Chin tuck and lie on side/back, supersupraglottic swallow, Mendelssohn manoeuvre, clearing swallows	Falsetto voicing, Mendelssohn manoeuvre, shaker technique, surface electromyography (EMG)

Table 5.3 *Continued*

Stage of swallow	Swallow disorder	Compensatory strategy	Restorative/rehabilitative exercises/therapy
Pharyngeal	Cricopharyngeal dysfunction/reduced anterior movement of hyolaryngeal structure	Head rotation, avoid mixed consistencies	Shaker technique
Fatigue		Nutritional supplements, decrease meal size, increase frequency of meals	

feel their larynx rising during the swallow, and at its highest point, to hold it in that position for several seconds. A double swallow may improve clearance of food remaining in the pharynx. Supraglottic swallowing is intended to max-imise closure of the laryngeal inlet. Breath is held before swallowing, with the aim of adducting the vocal cords and protecting the airway although video-nasoendoscopy has shown that breath-holding does not always result in the vocal cords coming together. The patient swallows twice and immediately afterwards coughs to expel anything that has penetrated the laryngeal vestibule. Exercises specific to individual impairments, e.g. of tongue, lips and facial muscles, are frequently recommended (Logemann 1998). However, evaluation of these techniques is limited.

Compensatory postures and strategies eliminate or reduce the volume of materials aspirated into the airway. These were initially designed for use with patients with oropharyngeal cancer and require that patients are able to under-stand and cooperate with instructions. Compensatory postures do not necessar-ily match with principles of normal neurological movement patterns and, whilst effective in the short term to ensure that respiration and nutrition are not com-promised, they should not be regarded as long-term management without con-sidering issues of environment, postural tone and stability to promote normal tone, reflexes and sensory integration, with a view to preventing abnormal pat-terns of movement and reflexes becoming established (Logemann 1998). Such strategies aim to compensate for specific impairments (Table 5.3). For example, head and neck may be deliberately positioned. With the chin down ('chin tuck') the epiglottis shifts backwards and may narrow the laryngeal entrance and increase airway protection. This may be helpful if the pharyngeal phase is delayed but does not eliminate aspiration in all patients. Where there is unilat-eral pharyngeal paralysis, lateral head rotation may open the upper oesopha-geal sphincter and direct the bolus away from the paralysed side. Excluding the flaccid oesophageal sidewall, which otherwise weakens pharyngeal pressure gradients, allows remaining peristaltic contractions to achieve faster, more complete bolus transit. Described in research but seldom used in clinical prac-tice, palatal prostheses reshape the oral cavity to address individual problems in bolus manipulation and triggering of swallowing (Logemann 1998).

Texture modification and fluid consistencies

As swallow physiology is dependent on consistencies consumed, modification of food, liquid and medication can be utilised therapeutically (Cook et al. 1989). Modifying taste, temperature, texture, viscosity and volume can affect bolus preparation and swallow performance (Bisch et al. 1994; Logemann et al. 1995; Rosenbek et al. 1996). Thicker fluids and modified consistency diets compensate for deficits in swallow physiology and improve efficient transit through the mouth and pharynx, thereby improving the safety of the swallow.

Thin liquids lose cohesion very rapidly, so if a delay exists, naturally thicker or artificially thickened drinks are indicated to improve swallow efficiency (Marks & Rainbow 2003). However, decisions regarding thickener need to be client specific, dictated by the length of delay. Prescription of thickened fluids is not without potential problems: patients often do not like them and may decline to drink them and become dehydrated (Whelan 2001). Longer-term adherence to thickener use is poor but education programmes for patients and carers have been linked with more consistent use and thereby improved patient safety (Rosenvinge & Starke 2005). Other work has indicated that offering free fluids without thickener may not increase patients' risk of developing aspiration pneumonia (Garon et al. 1997).

There are a number of different classifications of modified texture foods and fluids, using varying descriptors. Terminology varies between locations (for example, terms such as 'nectar', familiar in the US, are seldom used in the UK), as does interpretation of the same terms (for example, the consistency understood by 'custard'). The UK British Dietetic Association and the Royal College of Speech and Language Therapists developed a consensus taxonomy of descriptors (Tables 5.4 and 5.5); other countries have produced similar, with varying numbers of levels (BDA&RCSLT 2002). For example, the Dietitians' Association of Australian has defined four consistencies of diet: unmodified regular foods; Texture A, soft; Texture B, minced and moist; Texture C, smooth puree. Liquidising food increases the volume without a concomitant increase in calorific load. It is important that food, however prepared, should look colourful and appetising, which can be achieved by blending food separately, using food moulds and garnishes. Most community meal schemes (e.g. Meals on Wheels) are able to supply modified texture meals, although menu choice may be limited.

Nutritional supplementation

Fortified foods are an effective method of increasing the calorific load of food and drinks by adding extra calories using full fat products, sugars and fortified milk. Increasing the number of meals and introducing snacks between meals to approximately six per day will also increase nutritional intake. Supplements, available on prescription or 'over the counter', may augment normal intake or be nutritionally complete. Nutritional benefit and improved clinical outcomes were demonstrated in 42 acute non-dysphagic stroke patients with impaired nutrition by using nutritional supplements (Gariballa et al. 1998). These findings were supported by FOOD Trial Collaboration, who reiterated general

Table 5.4 Texture modification of fluids.

Texture	Description of fluid texture	Fluid example
Thin fluid	Still water	Water, tea, coffee without milk, diluted squash, spirits, wine
Naturally thick fluid	Product leaves a coating on an empty glass	Full cream milk, cream liqueurs, Complan, Build Up (made to instructions), Nutriment, commercial sip feeds
Thickened fluid	Fluid to which a commercial thickener has been added to thicken consistency	
Stage 1 =	Can be drunk through a straw Can be drunk from a cup if advised or preferred Leaves a thin coat on the back of a spoon	
Stage 2 =	Cannot be drunk through a straw Can be drunk from a cup Leaves a thick coat on the back of a spoon	
Stage 3 =	Cannot be drunk through a straw Cannot be drunk from a cup Needs to be taken with a spoon	

From the British Dietetic Association and Royal College of Speech and Language Therapists Joint Working Group (2002) National descriptors for texture modification in adults. Reproduced with permission.

nutritional recommendations that supplement use should be targeted at those with demonstrated need (Dennis et al. 2005b). However, patient preference, adherence and the potential for 'taste fatigue' as well as availability also need to be considered when recommending these.

Enteral nutrition

Enteral feeding may be used to provide nutritional support for patients with a functioning gastrointestinal tract who are unable to eat orally; dysphagia as a result of stroke was the most common reason for enteral tube feeding (ETF) in the UK between 1996 and 1999, accounting for 72% of ETF registrations. An estimated 1.7% of all patients who suffered a stroke in the UK during this period received home ETF (Elia et al. 2001). Following a decade of increasing numbers, new adult ETF patients in the stroke population declined between 2000 and 2006, from 2308 to 1260 (BANS 2007). ETF may also be used, less commonly, to augment inadequate oral intake; in long-term management it may be appropriate to have complementary routes of intake with quality of life being the focus (Rabeneck et al. 1997).

A naso-gastric tube (NGT) is normally a short-term solution (up to around 28 days) for individuals with nutritional difficulties. Potential complications include oesophagitis, ulceration, most commonly nasal or gastric, inadvertent removal and tube displacement, blockage and poor patient compliance (Bath et al. 1999). Particular considerations are methods of checking accurate

Table 5.5 Texture modification of food.

Texture	Description of food texture	Food examples
A	A smooth, pouring, uniform consistency A food that has been pureed and sieved to remove particles A thickener may be added to maintain stability Cannot be eaten with a fork	Tinned tomato soup Thin custard
B	A smooth, uniform consistency A food that has been pureed and sieved to remove particles A thickener may be added to maintain stability Cannot be eaten with a fork Drops rather than pours from a spoon but cannot be piped and layered Thicker than A	Soft whipped cream Thick custard
C	A thick, smooth, uniform consistency A food that has been pureed and sieved to remove particles A thickener may be added to maintain stability Can be eaten with a fork or spoon Will hold its own shape on a plate, and can be moulded, layered and piped No chewing required	Mousse Smooth fromage frais
D	Food that is moist, with some variation in texture Has not been pureed or sieved These foods may be served or coated with a thick gravy or sauce Foods easily mashed with a fork Meat should be prepared as C Requires very little chewing	Flaked fish in thick sauce Stewed apple and thick custard
E	Dishes consisting of soft, moist food Foods can be broken into pieces with a fork Dishes can be made up of solids and thick sauces or gravies Avoid foods which cause a choking hazard (see list of high-risk foods*)	Tender meat casseroles (approx. 1.5 cm diced pieces) Sponge and custard
Normal	Any foods	Include all foods from 'high-risk foods' list*

From the British Dietetic Association and Royal College of Speech and Language Therapists Joint Working Group (2002) National descriptors for texture modification in adults. Reproduced with permission.

*High-risk foods: stringy fibrous texture, e.g. pineapple, runner beans, celery, lettuce; vegetable and fruit skins including beans, e.g. broad, baked, soya, black-eye, peas, grapes; mixed consistency foods, e.g. cereals which do not blend with milk such as muesli, mince with thin gravy, soup with lumps; crunchy foods, e.g. toast, flaky pastry, dry biscuits, crisps; crumbly items, e.g. bread crusts, pie crusts, crumb, dry biscuits; hard foods, e.g. boiled and chewy sweets and toffees, nuts and seeds; husks, e.g. sweetcorn, granary bread.

placement; pH testing of gastric aspirate is preferred, with chest X-ray where this is not possible (National Institute for Health and Clinical Excellence 2006). Auscultation, and many other previously common approaches, have not demonstrated acceptable levels of accuracy (Metheny et al. 1998). Management of intubated but confused patients also poses problems, with cultural, national and personal differences of opinion about the ethics of restraint, whether via sedation, bed clothes, tying hands to bed rails or mittens. A device known as a bridle shows promise and increasing popularity for minimising tube displacement amongst selected patient groups (Williams 2005). Naso-jejunal (NJ) tubes are uncommon; they can be used for patients with abnormal gastric function but there is a greater risk of aspiration due to reflux in this patient group.

Gastrostomies are a longer-term solution but patient selection is important owing to the impact on quality of life. They can be placed surgically, via percutaneous endoscopy (PEG) or inserted radiographically (RIG). For patients with abnormal gastric function, percutaneous endoscopic jejunostomy (PEJ) tubes are the preferred option although reflux may not be abolished (Lien et al. 2000). Gastrostomies with balloon retention devices are useful for some patients as they allow for rapid replacement by appropriately trained staff.

Symptoms associated with feeding may include diarrhoea, vomiting, infection of the PEG site and leakage. Further complications associated with PEG feeding may include infection and hypergranulation at the stoma site, and 'buried bumper' (where the gastric retaining device migrates into the gastric or abdominal wall). Blocked tubes are not uncommon but can be minimised by good management and patient and carer education (Colagiovanni 2000).

Parenteral nutrition (PN) is a means of supplying full nutritional support intravenously for individuals who have a non-functioning gastrointestinal tract. It is rarely required in the stroke population.

Local standards for PEG management have been developed and the British Association for Parenteral and Enteral Nutrition (BAPEN) has set standards for practice for home ETF (Elia 2000) which includes contact with a support group, such as Patients on Intravenous and Naso-gastric Nutrition Therapy (PINNT). Various systems of long-term support or back-up are provided, entailing, for example, hospital outreach, community nursing and/or support services contracted from commercial companies. For all patients with neurological damage who have nothing orally, oral stimulation programmes are essential in order to prevent hypersensitive oral defensive patterns becoming established, which may make oral hygiene routines difficult to maintain (http://www.fott.co.uk).

Smell and taste

Amongst groups of older adults, taste dysfunction has been linked with low body weight and lower energy intake, reduced appetite and poorer immune function; dietary intervention with flavour-modified meals increased dietary intake and improved immunity and muscle function. Hence smell and taste are intimately linked with when and why people want to start and stop eating, the quantity and qualities of food eaten and outcomes related to this (de Jong et al. 1999; Schiffman & Graham 2000; Schiffman & Warwick 1993). It has not been established whether taste impairment in stroke patients affects dietary intake, or whether similar approaches to flavour modification for taste-impaired stroke patients might enhance nutritional intake. Currently, taste and smell dysfunction are seldom sought as part of neurological assessment of stroke patients, but questions could be included as part of nursing nutritional assessment, with a view to tailoring menu choices to sensory abilities and preferences.

Management of other eating-related disabilities

Posture and head control, upper limb impairment, cognitive, communication, visual and perceptual deficits all impact on ability to eat safely and recognise and communicate dietary wants and needs. Clearly, eating is a complex activity requiring integration of multiple skills. The same can be said of skilled feeding. This requires sensitive management, should in no way attract attention to what is occurring, and when done well, has been described as a 'silent dance', in which the person fed sees their own actions reflected in those of their helper (Martinsen et al. 2008). At the other extreme, self-management of artificial nutritional support (home ETF) may be facilitated with local support programmes and clinicians.

For many stroke patients focus on more than single actions affects performance; for example, Harley et al. (2006) reported that the effort of just speaking could be sufficient to disturb postural control early after stroke. Rehabilitation interventions are normally related to the activities of daily living in which actions are applied. Rehabilitation interventions are available and used for eating-related deficits (refer to Chapters 7, 8, 9 and 11), the relevance of rehabilitation in relation to ability to eat is recognised (Koltin & Rosen 1996), but little work has focused specifically on this. Meal-times present rehabilitation opportunities, where patients may practise application of a range of skills worked on during therapy sessions.

A wide range of assistive devices may be helpful; for example, plate-guards, non-slip mats, adapted cutlery. Many others can also be useful in relation to meal preparation. Reviewing patients at three to five years post-stroke, Sorensen et al. (2003) found a significant increase in use of aids for cooking and eating, flagging either changing patterns of need or limited understanding of what was available during early stages. Either interpretation highlights the importance of information-giving and good preparation of patients and families.

Psychosocial effects

Mood disorder and appetite

Identification and treatment of mood disorder post-stroke is now widely accepted as an important component of standard stroke care. Treatment of depression in patients with physical illness resulted in beneficial effects upon symptoms (Gill & Hatcher 2000). However, in stroke patients treatment has not always improved outcomes despite alleviation of depressive symptoms (Age Concern 2006; Gall 2001). Similarly, it is not known whether treatment of depression will relieve depression-related appetite dysfunction, whether of suppression or carbohydrate craving. In high-risk situations such as cachexia, appetite stimulants such as prednisolone may be used: there is no evidence that such an approach may confer benefit for stroke patients.

The eating environment

However, there are non-pharmacological means whereby dietary intake may be enhanced. These include attention to the psychosocial dimension of eating by creating a pleasant, relaxed atmosphere in which food is eaten as a shared social experience. This is not easy in hospital wards where people eat in isolation at their bedsides with ward activities going on around them, limited by set meal delivery and collection times. However, given recognition of its importance, and particularly with the help of family and friends, this may be addressed and is, in part, the topic of a UK initiative (Protected Mealtimes: http://195.92.246.148/nhsestates/better_hospital_food/bhf_content/protected_mealtimes/overview.asp). Such an approach also entails ensuring meal systems are able to meet individual food preference, so that patients are able to choose what they eat. This is not just an issue for those of ethnic minorities, for whom choice is often more limited, especially when combined with need for texture modification. In hospital systems where patients experience transfers between wards, catering systems do not always have flexibility to keep track of patient movements. Ensuring out-of-hours availability of palatable snacks is also important; given decreasing lengths of stay and increasing investigations, it is increasingly important that food is available not just at set meal-times. Such an approach may not fit easily within systems that regard food as hotel services, targeted for cost-containment.

Conclusion

A considerable proportion of stroke patients demonstrate evidence of malnutrition or nutritional risk at admission to hospital; many will experience a wide range of eating-related disabilities that will prevent or deter them from eating for at least some part of their recovery period. Depression, common at all stages post-stroke, is also linked with appetite changes, and for some, reduced dietary intake, although the sequence of events is unclear, i.e. whether depression causes or follows appetite changes. This is important, because malnutrition has been linked with increased complication rates, poorer rehabilitation outcomes and more deaths amongst stroke patients. Eating is also an important component of quality of life, and nutritional status and ability to eat have long-term effects for stroke survivors, their families and social circles.

Nutritional screening and assessment is the essential first stage towards identifying individual needs, goals, care plans and programmes. However, whilst nutritional screening for all patients is widely advocated (unless a good case for exemption can be made), this does not always occur. In part this may be attributed to the challenges posed to undertake screening with immobile, possibly aphasic or cognitively-impaired, acutely unwell people. Nonetheless, without some form of screening and assessment, this important component of rehabilitation may be neglected or ineffectively addressed.

Many eating-related disabilities are already the subject of rehabilitation interventions, although meal-times may be under-utilised as opportunities to practise skills addressed during therapy sessions. Others, such as smell and taste dysfunction, remain under-explored. Decision-making in relation to provision of artificial nutrition support may pose challenges, and require active involvement and collaboration of the whole team with the patient (insofar as this is possible), family and carers. Decision-making for severely disabled patients presents particular difficulties, and may require engagement with family members with power of attorney and independent advocates.

Nutrition may be provided to patients through a range of means; care planning and goal-setting need to be established collaboratively, monitored and reviewed regularly. Methods to address long-term problems, enduring beyond hospital discharge, need to be discussed in relation to what is available within and through community resources. The need for ongoing review should be borne in mind. Education and training for patients and carers is important at all stages, but perhaps especially in relation to long-term management. Ultimately, patients may make decisions to take risks within their context of overall quality of life which health care professionals would not sanction, based on differing perceptions of the balance of benefit and risk.

> *I manage to do a bit of cooking but sometimes I can't, because I can't do it or because of safety reasons. My husband does all the shopping, when he comes in the evening. I go in the kitchen and I just help him, because I feel I want to be part of it. I manage some things, if there's no limited time for it I can do it. So it's OK to do those things, and I feel more myself, don't feel so hopeless.*
>
> (56-year-old female stroke survivor, six months post-stroke, London)

S1:   *Sheila usually prepares my meal, dishes it up and cuts it up for me.*
I: *Right.*
S2:   *But if I've missed bits, then he can manage it unless it was something like a lamb chop, he couldn't manage the meat on a chop, but he could, he could certainly manage his eggs. Fried egg and softer things, can't you?*
S1:   *Yes. Oh yes.*
I: *And how about chewing and swallowing?*
S1:   *No, no difficulties there, I'm doing quite well.*
S2:   *Actually I would, I would dispute that slightly. Again, we decided that if we felt differently we'd say something to you.*
I: *Yes?*
S2:   *Um, I think he does have some difficulties sometimes, in swallowing. Remember when the tablets don't go down? And then you discover they're still in your mouth?*
S1:   *Yes. In fact I –*
S2:   *And –*
S1:   *I've lost one once or twice haven't I?*
S2:   *Well we've had a bit of a laugh over it haven't we. The other thing is, he has what I call nursery food a lot of the time, although that's a bit of an exaggeration, spaghetti bolognese, shepherds pie, and a normal stir fry that I would enjoy eating is beyond Bernard to eat.*

So if I decide I want a stir fry I do him peas or something. Salad, even if it's cut very small, is not easy for Bernard to swallow, it doesn't go down very well, so you avoid eating it don't you, and we've quietly adjusted to that, so I would say that his swallowing isn't as good as it used to be. Um, I wouldn't dream of giving him steak, and we don't have any roast meats any more, rather casserole meats, cause they're easier to slip down, so I do think that his swallowing is slightly impaired.

S1: *I mean it's my preference, isn't it?*

S2: *It's your preference now Bernard yes, I certainly wouldn't make an issue of it with you.*

S1: *No. I think I've adapted fairly well to it, my liking fits in very well with what we're eating now.*

(Interviewer (I); 75-year-old male stroke survivor (S1); stroke survivor's wife (S2); six months post-stroke, London)

References

Age Concern, 2006, *Hungry To Be Heard: The Scandal of Malnourished Older People in Hospital*, Age Concern.

Aquilani, R, Galli, M, Guarnaschelli, C, Fugazza, G, Lorenzoni, M et al., 1999, Prevalence of malnutrition and inadequate food intake in self-feeding rehabilitation patients with stroke, *Europa Medicophysica*, vol. 35, no. 2, pp. 75–81.

Axelsson, K, Asplund, K, Norberg, A, & Eriksson, S, 1989, Eating problems and nutritional status during hospital stay of patients with severe stroke, *Journal of the American Dietetic Association*, vol. 89, no. 8, pp. 1092–1096.

BANS, 2007, *Personal Communication: British Artificial Nutrition Survey (BANS), a committee of BAPEN (The British Association for Parenteral and Enteral Nutrition)*, BANS, Redditch, Worcs.

Bath, PMW, Bath-Hextall, FJ, & Smithard, DG, 1999, *Interventions for dysphagia in acute stroke*, Cochrane Database of Systematic Reviews, Issue 4, CD000323.

BDA&RCSLT, 2002, *National Descriptors for Texture Modification in Adults*, British Dietetics Society and the Royal College of Speech and Language Therapy, London.

Beck, AM, & Ovesen, L, 1998, At which body mass index and degree of weight loss should hospitalized elderly patients be considered at nutritional risk? *Clinical Nutrition*, vol. 17, no. 5, pp. 195–198.

Bisch, EM, Logemann, JA, Rademaker, AW, Kahrilas, PJ, & Lazarus, CL, 1994, Pharyngeal effects of bolus volume, viscosity, and temperature in patients with dysphagia resulting from neurologic impairment and in normal subjects, *Journal of Speech and Hearing Research*, vol. 37, no. 5, pp. 1041–1059.

Boaden, E, Davies, S, Storey, L, & Watkins, C, 2006, *Inter-professional Dysphagia Framework*, University of Central Lancashire, Preston.

Broom, J, 1993, Sepsis and trauma, in *Human Nutrition and Dietetics*, 9th edn, JS Garrow & WPT James, eds., Churchill Livingstone, Edinburgh, pp. 456–463.

Brott, T, Adams, HP, Jr, Olinger, CP, Marler, JR, Barsan, WG et al., 1989, Measurements of acute cerebral infarction: a clinical examination scale, *Stroke*, vol. 20, no. 7, pp. 864–870.

Brozek, J, 1985, *Malnutrition and Human Behaviour: Experimental, Clinical and Community Studies*, Van Nostrand Reinhold Co., New York.

Bruinsma, KA, & Taren, DL, 2000, Dieting, essential fatty acid intake, and depression, *Nutrition Reviews*, vol. 58, no. 4, pp. 98–108.

Bulow, M, Olsson, R, & Ekberg, O, 2003, Videoradiographic analysis of how carbonated thin liquids and thickened liquids affect the physiology of swallowing in subjects with aspiration on thin liquids, *Acta Radiologica*, vol. 44, no. 4, pp. 366–372.

Chalela, JA, Haymore, J, Schellinger, PD, Kang, DW, & Warach, S, 2004, Acute stroke patients are being underfed: a nitrogen balance study, *Neurocritical Care*, vol. 1, no. 3, pp. 331–334.

Chen, CC, Schilling, LS, & Lyder, CH, 2001, A concept analysis of malnutrition in the elderly, *Journal of Advanced Nursing*, vol. 36, no. 1, pp. 131–142.

Chen, ZY, Sea, MM, Kwan, KY, Leung, YH, & Leung, PF, 1997, Depletion of linoleate induced by weight cycling is independent of extent of calorie restriction, *American Journal of Physiology*, vol. 272, no. 1 Pt 2, p. R43–R50.

Choi-Kwon, S, Yang, YH, Kim, EK, Jeon, MY, & Kim, JS, 1998, Nutritional status in acute stroke: undernutrition versus overnutrition in different stroke subtypes, *Acta Neurologica Scandinavica*, vol. 98, no. 3, pp. 187–192.

Colagiovanni, L, 2000, Preventing and clearing blocked feeding tubes, *Nursing Times Plus*, vol. 96, no. 17 Suppl, pp. 3–4.

Cook, IJ, Dodds, WJ, Dantas, RO, Massey, B, Kern, MK et al., 1989, Opening mechanisms of the human upper esophageal sphincter, *American Journal of Physiology*, vol. 257, no. 5 Pt 1, pp. G748–G759.

Davalos, A, Ricart, W, Gonzalez-Huix, F, Soler, S, Marrugat, J et al., 1996, Effect of malnutrition after acute stroke on clinical outcome, *Stroke*, vol. 27, no. 6, pp. 1028–1032.

Davis, JP, Wong, AA, Schluter, PJ, Henderson, RD, O'Sullivan, JD et al., 2004, Impact of premorbid undernutrition on outcome in stroke patients, *Stroke*, vol. 35, no. 8, pp. 1930–1934.

de Groot, CP, van den Broek T, & van Staveren W, 1999, Energy intake and micronutrient intake in elderly Europeans: seeking the minimum requirement in the SENECA study, *Age and Ageing*, vol. 28, no. 5, pp. 469–474.

de Jong, N, Mulder, I, de Graaf, C, & van Staveren, WA, 1999, Impaired sensory functioning in elders: the relation with its potential determinants and nutritional intake, *Journal of Gerontology Series A – Biological Sciences, Medical Sciences*, vol. 54, no. 8, pp. B324–B331.

Dennis, MS, Lewis, SC, & Warlow, C, 2005a, Effect of timing and method of enteral tube feeding for dysphagic stroke patients (FOOD): a multicentre randomised controlled trial, *Lancet*, vol. 365, no. 9461, pp. 764–772.

Dennis, MS, Lewis, SC, & Warlow, C, 2005b, Routine oral nutritional supplementation for stroke patients in hospital (FOOD): a multicentre randomised controlled trial, *Lancet*, vol. 365, no. 9461, pp. 755–763.

Department of Health, 2004, *Standards for Better Health*, Department of Health, London.

Duffy, VB, Backstrand, JR, & Ferris, AM, 1995, Olfactory dysfunction and related nutritional risk in free-living, elderly women, *Journal of the American Dietetic Association*, vol. 95, no. 8, pp. 879–884.

Ebrahim, S, Barer, D, & Nouri, F, 1987, An audit of follow-up services for stroke patients after discharge from hospital, *International Disability Studies*, vol. 9, no. 3, pp. 103–105.

Edington, J, Kon, P, & Martyn, CN, 1996, Prevalence of malnutrition in patients in general practice, *Clinical Nutrition*, vol. 15, no. 2, pp. 60–63.

Elia, M, 2000, *Guidelines for Detection and Management of Malnutrition: A Report by the Malnutrition Advisory Group*, BAPEN, Maidenhead.

Elia, M, Stratton, RJ, Holden, C, Meadows, N, Micklewright, A et al., 2001, Home enteral tube feeding following cerebrovascular accident, *Clinical Nutrition*, vol. 20, no. 1, pp. 27–30.

Elter, JR, Offenbacher, S, Toole, JF, & Beck, JD, 2003, Relationship of periodontal disease and edentulism to stroke/TIA, *Journal of Dental Research*, vol. 82, no. 12, pp. 998–1001.

Esper, DH, Coplin, WM, & Carhuapoma, JR, 2006, Energy expenditure in patients with nontraumatic intracranial hemorrhage, *Journal of Parenteral and Enteral Nutrition*, vol. 30, no. 2, pp. 71–75.

Farrell, JF, 1956, The effect of mastication on the digestion of foods, *British Dental Journal*, vol. 100, pp. 149–155.

Finch, S, Doyle, W, Lowe, C, Bates, CJ, Prentice, A, Smithers, G, & Clarke, PC, 1998, *National Diet and Nutrition Survey: People Aged 65 Years and Over: Volume 1: Report of the Diet and Nutrition Survey*, The Stationery Office, London.

Finestone, HM, Greene-Finestone, LS, Foley, NC, & Woodbury, MG, 2003, Measuring longitudinally the metabolic demands of stroke patients: resting energy expenditure is not elevated, *Stroke*, vol. 34, no. 2, pp. 502–507.

Finestone, HM, Greene-Finestone, LS, Wilson, ES, & Teasell, RW, 1996, Prolonged length of stay and reduced functional improvement rate in malnourished stroke rehabilitation patients, *Archives of Physical Medicine and Rehabilitation*, vol. 77, no. 4, pp. 340–345.

Finsterer, J, Stollberger, C, & Kopsa, W, 2004, Weight reduction due to stroke-induced dysgeusia, *European Neurology*, vol. 51, no. 1, pp. 47–49.

FOOD Trial Collaboration, 2003, Poor nutritional status on admission predicts poor outcomes after stroke: observational data from the FOOD trial, *Stroke*, vol. 34, no. 6, pp. 1450–1456.

Foundas, AL, Macauley, BL, Raymer, AM, Maher, LM, Heilman, KM et al., 1995, Ecological implications of limb apraxia: evidence from mealtime behavior, *Journal of International Neuropsychology*, vol. 1, no. 1, pp. 62–66.

Gall, A, 2001, Post-stroke depression, *British Journal of Therapy and Rehabilitation*, vol. 8, no. 7, pp. 252–257.

Gariballa, SE, Parker, SG, Taub, N, & Castleden, CM, 1998, A randomized, controlled, a single-blind trial of nutritional supplementation after acute stroke, *Journal of Parenteral and Enteral Nutrition*, vol. 22, no. 5, pp. 315–319.

Gariballa, SE, & Sinclair, AJ, 1998, Assessment and treatment of nutritional status in stroke patients, *Postgraduate Medical Journal*, vol. 74, no. 873, pp. 395–399.

Garon, BR, Engle, M, & Ormiston, C, 1997, A randomised control study to determine the effects of unlimited oral intake of water, *Journal of Neurological Rehabilitation*, vol. 11, pp. 139–148.

Gill, D, & Hatcher, S, 2000, *Antidepressants for depression in medical illness*, Cochrane Database of Systematic Reviews, Issue 4. Art No: CD001312.

Gillen, R, Tennen, H, McKee, TE, Gernert-Dott, P, & Affleck, G, 2001, Depressive symptoms and history of depression predict rehabilitation efficiency in stroke patients, *Archives of Physical Medicine and Rehabilitation*, vol. 82, no. 12, pp. 1645–1649.

Harley, C, Boyd, JE, Cockburn, J, Collin, C, Haggard, P et al., 2006, Disruption of sitting balance after stroke: influence of spoken output, *Journal of Neurology, Neurosurgery and Psychiatry*, vol. 77, no. 5, pp. 674–676.

Heckmann, JG, Stossel, C, Lang, CJ, Neundorfer, B, Tomandl, B et al., 2005, Taste disorders in acute stroke: a prospective observational study on taste disorders in 102 stroke patients, *Stroke*, vol. 36, no. 8, pp. 1690–1694.

Hiiemae, KM, & Palmer, JB, 1999, Food transport and bolus formation during complete feeding sequences on foods of different initial consistency, *Dysphagia*, vol. 14, no. 1, pp. 31–42.

Hochstenbach, J, & Mulder, T, 1999, Neuropsychology and the relearning of motor skills following stroke, *International Journal of Rehabilitation Research*, vol. 22, no. 1, pp. 11–19.

Jacobsson, C, Axelsson, K, Norberg, A, Asplund, K, & Wenngren, BI, 1997, Outcomes of individualized interventions in patients with severe eating difficulties, *Clinical Nursing Research*, vol. 6, no. 1, pp. 25–44.

Jacobsson, C, Axelsson, K, Osterlind, PO, & Norberg, A, 2000, How people with stroke and healthy older people experience the eating process, *Journal of Clinical Nursing*, vol. 9, no. 2, pp. 255–264.

Kalra, L, Smith, DH, & Crome, P, 1993, Stroke in patients aged over 75 years: outcome and predictors, *Postgraduate Medical Journal*, vol. 69, no. 807, pp. 33–36.

Kalra, L, Perez, I, Gupta, S, & Wittink, M, 1997, The influence of visual neglect on stroke rehabilitation, *Stroke*, vol. 28, no. 7, pp. 1386–1391.

Kayser-Jones, J, & Schell, E, 1997, The effect of staffing on the quality of care at mealtime, *Nursing Outlook*, vol. 45, no. 2, pp. 64–72.

Keller, HH, 1993, Malnutrition in institutionalized elderly: how and why? *Journal of the American Geriatrics Society*, vol. 41, no. 11, pp. 1212–1218.

Kim, JS, & Choi, S, 2002, Altered food preference after cortical infarction: Korean style, *Cerebrovascular Diseases*, vol. 13, no. 3, pp. 187–191.

Koltin, SE, & Rosen, HS, 1996, Hemiplegia and feeding: an occupational therapy approach to upper extremity management, *Topics in Stroke Rehabilitation*, vol. 3, no. 3, pp. 69–86.

Krall, E, Hayes, C, & Garcia, R, 1998, How dentition status and masticatory function affect nutrient intake, *Journal of the American Dental Association*, vol. 129, no. 9, pp. 1261–1269.

Kuhlemeier, KV, Rieve, JE, Kirby, NA, & Siebens, AA, 1989, Clinical correlates of dysphagia in stroke patients, *Archives of Physical Medicine and Rehabilitation*, vol. 70, p. A-56.

Lennard-Jones, JE, 1998, *Ethical and Legal Aspects of Clinical Hydration and Nutritional Support*, The British Association for Parenteral and Enteral Nutrition, Maidenhead.

Lien, HC, Chang, CS, & Chen, GH, 2000, Can percutaneous endoscopic jejunostomy prevent gastroesophageal reflux in patients with preexisting esophagitis? *American Journal of Gastroenterology*, vol. 95, no. 12, pp. 3439–3443.

Logemann, J, 1998, *Evaluation and Treatment of Swallowing Disorders*, 2nd edn, Pro-Ed, Austin, Texas.

Logemann, JA, Pauloski, BR, Colangelo, L, Lazarus, C, Fujiu, M et al., 1995, Effects of a sour bolus on oropharyngeal swallowing measures in patients with neurogenic dysphagia, *Journal of Speech and Hearing Research*, vol. 38, no. 3, pp. 556–563.

Lupton, D, 1996, *Food, the Body and the Self*, Sage Publications, London.

Marik, PE, 2001, Aspiration pneumonitis and aspiration pneumonia, *New England Journal of Medicine*, vol. 344, no. 9, pp. 665–671.

Marks, L, Rainbow, D, 2003, *Working with Dysphagia*, Speechmark Publishing Ltd, Oxon.

Martinsen, B, Harder, I, & Biering-Sorensen, F, 2008, The meaning of assisted feeding for people living with spinal cord injury: a phenomenological study, *Journal of Advanced Nursing*, vol. 62, no. 5, pp. 533–540.

McLaren, SMG, & Dickerson, JWT, 2000, Measurement of eating disability in an acute stroke population, *Clinical Effectiveness in Nursing*, vol. 4, pp. 109–120.

Metheny, N, Wehrle, MA, Wiersema, L, & Clark, J, 1998, Testing feeding tube placement: Auscultation vs. pH method, *American Journal of Nursing*, vol. 98, no. 5, pp. 37–42.

Millns, B, Gosney, M, Jack, CI, Martin, MV, & Wright, AE, 2003, Acute stroke predisposes to oral gram-negative bacilli – a cause of aspiration pneumonia? *Gerontology*, vol. 49, no. 3, pp. 173–176.

National Institute for Health and Clinical Excellence, 2006, *Nutrition Support in Adults: Oral Nutrition Support, Enteral Tube Feeding and Parenteral Nutrition*, NICE, Clinical Guideline 32.

Nip, WRF, 2007, *Mood and food: an investigation of mood state and nutritional status after stroke*, London, Doctoral thesis, St George's, University of London.

Perry, L, 2002, *Eating after stroke: natural history and investigation of an evidence-based intervention*, Doctoral thesis, University of London.

Perry, L, & Love, CP, 2001, Screening for dysphagia and aspiration in acute stroke: a systematic review, *Dysphagia*, vol. 16, no. 1, pp. 7–18.

Perry, L, & McLaren, S, 2003a, Eating difficulties after stroke, *Journal of Advanced Nursing*, vol. 43, no. 4, pp. 360–369.

Perry, L, & McLaren, S, 2003b, Nutritional support in acute stroke: the impact of evidence-based guidelines, *Clinical Nutrition*, vol. 22, no. 3, pp. 283–293.

Perry, L, & McLaren, S, 2004, An exploration of nutrition and eating disabilities in relation to quality of life at 6 months post-stroke, *Health and Social Care in the Community*, vol. 12, no. 4, pp. 288–297.

Platts, MM, Rafferty, D, & Paul, L, 2006, Metabolic cost of over ground gait in younger stroke patients and healthy controls, *Medicine and Science in Sports and Exercise*, vol. 38, no. 6, pp. 1041–1046.

Power, ML, Fraser, CH, Hobson, A, Singh, S, Tyrrell, P et al., 2006, Evaluating oral stimulation as a treatment for dysphagia after stroke, *Dysphagia*, vol. 21, no. 1, pp. 49–55.

Pritchard, TC, Macaluso, DA, & Eslinger, PJ, 1999, Taste perception in patients with insular cortex lesions, *Behavioural Neuroscience*, vol. 113, no. 4, pp. 663–671.

Rabeneck, L, McCullough, LB, & Wray, NP, 1997, Ethically justified, clinically comprehensive guidelines for percutaneous endoscopic gastrostomy tube placement, *Lancet*, vol. 349, no. 9050, pp. 496–498.

Reilly, HM, 1996, Nutrition in clinical management: malnutrition in our midst, *Proceedings of the Nutrition Society*, vol. 55, pp. 841–853.

Rosenbek, JC, Roecker, EB, Wood, JL, & Robbins, J, 1996, Thermal application reduces the duration of stage transition in dysphagia after stroke, *Dysphagia*, vol. 11, no. 4, pp. 225–233.

Rosenvinge, SK, & Starke, ID, 2005, Improving care for patients with dysphagia, *Age and Ageing*, vol. 34, no. 6, pp. 587–593.

Royal College of Speech and Language Therapy, 2006, *Communicating Quality 3: RCSLT's Guidance on Best Practice in Service Organisation and Provision*, RCSLT, 2 White Hart Yard, London, SE1 1NX.

Sala, R, Munto, MJ, de la, CJ, Preciado, I, Miralles, T et al., 1998, Swallowing changes in cerebrovascular accidents: incidence, natural history, and repercussions on the nutritional status, morbidity, and mortality, *Revista de Neurologia*, vol. 27, no. 159, pp. 759–766.

Schiffman, SS, & Graham, BG, 2000, Taste and smell perception affect appetite and immunity in the elderly, *European Journal of Clinical Nutrition*, vol. 54 Suppl 3, pp. S54–S63.

Schiffman, SS, & Warwick, ZS, 1993, Effect of flavor enhancement of foods for the elderly on nutritional status: food intake, biochemical indices, and anthropometric measures, *Physiology and Behavior*, vol. 53, no. 2, pp. 395–402.

Selley, WG, Flack, FC, Ellis, RE, & Brooks, WA, 1989, Respiratory patterns associated with swallowing. Part 2: Neurologically impaired dysphagic patients, *Age and Ageing*, vol. 18, no. 3, pp. 173–176.

Sheiham, A, Steele, JG, Marcenes, W, Lowe, C, Finch, S et al., 2001, The relationship among dental status, nutrient intake, and nutritional status in older people, *Journal of Dental Research*, vol. 80, no. 2, pp. 408–413.

Sidenvall, B, Fjellstrom, C, & Ek, AC, 1996, Cultural perspectives of meals expressed by patients in geriatric care, *International Journal of Nursing Studies*, vol. 33, no. 2, pp. 212–222.

Siebens, H, Trupe, E, Siebens, A, Cook, F, Anshen, S et al., 1986, Correlates and consequences of eating dependency in institutionalized elderly, *Journal of the American Geriatric Society*, vol. 34, no. 3, pp. 192–198.

Smithard, DG, O'Neill, PA, Parks, C, & Morris, J, 1996, Complications and outcome after acute stroke. Does dysphagia matter? *Stroke*, vol. 27, no. 7, pp. 1200–1204.

Sorensen, HV, Lendal, S, Schultz-Larsen, K, & Uhrskov, T, 2003, Stroke rehabilitation: assistive technology devices and environmental modifications following primary rehabilitation in hospital – a therapeutic perspective, *Assistive Technology*, vol. 15, no. 1, pp. 39–48.

Stone, SP, Wilson, B, Wroot, A, Halligan, PW, Lange, LS et al., 1991, The assessment of visuo-spatial neglect after acute stroke, *Journal of Neurology, Neurosurgery and Psychiatry*, vol. 54, no. 4, pp. 345–350.

Taub, NA, Wolfe, CD, Richardson, E, & Burney, PG, 1994, Predicting the disability of first-time stroke sufferers at 1 year: 12-month follow-up of a population-based cohort in southeast England, *Stroke*, vol. 25, no. 2, pp. 352–357.

Touho, H, Karasawa, J, Shishido, H, Morisako, T, Numazawa, S et al., 1990, Measurement of energy expenditure in acute stage of cerebrovascular diseases, *Neurologia Medico-Chirurgica (Tokyo)*, vol. 30, no. 7, pp. 451–455.

Unosson, M, Ek, AC, Bjurulf, P, von Schenck, H, & Larsson, J, 1994, Feeding dependence and nutritional status after acute stroke, *Stroke*, vol. 25, no. 2, pp. 366–371.

Vir, SC, & Love, AH, 1979, Nutritional status of institutionalized and noninstitutionalized aged in Belfast, Northern Ireland, *American Journal of Clinical Nutrition*, vol. 32, no. 9, pp. 1934–1947.

Wade, DT, Legh-Smith, J, & Hewer, RA, 1987, Depressed mood after stroke: A community study of its frequency, *British Journal of Psychiatry*, vol. 151, pp. 200–205.

Wayler, AH, & Chauncey, HH, 1983, Impact of complete dentures and impaired natural dentition on masticatory performance and food choice in healthy aging men, *Journal of Prosthetic Dentistry*, vol. 49, no. 3, pp. 427–433.

Weekes, E, & Elia, M, 1992, Resting energy expenditure and body composition following cerebro-vascular accident, *Clinical Nutrition*, vol. 11, no. 1, pp. 18–22.

Westergren, A, Karlsson, S, Andersson, P, Ohlsson, O, & Hallberg, IR, 2001, Eating difficulties, need for assisted eating, nutritional status and pressure ulcers in patients admitted for stroke rehabilitation, *Journal of Clinical Nursing*, vol. 10, no. 2, pp. 257–269.

Whelan, K, 2001, Inadequate fluid intakes in dysphagic acute stroke, *Clinical Nutrition*, vol. 20, no. 5, pp. 423–428.

Wilkinson, PR, Wolfe, CD, Warburton, FG, Rudd, AG, Howard, RS et al., 1997, A long-term follow-up of stroke patients, *Stroke*, vol. 28, no. 3, pp. 507–512.

Williams, J, 2005, Using an alternative fixing device for nasogastric tubes, *Nursing Times*, vol. 101, no. 35, pp. 26–27.

Yoneyama, T, Yoshida, M, Ohrui, T, Mukaiyama, H, Okamoto, H et al., 2002, Oral care reduces pneumonia in older patients in nursing homes, *Journal of the American Geriatrics Society*, vol. 50, no. 3, pp. 430–433.

Chapter 6

Promoting continence

Kathryn Getliffe and Wendy Brooks

Key points

- Urinary incontinence is common in the community, with more than one in three people over 40 years reporting symptoms of bladder problems. Many stroke patients may have experienced problems before their stroke.
- Urinary incontinence is common after a stroke, reported to affect 32–79% of patients.
- Bowel function is often affected by a stroke; up to 60% of those in rehabilitation wards experience constipation. Faecal incontinence is often related to functional disability, and more than 30% of stroke patients are incontinent of faeces at 7–10 days, 11% at three months and later.
- Mobility and manual dexterity problems can compound bladder and bowel symptoms because they can make toileting access difficult. Other problems such as visual disturbances, dysphagia and cognition also contribute indirectly to continence difficulties.
- All nurses should be trained in basic assessment and management of bladder and bowel problems; should know where to get further advice and help.
- Bladder and bowel care requires active management – this includes a written personalised plan, taking into consideration required assistance, personal needs and goals.

I don't go out, I don't even ask anyone round ... I'm so embarrassed about the smell. I do try and keep myself clean but it gets onto your clothes and furniture. Sometimes I wish that I hadn't survived because it's no life I'm leading now.

(Female stroke survivor)

Introduction

Bladder and bowel problems are common following stroke and can have a huge impact on physical and psychological aspects of quality of life, for both patients and carers. The stroke survivor quoted above shows powerfully the devastating nature of incontinence and it is known that depression is twice as likely in survivors who are incontinent compared with those who are not (Brittain 1998). Health care professionals can do much to help improve and manage bladder and bowel problems in stroke patients and this starts with a good understanding of key issues. This chapter examines the causes and contributing factors, and discusses assessment and management protocols together with the evidence base which underpins them.

The reported prevalence of urinary incontinence after stroke is high, varying between 32% and 79% in population- and hospital-based studies (Brittain et al. 1999; Patel et al. 2001). Differences in defining urinary incontinence and time of measurement post-stroke (e.g. at admission, one week, one month) contribute to this wide range. In the UK, the National Sentinel Audit of Stroke (Royal College of Physicians 2002) reported that 44% of patients hospitalised following stroke suffer with urinary incontinence at one week post-stroke. Many stroke patients (25–50%) are still suffering from urinary incontinence on discharge (Barratt 2002; Patel et al. 2001) and prevalence of incontinence two years post-stroke is still around 10% (Patel et al. 2001). The causes of urinary incontinence can be varied and complex including pathophysiological effects of stroke on neural pathways involved in bladder control and/or a consequence of functional disability. Urinary incontinence is widely recognised as an important prognostic indicator of mortality and poor outcome, in terms of functional disability, cognition and discharge destination – home or institutional care (Patel et al. 2001; Thomas et al. 2005). In one study, urinary incontinence was significantly associated with age over 75 years, dysphagia, visual field defect and motor weakness (Patel et al. 2001). Other studies have also shown that poorer stroke survival, increased disability and institutionalisation rates are linked with post-stroke urinary incontinence, particularly in patients with impaired awareness of the need to void (Brittain et al. 1999).

Urinary incontinence is common in the general population and can affect people of all ages. More than one in three people over 40 years reported symptoms of bladder problems in a large survey (Perry et al. 2000), although most did not find their symptoms sufficiently bothersome to seek help. This high prevalence of urinary incontinence symptoms in the general population suggests that many stroke survivors may be vulnerable to exacerbation of pre-existing urinary incontinence and this should be borne in mind during assessment of continence problems. The major types of urinary incontinence are characterised by different patterns of symptoms and are summarised in Box 6.1.

Bowel problems, including faecal incontinence (FI), are more likely to be related to resultant functional disability than direct effects of the stroke. Bowel function is recognised as a considerable problem following a stroke, with constipation affecting 60% of those in rehabilitation wards (Robain et al. 2002). FI has been reported to affect more than 30% of stroke patients at 7–10 days,

---

Box 6.1   Main types of urinary incontinence (UI).

- *Urge UI:* characterised by urinary leakage accompanied by, or immediately preceded by, urgency (little warning of an urgent need to void, unable to hold on). May result in major leakage with complete bladder emptying, or in frequent small leaks. Where the bladder is not emptying completely, patients may complain of a frequent need to urinate because the bladder fills up so quickly due to residual urine. Most common type of UI in stroke patients.
- *Stress UI:* characterised by urinary leakage associated with increased abdominal pressure, e.g. coughing, sneezing, effort or exertion. No post-void residual urine. Caused by weakness of pelvic floor, therefore unlikely to be a direct result of stroke but symptoms of pre-existing stress UI may be exacerbated.
- *Mixed UI:* involuntary leakage associated with urgency and also with exertion, effort, sneezing or coughing.
- *Functional UI:* failure to manage toileting is due to factors other than physiological bladder control, e.g. poor mobility (unable to reach toilet alone), poor manual dexterity (unable to manage clothing or hold a urinal), poor communication (unable to ask for help or express inability to hold on).
- *Voiding difficulties:* caused by outlet obstruction or detrusor hypoactivity. Large residual urine volume with or without overflow. May have frequent urinary tract infections (UTIs).

11% at three months, 11% at one year and 15% at three years (Harari et al. 2003). In this study of over 800 stroke patients, those with FI at three months were at increased risk of long-term placement in a nursing home and death within one year. FI may be due to impaction and overflow and/or may be associated more with disability-related factors such as ability to self-toilet and medication, rather than the actual stroke brain injury (Harari et al. 2004). Other impairments that are common following a stroke, such as aphasia, dysphagia, cognitive problems or mood changes, may also indirectly affect bowel function.

Importance of good continence care

Good continence care can help to militate against the effects of stroke, including reducing risks of falls as ambulant patients try to get to a toilet quickly (Brown et al. 2000). Good continence care also plays a key role in helping to restore self-esteem and promote independence (Department of Health 2000). Because of the very personal nature of continence problems many people are embarrassed and find bladder or bowel problems difficult subjects to talk about. The attitudes of health professionals can exert a major influence and it is important to take a proactive, positive and well-informed approach. Since urinary incontinence is known to increase with advancing age and many stroke patients are also elderly it is particularly important that health care professionals do not adhere to a belief that incontinence is inevitable and a non-reversible part of the ageing process. 'Mary' (Case example 6.1) provides an example of someone with urinary symptoms both related to and exacerbated by her stroke, but who had previously been independently continent.

Failure to adequately assess, treat and support people with a continence problem robs them of their dignity and imposes limitations on lifestyles,

Case example 6.1 Mary.

Mary was a 79-year-old woman admitted to hospital with right middle cerebral artery infarction. She had left arm and leg weakness, left-sided sensory inattention and urinary incontinence. She had been registered blind for the past four years but otherwise was able-bodied, independent and continent prior to her stroke.

Box 6.2   UK National Clinical Guidelines for Stroke (Intercollegiate Stroke Working Party 2008a) recommendations.

Acute phase:

- The acute admitting ward should have a documented policy on detection and management of bowel and bladder function in the acute phase.
- Patient should not have an indwelling (urethral) catheter inserted in the first 48 hours unless indicated to relieve urinary retention.
- Urinary and faecal incontinence should be managed by high levels of nursing care in the acute phase.

Rehabilitation phase:

(A) All wards and stroke units should have established assessment and management protocols for both urinary and faecal incontinence, and for constipation.
(B) All patients with loss of control of the bladder at two weeks should:
  - Be assessed for other causes of incontinence, which should be treated if identified.
  - Have an active plan of management documented.
  - Be offered simple treatments such as bladder re-training, pelvic floor exercises and external equipment first.
  - Only be given an indwelling urethral catheter after other methods of management have failed.
  - Only be discharged home with continuing incontinence after the carer (family member) or patient has been fully trained and adequate arrangements for continuing supply of continence aids and services are confirmed and in place.
(C) All patients with a loss of control over their bowels at two weeks should:
  - Be assessed for other causes of incontinence, which should be treated if identified.
  - Have a documented, active plan of management.
  - Be referred for specialist treatments if the patient is able to participate in treatments.

employment opportunities and social functioning. Even if continence cannot be fully restored, there is always potential for improvement to overall quality of life. UK National Clinical Guidelines for Stroke (Intercollegiate Stroke Working Party 2008a) specify that all wards should have management protocols for urinary incontinence (Box 6.2), yet many wards do not have this information available. In 2008 the UK National Sentinel Audit for Stroke found that 30% of patients audited should have had a continence plan, but of these, there was indication of active management of the problem in only 60% of notes (Intercollegiate Stroke Working Party 2008b). In 2004 the same national audit demonstrated that provision of guidelines and protocols for continence management varied hugely depending on the type of ward that stroke patients were treated on, with only 45% of general wards and 81% of stroke units compliant with this standard.

Bladder problems and urinary incontinence

Control of micturition

Before considering assessment and management of bladder problems and urinary incontinence it is important to understand the normal control of micturition. The bladder has two main functions: storage of urine at low pressure, and periodic elimination of urine under voluntary control. The major anatomical structures involved in both functions are the:

- Bladder (detrusor muscle) and bladder neck
- Urethra, and urethral sphincter mechanism (striated muscle)
- Pelvic floor

During storage of urine the bladder neck and external sphincter are closed and the detrusor muscle is relaxed (via inhibitory control from higher centres). The bladder stretches to accommodate the increasing volume of urine produced by the kidneys, whilst allowing pressure inside to remain low as the volume increases. During the filling cycle stretch receptors within the detrusor muscle pass impulses to the spinal micturition centre (via sacral level nerves S2–S4) and then, via the spinal cord (lateral spino-thalamic tracts), to the pontine micturition centre and the frontal cortex. At a bladder volume of around 150–250 ml these impulses are perceived as the desire to void but are effectively suppressed by the higher centres until a convenient time to do this. A 'normal' bladder will hold around 400–500 ml of urine before needing to empty. Voluntary voiding requires coordinated relaxation of the external sphincter and bladder neck, followed by detrusor muscle contraction (via parasympathetic stimulation). These two different sets of activities are mediated by three sets of peripheral nerves: pelvic nerves (parasympathetic, cholinergic); hypogastric nerves (sympathetic, adrenergic); pudendal nerves (somatic). The necessary coordination is achieved via the spinal-pontine spinal reflex, involving the spinal micturition centre (S2–S4) and the pontine micturition centre (the main switching centre between filling and voiding cycles). Voluntary control of voiding appears to be dependent on connections between the frontal cortex and regions within the hypothalamus as well as the brainstem (Yoshimura et al. 2004).

Causes of urinary incontinence post-stroke

There are three mechanisms that are likely to contribute to symptoms of urinary incontinence post-stroke (Gelber et al. 1993):

- Disruption of the neuro-micturition pathways resulting in detrusor overactivity and symptoms of urgency and frequency (common terms: bladder hyperreflexia; overactive bladder syndrome, urge incontinence)
- Incontinence due to stroke-related cognitive, language or mobility deficits (functional incontinence)

- Concurrent neuropathy or medication use resulting in bladder hyporeflexia (causing urinary retention and incomplete bladder emptying)

Main types of urinary incontinence

The main types of urinary incontinence are summarised in Box 6.1 and discussed below.

Urge incontinence

Urge incontinence is the most common type of urinary incontinence in stroke patients (Khan et al. 1990; Wyndaele et al. 2005) and is characterised by a sudden, compelling urge to void that is difficult or impossible to defer. The problem is caused by overactivity of the detrusor muscle of the bladder, often termed overactive bladder syndrome (OAB) or more specifically 'bladder hyper-reflexia' where there is a known neurological cause. The neurological damage resulting from strokes may cause loss of inhibitory impulses from the brain, allowing inappropriate activation of the sacral reflex arc so that the bladder begins to contract before micturition is voluntarily initiated. Damage above the pons leaves the spinal-bulbar-spinal reflex intact. Coordinated sphincter relaxation and detrusor contraction for voiding is therefore preserved but the inhibitory input to delay micturition may be lost or impaired. This results in detrusor overactivity, characterised by symptoms of urinary frequency and urgency, with or without urge incontinence. Bladder contractions may occur spontaneously or on provocation (e.g. with coughing or vigorous exercise), or while the patient is attempting to inhibit micturition. Contractions may be sufficiently strong to cause major leakage (complete bladder emptying) or may only cause partial emptying (frequent small leaks). If the bladder is not emptied effectively large residual volumes of urine (100 ml and more) are common. The bladder's capacity also decreases since it no longer has the opportunity to fill completely. Patients with OAB or hyperreflexia usually complain of urgency with little or no warning of the need to void, and may be incontinent of urine before reaching the toilet. In addition, they commonly experience persistent frequency and nocturnal enuresis. Overactivity of the bladder can be objectively demonstrated by urodynamic studies, which measure pressure changes as they occur within the bladder and urethra during filling of the bladder. Overactivity is the most frequent urodynamic finding in people who have had a stroke, but the procedure is invasive and is not routinely required for all patients. Nursing management of urge incontinence is outlined in Table 6.1. Recent reviews indicate that bladder training may be a useful intervention (Wallace et al. 2007) and this is discussed further below.

Stress incontinence

Stress incontinence is characterised by urinary incontinence upon exertion. Stress incontinence does not occur as a direct consequence of stroke because

Table 6.1 Urge incontinence.

Nursing intervention	Rationale
Start bladder retraining at a length of time the patient can manage (based on the frequency volume chart)	This intervention may be useful for urge incontinence (Wallace et al. 2007). It encourages the bladder to progressively hold more and more urine until a 'normal' time interval is reached
Body-worn pads of appropriate size if required (bearing in mind that this may compound the problem by slowing down access to the toilet/bedpan/bottle)	To provide confidence and comfort until continent
Exclude or reduce caffeine (tea, coffee, coca cola, chocolate) and citrus fruits (oranges, lemons and limes) from the patient's diet (following explanation and agreement with the patient or relevant other)	These substances may exacerbate symptoms (Bryant et al. 2002)
If the patient reaches a plateau with the bladder retraining programme, discuss with medical staff regarding drugs for urinary frequency (e.g. oxybutynin, tolterodine, solifenacin succinate). NB. Some medications are tolerated better and cause fewer side-effects, such as dry mouth, than others	This may help the patient to progress further with bladder training

Table 6.2 Stress incontinence (Bo et al. 1999).

Nursing intervention	Rationale
The patient should be assessed for ability to undertake pelvic floor education	Pelvic floor exercise has been shown to be effective in reducing the amount of leakage caused by stress incontinence (Bo et al. 1999)
A patient diary recording episodes of wetness should be commenced	This will help monitor progress and highlight activities resulting in wetness

its primary cause is weakness of the pelvic floor; however, it is fairly common in the elderly female population and may also present as mixed incontinence, with symptoms of both stress and urge incontinence. Weakness of the pelvic floor muscles (or prostatectomy in some men) can result in urine leakage on exertion (standing, coughing and sneezing). Stroke may exacerbate any existing stress incontinence due to increased weakness, reduced muscle tone and additional mobility problems, which may increase the amount of exertion required to move. Treatment strategies are aimed at improving pelvic floor muscle strength and tone (Bo et al. 1999, 2005; National Institute for Health and Clinical Effectiveness (NICE) 2006). However, the exercises involved require concentration, effort and persistence, and are therefore probably best initiated after the acute period when some recovery has taken place. Patients should be referred to a continence specialist for assessment of muscle floor strength, development of an individualised exercise regime and ongoing support. Nursing management of stress incontinence is outlined in Table 6.2.

Table 6.3 Functional incontinence.

Nursing intervention	Rationale
Ensure all aids to communication are employed. Nurse call bell within easy reach, printed picture/text cards at bedside if required	To help the patient express elimination needs
Body-worn pads and pants of appropriate size if required (bearing in mind that this can sometimes compound the problem if the problem is poor manual dexterity)	To provide confidence and comfort until continent
Hand-held urinals (with absorbent gel if required)	Can be used in a bed or chair, may help prevent episodes of incontinence due to poor mobility. Absorbent gels helps to prevent spills
Advice to patient or relevant other on adapted or easy to remove clothing (loose jogging trousers, Velcro fly fastening, hold up stockings, wrap around skirts)	To provide quick, easy access to toileting
Frequency volume chart to monitor episodes of incontinence	To monitor progress and aid planning of treatment (patient may be consistently wet at lunch time when staff are giving out meals; taking the patient to the toilet prior to lunch may solve the problem)
Regular toileting regime based on results of intake/output monitoring	Ensures that the patient is given the opportunity to use the toilet on a regular basis

Functional incontinence

Impaired functional status can contribute to urinary incontinence by inhibiting effective toileting skills even in the absence of physiological bladder dysfunction (Ouslander & Schnelle 1993) and is a common outcome of stroke. The type and amount of help or intervention required to resolve or minimise problems will vary between individuals and will need detailed assessment. Nursing management of functional urinary incontinence is outlined in Table 6.3.

Voiding difficulties: retention of urine – hyporeflexia

Accumulation of urine in the bladder can result from voiding difficulties and incomplete emptying. It is important that urinary retention is identified and treated because it can lead to urinary tract infection (UTI), hydronephrosis, pyelonephritis and renal failure. The following symptoms are common indicators of retention:

- Constant wetness (dribbling) caused by urinary overflow
- Distended abdomen
- Feeling of incomplete bladder emptying
- Recurrent urine infections
- Residual volume of more than 100 ml

Nursing management of incomplete bladder emptying is outlined in Table 6.4.

Table 6.4 Incomplete bladder emptying.

Nursing intervention	Rationale
Exclude faecal impaction	The bowel may be causing obstruction to the urethra
Consider drugs that the patient is taking	Some drugs may have an effect on bladder tone resulting in retention
Intermittent catheterisation where post-micturition bladder scan shows residual of >100 ml. This may be undertaken by the patient, nurses or carer as appropriate	Less traumatic to urethra than an indwelling catheter Less risk of infection than with an indwelling catheter Preserves normal bladder function of filling/emptying Often acts as a treatment producing normal bladder emptying

Table 6.5 Acute retention (with or without overflow incontinence).

Nursing intervention	Rationale
Exclude faecal impaction	The bowel may be causing obstruction to the urethra
Consider drugs that the patient is taking	Some drugs may have an effect on bladder tone resulting in retention
Intermittent catheterisation using low-friction hydrophilic catheter 2–4 times a day or whenever bladder scan shows volume >500 ml. This may be undertaken by the patient, nurses or carer as appropriate	Less traumatic to urethra than an indwelling catheter Less risk of infection than with an indwelling catheter Preserves normal bladder function of filling/emptying Often acts as a treatment producing normal bladder emptying
In some cases (severe obstruction due to enlarged prostrate or urethral trauma, for example) intermittent catheterisation may not be appropriate. In these cases refer to medical staff/or appropriate person	An indwelling urethral catheter or suprapubic catheter may need to be inserted if intermittent catheterisation cannot be used

When urinary retention is acute, developing over a short time frame, it can also be extremely painful. By contrast, chronic retention due to incomplete emptying can develop over a longer period and may not be associated with pain. In either case the first consideration is to review the patient's medication because some drugs (e.g. sedatives, anticholinergics) may affect bladder tone. It is also wise to consider whether the patient may be constipated because this can cause urinary retention. A digital rectal examination may be necessary to confirm constipation but should only be performed by someone trained in this skill (RCN 2000). Nursing management of acute urinary retention is outlined in Table 6.5.

Assessment of incontinence and bladder dysfunction

Initial assessment on admission

All patients admitted to hospital with stroke should have a basic nursing assessment including urine testing within 24 hours of admission, to identify individuals with urinary incontinence and detect the presence or absence of UTI or other abnormality. At this early stage it is important to ensure that aids to communication are available, such as the nurse call bell being within easy reach and picture or text cards at bedside if appropriate. Body-worn pads may be used to provide confidence and comfort if required. Hand-held urinals are available for male and female use and can be used in bed or in a chair. They can help prevent episodes of incontinence due to reduced mobility. Absorbent gel used within the urinal can prevent spillage where manual dexterity is a problem.

Patients with bladder problems should have a full continence assessment within seven days of admission (see locally agreed guidelines and standards) and it should be recognised that this requires time and privacy, because it can be difficult for patients to feel comfortable talking about bladder and bowel activity. Nursing assessment of urinary incontinence is outlined in Table 6.6.

Frequency and volume charting

All patients with urinary incontinence should have frequency and volume of fluid intake and output recorded for a minimum of three to five days (preferably five to seven days) following admission or onset of urinary incontinence. This will indicate:

- The current pattern of voiding (how often and how much), and determine if particular times are more problematic than others (e.g. dry during the day but wet at night)
- Bladder capacity (indicated by the maximum volume voided)
- Maximum length of time the patient can hold on between voids during day and night
- The number, type and timing of drinks taken

All of these data can help to confirm the type of urinary incontinence and where appropriate, the optimum schedule for bladder training interventions. This information also provides a baseline from which to measure improvement once interventions have been initiated. Where possible, patients should be responsible for keeping their own chart, but cognitively impaired people and those with upper limb involvement may be unable to do so. In this case, health care staff may be able to check pads hourly to record the information. It is essential to include clear, simple instructions at the top of the chart, especially if it is to be used in a ward situation where multidisciplinary health care staff will be involved in recording.

Full assessment of incontinence

A full assessment of urinary incontinence should be undertaken as soon as possible and certainly within seven days from admission or onset of urinary incontinence. There are three basic questions to consider during the assessment:

- Is there a failure of bladder storage?
- Is there a failure of bladder emptying?
- Is the problem due to functional disability?

Table 6.6 Nursing assessment of urinary incontinence.

Intervention	Rationale
Basic nursing assessment: all patients admitted to hospital with stroke will receive a basic nursing assessment within 24 hours of admission	To identify individuals who are incontinent of urine
Urine testing: all patients will have their urine tested within 24 hours of admission	To identify presence of leucocytes, nitrites and protein which indicate a urinary tract/ kidney infection
If results are positive for leucocytes, nitrites and protein, an MSU will be sent to the laboratory for culture and analysis	To identify appropriate antibiotic treatment
If there are other abnormal findings (e.g. glucose) complete assessment as appropriate (e.g. check blood glucose) and refer to medical team	Other disease processes may be present
Frequency/volume chart: all patients with UI (including those with a urinary catheter) will have frequency and volume of fluid intake and output recorded for a minimum of 5–7 days (following admission or from onset of UI)	To assess: • current pattern of voiding • bladder capacity • maximum length of time the patient can hold on between voids during day/night • number/type of drinks taken This information will show if particular times are problematic (e.g. dry during day but wet at night); help determine best schedule for prompted voiding or bladder training
Full assessment of UI will be undertaken within 7 days (from admission or from onset of UI)	To identify problems caused by and/or contributing to UI
(see main text)	To determine the type of incontinence and plan appropriate treatment/management
Treatment options will be discussed and agreed with the patient or relevant other person	To promote patient-centred care and reduce anxiety for patient/carer
A plan of care for the treatment and management of urinary incontinence will be documented in the patient's notes within 7 days of admission, and treatment initiated	To improve or manage symptoms of UI and to promote ongoing continuity of care
Reassessment/evaluation will be undertaken and documented at regular intervals according to the plan of care	To identify improvement (and provide positive feedback to patients/carers) and/or need to change plan of care

The pattern of symptoms described and the results of the frequency and volume charting will provide a good indication of the type of continence problem and this will guide the treatment and management strategy. Many organisations have developed their own assessment forms and/or care guidelines or patient pathways but the key components of assessment are summarised in Table 6.7 and Box 6.3 and discussed below.

Transient causes of urinary incontinence, including UTI

Although urinary incontinence is common after stroke it is always important to exclude transient causes early on in the assessment process. Urinary tract

Table 6.7 Key components of assessment of urinary incontinence (NB: patients may be suffering from more than one type of UI).

History taking and recording symptoms	• Relevant medical, surgical and obstetric history • Urinary/bowel symptoms and how they differ now from normal patterns • Onset of symptoms and whether related to specific activities • Medications, both prescribed and over-the-counter medicines (OTCs) • Cognitive ability and communication skills • Functional capacity (mobility, dexterity, hearing, vision etc.) • Aids and appliances used/needed (for mobility/dexterity) • Attitude to problem, how symptoms affect daily living and desire for treatment (consider use of a simple quality of life measure/scale) • Social and environmental factors
Clinical assessment	• Urinalysis • Urinary frequency/volume chart, recorded for 3–5 days • Fluid intake • Constipation
Physical examinations and tests	• Abdominal palpation (urinary retention; constipation) • Post-voiding residual urine (bladder scan) • Skin health/soreness/rash in perianal, genital, groin area • Functional assessment of toileting skills

---

Box 6.3 Examples of questions to help determine a pattern of symptoms and the type of urinary incontinence.

Basic questions:

• Onset: when did UI start?
• Degree: mild, moderate, severe?
• Frequency: how often in 24 hours?
• Urgency: able to reach toilet in time?
• Leaking on exertion: on getting up, coughing, sneezing
• Nocturia: need to get up for toilet at night?
• Dysuria: does it hurt to pass urine? (check for UTI)

Voiding difficulties:

• Poor stream: Is the urine flow slow/intermittent?
• Hesitancy: Trouble starting urine flow?
• Straining: Straining to empty the bladder?
• Residual: Is the bladder emptying completely?

---

infection is a frequent cause of urinary incontinence and urine should be tested for leucocytes and nitrites within 24 hours of admission. Other transient causes of urinary incontinence may include chest infection and acute or chronic cough; confusion and disorientation; unfamiliar surroundings; and depression and emotional distress (particularly in frail elderly patients). A useful mnemonic for causes of transient incontinence is that of DIAPPERS – provided by Resnick (1990) (Table 6.8).

Table 6.8 Causes of transient incontinence – DIAPPERS (Resnick 1990).

Delirium	May result from drugs, surgery or an acute illness
Infection	Symptomatic urinary tract infections can cause urinary incontinence
Atrophic urethritis/vaginitis	Thinning, friable, irritated tissues that may cause or contribute to incontinence
Pharmaceuticals	Drugs include sedatives, narcotics, antimuscarinics, calcium channel blockers, loop diuretics, angiotensin-converting enzyme inhibitors, non-steroidal anti-inflammatory drugs and alpha-receptor agonists/antagonists
Psychiatric	Can cause incontinence if severe depression
Excess urine output	Can result from large fluid intake, caffeinated drinks and endocrine problems
Restricted mobility	Arthritis, pain, postprandial hypotension, poor use of assistive devices or fear of falling
Stool impaction	Can cause both urinary and faecal incontinence that can be corrected with disimpaction

Relevant history and recording symptoms

People with stroke may have a non-neurological cause for their bladder and bowel symptoms and if symptoms existed pre-stroke the underlying cause will need to be investigated. Co-morbid conditions which exacerbate urinary incontinence include asthma and chronic chest conditions, because continual strain is exerted on the urethral sphincter mechanism by coughing, which increases abdominal pressure. Other conditions that can contribute to urinary incontinence include neurological conditions such as multiple sclerosis and spinal injuries, diabetes (mellitus and insipidus), dementia, learning disabilities, and back pain. If urinary incontinence is post-stroke it is most likely to be stroke related but it should be noted that recent onset urinary incontinence can also be caused by transitory conditions (see above).

Previous gynaecological or urological interventions need to be noted and their impact on urinary incontinence considered; for example, obstetric difficulties can contribute to weak pelvic floor muscles; prostatectomy may leave a man with a post-micturition dribble, possibly due to a weak detrusor contraction or a weak sphincter.

Functional capacity and assessment of toileting skills

Physical and cognitive disabilities present before stroke or resulting from stroke often have a severe effect on toileting, which may be a crucial factor in losing or gaining continence. Particular issues to examine include ability to:

- Find and get to a toilet or to request help
- Manage clothing
- Maintain appropriate posture for micturition or bowel movement

The extent and nature of disabilities are likely to affect the implementation and success of management strategies and therefore, a functional assessment of toileting skills is important. This may include use of a standardised cognitive function test on all patients, such as the Abbreviated Mental Test Score – AMTS (Hodkinson 1972). Where there appears to be a problem, further testing will be required. The Mini Mental State Examination – MMSE (Folstein et al. 1975) is the most commonly used instrument for screening cognitive functioning. The test takes only about 10 minutes, but is limited because it will not detect subtle memory losses, particularly in well-educated patients (Tombaugh & McIntyre 1992; see Chapter 9 for further detail of cognitive functioning). Scores of 25–30 out of 30 are considered normal, 18–24 indicate mild to moderate impairment, and scores of 17 or less indicate severe impairment (Crum et al. 1993).

Medications

Many drugs can disturb bladder and bowel function. Polypharmacy can often be a contributing factor to bladder and bowel problems, particularly in elderly people with several co-morbid conditions. Some of the most common drug groups that may affect bladder function are diuretics, anticholinergics, sympathomimetics, some antihypertensives, and antiparkinsonism drugs (Rigby 2007).

Social and environmental factors

This is an important part of assessment that can be overlooked while patients are in an acute stage of care in hospital. However, it is essential that patients with continuing urinary incontinence receive continuity of care when they are discharged. The impact of incontinence on working life, sexual relationships, and family and friends may be dramatic; the workplace, home or institutional setting may contribute to difficulties in maintaining continence, particularly in older people.

Physical examinations and tests

Simple palpation of the abdomen is useful to assess for bladder distension or constipation. Observation of skin condition around the symphysis pubis and groin may reveal soreness from urinary incontinence or the wearing of pads. A rectal examination may be used to feel for a faecally loaded rectum but this is considered an invasive procedure and should not be undertaken without permission and appropriate training (RCN 2000).

Retention of urine can result from voiding difficulties. If retention is suspected the simplest and most accurate non-invasive investigation is an ultrasound scan of the bladder. Training is required before undertaking bladder scanning and interpreting results because it is sometimes hard to get a good image. Obesity can make scanning a patient difficult or impossible, and constipation or bowel gas can blur the image. If a portable bladder scan is not available the bladder can be drained via an intermittent catheter and the volume measured. However, wherever possible the non-invasive method (bladder scanner) is preferable, to promote patient dignity, comfort and safety.

There is no universal agreement on the amount of post-void residual (PVR) that requires intervention and some people retain a small amount of urine with no deleterious effects. However, where a residual is symptomatic, i.e. there is urinary incontinence, urgency, frequency or urinary tract infection, then action should be taken to address the problem. Tam et al. (2006) found an increased risk of UTI when the PVR was more than 100 ml and this appears to be a reasonable and practical cut-off value for patients that should prompt further investigation and possible intervention.

Figure 6.1 demonstrates an example of a simple assessment tool to help guide diagnosis.

Treatment strategies and care planning for urinary incontinence

Staffing levels and nursing skill mix varies greatly across stroke units. In 2008 the UK National Sentinel Audit noted, 'The striking statistic for nurse staffing in acute stroke units is that there is a median of 1.8 (IQR 1.5–2.5) qualified nurses per 10 acute stroke unit beds. This is far too low for a group of patients who should be receiving level 2 (equivalent to HDU) nursing care .... There are wide variations between units which are unlikely to be explained solely by differences in case mix' (Intercollegiate Stroke Working Party 2008b). Although many of the interventions for promoting continence in stroke patients are simple, they can be labour intensive and the success of any continence promotion programme will be dependent on availability of adequate staff with appropriate skills.

Whilst the ultimate aim of treatment intervention is to achieve continence, this may not always be realistic and it is important to determine the patient's own goals and motivation when planning a care programme. Whilst independent continence may be achievable for many, for some the goal will be dependent continence, i.e. dry with toileting assistance, medication, pads or appliances. A paradigm for continence has been described (Fonda et al. 2005), including dependent and independent continence, incontinence and contained incontinence (Figure 6.2).

In the early stages post-stroke it may help patient comfort and confidence to use a body-worn absorbent pad if they are unable to get to the toilet or hold a urinal. However, pad use should be frequently reassessed because the presence of a pad can slow down access to the toilet, bedpan or urine bottle and inhibit other treatment effects. The treatment strategy adopted will be dependent on the type of urinary incontinence problem and the patient's capacity to undertake what is required.

Scheduled voiding regimens
Scheduled toileting programmes can be beneficial in reducing episodes of incontinence for a range of patients with varying degrees of difficulty in bladder management following stroke (summarised in Table 6.9). The evidence to support these programmes has been the subject of a series of Cochrane reviews.

Patient name:_____ Hospital no._____

Date of assessment:_____   Name of assessor:_____

Date of onset of urinary incontinence:_____

1. Review the patient's drug chart for drugs that may be implicated in urinary incontinence (diuretics, sedatives etc.)

2. Urine test result (using dipstix)

Leucocytes   positive   [ ]   negative   [ ]

Nitrites   positive   [ ]   negative   [ ]

If positive send Mid Stream Urine sample to lab for culture and sensitivity

3. Does the patient have any pain/discomfort related to passing urine?

                    Yes   [ ]   No   [ ]

If yes document in notes, inform medical staff and consider analgesia

4. Does the patient have any of the following indications in the perianal/genital/groin area

Soreness   Yes   [ ]   No   [ ]

Rash   Yes   [ ]   No   [ ]

Candida   Yes   [ ]   No   [ ]

If yes document in notes and inform medical staff

5. Can the patient hold the urine in the bladder once the desire to pass urine is felt?

                    Yes   [ ]   No   [ ]

If no treat as overactive bladder

6. Is the urinary incontinence initiated or aggravated by coughing, sneezing or standing?

                    Yes   [ ]   No   [ ]

If yes treat as stress incontinence

7. Is the patient independently mobile

                    Yes   [ ]   No   [ ]

Can the patient use a hand-held urinal unaided

                    Yes   [ ]   No   [ ]

Can the patient communicate their need to pass urine

                    Yes   [ ]   No   [ ]

If no to one or more of the last three questions treat as functional incontinence

8. Is the patient able to pass urine spontaneously (bladder scan >500 ml)?

                    Yes   [ ]   No   [ ]

If no treat as acute retention

If yes   **Post-micturition bladder scan result ....ml**

        More than 100 ml [ ]   Less than 100 ml   [ ]

If more than 100 ml treat as incomplete bladder emptying

9. Patient's normal bowel pattern_____

Date of patient's last bowel movement_____

Consider whether the patient may be suffering from constipation.

NB: Patients may be suffering with more than one type of incontinence. A 48-hour frequency/volume chart will help with diagnosis.

Figure 6.1 An example of a simple assessment tool to guide diagnosis.

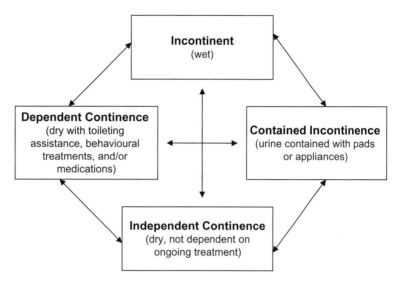

Figure 6.2 A paradigm for continence. From Fonda et al. (2005), reproduced with permission.

Table 6.9 Scheduled voiding regimes.

Regimen	Possible patients	Approach
Bladder training (Wallace et al. 2007)	Overactive bladder syndrome, bladder hyperreflexia Well-motivated, physically and mentally able to manage own toileting	Gradual increase in interval between voiding (often only 15–30 min at a time) until satisfactory pattern achieved
Habit training (Ostaszkiewicz et al. 2004a)	Some mental awareness. May also have physical disabilities	Assigned toileting schedule (e.g. 2-hourly). Schedule adjusted to fit patient's voiding pattern
Prompted voiding (Eustice et al. 2003)	Severe cognitive and physical disabilities	Prompted to void at regular intervals; only taken to toilet if response is positive
(Ostaszkiewicz et al. 2004b)	Spinal cord injury; cognitive and physical disabilities	Fixed times which may include techniques to trigger voiding

Overactive bladder and bladder training

Bladder training is the major approach to improving control over frequency, urgency and urge incontinence (Wallace et al. 2007), although its value in patients with neurogenic detrusor overactivity, rather than idiopathic detrusor instability, is less well established. The first step is to identify the minimum time the patient can hold on between voiding episodes. This can be done by completing an initial baseline frequency/volume chart. The patient then aims to empty their bladder regularly at these intervals (e.g. every hour) throughout

---

Case example 6.2 Assessment and management of Mary's stroke-related continence problems.

Mary's urinary function was assessed (see Tables 6.1, 6.6, 6.7, Box 6.3, Figure 6.1). Mary reported that she had little or no warning that she needed to pass urine and monitoring of fluid intake and output showed that she was passing urine every two hours on average.

She was treated according to the guidelines for urge incontinence and commenced on a bladder retraining programme (Table 6.9). She progressed over a period of two weeks and had managed to reach three and a half hours between trips to the toilet and was dry during the day.

The problem at night time was caused by her waking and needing to use the toilet quickly. During the day she was able to transfer independently onto a commode from her chair; however, at night when she woke she was not safe to transfer on her own from the bed and by the time nurses responded she had often already been incontinent.

She was assessed using a female urinal with a drainage bag and was able to use it well despite her problems of poor sight, hemiparesis and sensory inattention. The care plan specified that the urinal was to be put within her reach on her unaffected side (to the right).

From this point she was dry both day and night and was able to be discharged home with the female urinal.

---

the day. If the patient remains dry on this schedule the interval is then increased by a small amount (usually by 15–30 minutes); progress is monitored and intervals are then gradually increased until a two- to three-hour voiding schedule is achieved and incontinence is improved or absent. This technique requires patients to be strongly motivated and able to manage their own toileting. During hospital admission this technique can be used with patients who may not necessarily be able to manage their own toileting. Nurses can assist patients with bladder retraining despite dysphasia, functional disability and even cognitive problems. Ongoing use of frequency and volume charting helps to demonstrate progress compared with baseline. Bladder training was successfully used to overcome Mary's urge incontinence during the day (Case example 6.2).

Medications

If bladder training alone is ineffective, a combined approach of bladder training with an anticholinergic medication should be considered. Guidance (NICE 2006) recommends oxybutynin as first-line treatment but darifenacin, solifenacin, tolterodine and trospium may also be beneficial. Anticholinergics interfere with the parasympathetic innervation of the detrusor muscle by blocking the neurotransmitter acetylcholine, resulting in fewer involuntary contractions. This drug group can cause unpleasant side-effects, including dry mouth, constipation and blurred vision. Patients often find these difficult to tolerate and so adherence to medication regimens can be a problem. Prior to prescribing this type of medication a bladder scan should be carried out to ensure residual of less than 100 ml. This is because of the possible effect of exacerbating or causing urinary retention.

Lifestyle changes

Although there is no strong research evidence, clinical experience suggests that caffeine (tea, coffee, cola and chocolate) and citrus fruits can exacerbate urge incontinence and patients may benefit from excluding or reducing these from their diet.

Nocturia

Nocturia is a common problem, particularly in older people, and is character-ised by waking one or more times during sleep to void, which is preceded and followed by sleep (Van Kerrebroeck et al. 2002). Whilst poor sleep is also common for patients in hospital, nocturia is often an accompaniment to an overactive bladder (Marinkovic et al. 2004). Nocturia can be defined as the need to wake and pass urine at night (in contrast to nocturnal enuresis where urine is passed unintentionally during sleep). One episode of nocturia per night is considered within normal limits. Treatment for nocturia and nocturnal enu-resis should start with management of fluid intake, particularly avoiding drink-ing large volumes within one to two hours of going to bed. Problems may also be reduced by careful timing of diuretic use to ensure the resultant diuresis is completed during the day. Afternoon naps with elevation of the legs can help to maintain good blood supply to the kidneys during the day and avoid pooling of fluid in the legs (Eustice & Wragg 2005). Nocturia can also be helped by medication with desmopressin acetate (DDAVP), a synthetic antidiuretic hormone (ADH). ADH causes less urine to be excreted by the kidneys and as a result the volume of urine in the bladder is reduced for some hours. Desmo-pressin can be taken as an oral tablet, but should only used once in a 24-hour period (Eckford et al. 1994). Desmopressin nasal spray is no longer available for nocturnal enuresis in the UK (http://www.mhra.gov.uk). Blood pressure and blood electrolytes should be monitored regularly since desmopressin also leads to sodium retention.

Functional incontinence – scheduled voiding regimes

Management of functional incontinence should be directed towards recognition and treatment of transient conditions, for example, UTI in the first instance. Physical disability may mean that toileting cannot be managed independently and a range of aids and strategies may be helpful to facilitate mobility, toilet access (including wheelchair access), maintenance of balance and adjustment of clothing. Advice on easy to remove clothing (loose jogging trousers, Velcro fly fastening etc.) can facilitate quick and easy access to toileting but patients should be referred to a continence specialist for more detailed help with aids and appliances. Poor eyesight, confusion or cognitive impairment may mean that the person cannot identify the toilet facilities; does not recognise the need to pass urine; and/or is not aware of the appropriate places where urine (or faeces) should be passed. Practical help may include good signposting and clearly identified toilets (e.g. large pictures of a toilet on the door, colour coded doors). Training in the use of a female urinal resolved Mary's nocturia (see Case example 6.2).

A scheduled toileting programme (Table 6.9 – habit training, prompted voiding, timed voiding) can be beneficial in reducing episodes of incontinence by ensuring that there is regular opportunity to use the toilet.

- *Habit training* is a toileting schedule based on the patient's usual pattern of voiding, determined from frequency and volume charting. Intervals are selected which are shorter than the patient's normal pattern and toileting is planned prior to the time when incontinence episodes are expected. Habit training has been used primarily in institutional settings with cognitively and physically impaired adults and has also been used in home settings (Colling et al. 2003; Ostaszkiewicz et al. 2004a).
- *Prompted voiding* is a voiding regime that can be used to teach people with or without cognitive impairment to initiate their own toileting through requests for help and positive reinforcement from carers when they do so. The individual is prompted to void at regular intervals, commonly every two hours, but is only taken to the toilet if response is positive (Eustice et al. 2003).
- *Timed voiding* is a fixed voiding schedule that remains unchanged (usually every two to four hours). It is used mainly to manage incontinence associated with neuropathic conditions, to prevent incontinence by regular bladder emptying before bladder capacity is exceeded (Ostaszkiewicz et al. 2004b).

Management and containment of incontinence

Despite the many advances in the treatment of bladder problems, incontinence (or the worry of incontinence) commonly persists and some form of containment using aids or appliances may be necessary. For men there are two main options, a penile sheath or absorbent pads and pants; for women, pads and pants are the main method available. Absorbent pads have a role to play in the management of urinary incontinence and can increase patient comfort and confidence during a treatment programme. The variety of pads on the market is wide, although choice may be limited in hospital settings (Getliffe & Fader 2007). However, it is important to use the correct size and absorbency level, and to ensure that they are fitted according to the manufacturer's instructions. For patients at home or in long-stay institutional settings there may be additional choices in terms of pad design (e.g. inserts placed inside tight fitting pants; pull-ups; all-in-ones which are rather like a large nappy). Some designs are more suitable for individual patients' lifestyles than others and it is important that they are aware of the alternatives, not least because management of urinary incontinence has such a large impact on quality of life. It is also important to bear in mind, particularly where urgency and reduced mobility are involved, that pads may present an additional delay in accessing the toilet and consequently could hamper progress in regaining continence.

Treatment and management of retention

A patient with *acute retention* may not be able to pass urine at all, or may be passing small amounts. In either case the bladder needs to be drained by in/out catheterisation as soon as the problem is identified. Frequent monitoring, aimed at preventing over-distension of the bladder, should continue with regular bladder scans, and further catheterisation for volumes over 400 ml. The frequency of the bladder scanning will depend on fluid intake and output, and clinical judgement will be required to determine how often this should be done. For patients with incomplete emptying, causing *chronic retention*, an intermittent catheterisation (IC) regime will need to be implemented. If IC is impractical or unsuccessful for any reason it may be necessary to insert an indwelling catheter. However, IC is the preferred option because it is associated with fewer catheter-related problems than indwelling catheterisation.

Intermittent catheterisation (IC)

In a hospital setting IC catheterisation is normally a sterile procedure but patients with sufficient dexterity can be taught to self-catheterise when they go home and to use a clean procedure. It is also possible for carers to learn the procedure if both parties agree to this, but this arrangement should not be undertaken lightly because it can have a profound impact on relationships.

The frequency of IC varies between individuals but as a general guide IC should be carried out sufficiently often to maintain the bladder volume below 500 ml. For many patients this will mean three to four times a day or even more but for those with incomplete emptying it may be only once daily, alternate days or even less. In the hospital setting, a common regime for patients with incomplete bladder emptying post-stroke is to perform IC twice a day (first thing in the morning and last thing at night). This will help to prevent UTI and promote continence during both day and night. However, IC should only be initiated after the patient has passed urine and if the patient has more than 100 ml residual urine and is symptomatic (experiences incontinence: urgency, frequency; or UTI). Residual volumes should be monitored by regular bladder scans and if the residual falls consistently below 100 ml, IC can be stopped.

All treatments should be discussed and agreed with the patient if possible. There are some cases where IC may be inappropriate; for example, if there is urethral trauma or obstruction; unusual anatomy, making IC difficult or painful; or if patients find the procedure unacceptable. In these cases it may be necessary to insert an indwelling catheter, but the reasons should be clearly documented in the patient's notes.

Indwelling catheterisation

It is important to emphasise that *urinary incontinence alone is not an indication for an indwelling catheter*. Problems with urinary incontinence cannot be assessed and treated while a catheter is in place, and many stroke patients are catheterised unnecessarily, usually in Emergency Departments or assessment wards. Often there is no record of why they were catheterised. The UK National Sentinel Audit of Stroke (Intercollegiate Stroke Working Party 2008b) found that overall 26% of patients were catheterised during the first week, and 26% of these (6% of all stroke admissions) were catheterised because of urinary incontinence. Although indwelling catheters can provide an effective way of draining the bladder, they are rarely completely trouble free and should only be used where other options are inappropriate or unsuccessful (Getliffe & Fader 2007). Common catheter-associated complications include:

- Leakage
- Tissue trauma and/or inflammatory reactions
- Catheter-associated infection (CAUTI)
- Recurrent blockage caused by mineral deposits (more common in long-term use)

In acute care settings urinary catheters are widely recognised as a major source of health care associated infections (Harbarth et al. 2003). Where an indwelling catheter is required, the catheter is usually inserted into the bladder via the urethra but an alternative route is suprapubically via a surgical incision in the abdominal wall. A variety of catheter materials are available, and selection is dependent on whether catheterisation is expected to be short term or long term (less than or more than 14 days). Patients who go home with a catheter will need a long-term catheter (made of silicone, hydrogel-coated latex or silicone elastomer-coated latex). These materials are designed to reduce friction during insertion and removal, and to be more comfortable *in situ*. Patients will also need appropriate education and ongoing support, including written guidance on how to manage the catheter and drainage equipment, how to get new supplies, when to seek help and who to contact.

Patients who have been using a catheter on free drainage may benefit from using a catheter valve for a period of time prior to potential catheter removal. The valve allows the bladder to fill and be emptied periodically, simulating normal bladder control. At night, the valve can be connected to a drainage bag to allow free drainage. Although there is a lack of published evidence, valves are widely considered to improve bladder tone and capacity and to help prevent urinary retention.

Some patients who need to remain catheterised may be able to use a valve at home but valves are generally unsuitable for patients with poor bladder capacity, detrusor overactivity, ureteric reflux or renal impairment. Patients must be able to manipulate the valve and empty the bladder regularly to avoid overfilling (Getliffe & Fader 2007).

Bowel problems and bowel care

As with bladder problems, bowel problems following stroke can arise from neurological damage or as a consequence of impaired functional capacity. Stroke patients may experience alterations in bowel function related to brain damage and loss of cortical inhibition, resulting in function akin to reflex bowel action (as seen after spinal cord injury). Cortical awareness of the urge to defecate and anal sphincter control may both be impaired, leading to urgency and faecal incontinence (FI), both of which can have highly detrimental effects on quality of life and social interactions. Stroke patients may also be prone to overflow FI due to constipation and faecal impaction. Constipation can occur through delayed colonic transit (Ho & Goh 1995); the general effect of reduced mobility and swallowing function on gut function; and the medication prescribed to ease symptoms (Craggs & Vaizey 1999; Winge et al. 2003). Constipation has no universally accepted definition (Richmond 2003) although it is characterised by persistent difficulty or seemingly incomplete defecation (Thompson et al. 1999). Although this definition can be difficult to use in practice because of the wide variation in bowel habits in the population and in what patients (and professionals) consider to be 'normal', it is generally acknowledged that constipation is multifactorial, and can be influenced by physical, psychological, physiological, emotional and environmental factors.

Bowel assessment

All patients with bowel problems should have a thorough bowel assessment to determine the type of problem, probable cause and contributing factors and treatment plan. A careful history of 'normal bowel habits' is important because there may have been pre-stroke constipation or other bowel problems. A history of long-term laxative use may suggest unresolved constipation problems. Laxative abuse may also be a contributory factor to current problems if the bowel is no longer responsive to laxative medication. Constipation is thought to regularly affect around 10% of the general population (Higgins & Johanson 2004) and although FI is far less common in the general population than urinary incontinence, the prevalence is generally accepted to be between 2% and 5% (Kenefick 2004).

A bowel habit diary kept over seven days will provide a good indication of the pattern of bowel activity or presence of constipation. Many people find it difficult to explain the type and consistency of their stools, and scales such as the Bristol Stool Form Scale (Figure 6.3) provide a helpful guide and classification (Heaton et al. 1992). A recording of dietary intake may also be useful because lack of fibre and/or poor fluid intake can contribute to constipation. Many medications can contribute to constipation and if the medication cannot be changed, the treatment plan will need to take this into account.

Examination

Abdominal palpation may help to identify a full bowel and for some patients a digital rectal examination (DRE) may be required to assess rectal loading/ faecal impaction and the constituency of the faecal material (which may be hard or soft). Nurses should have received suitable training before performing DRE or manual evacuation of faeces (RCN 2000). Any abnormalities of the

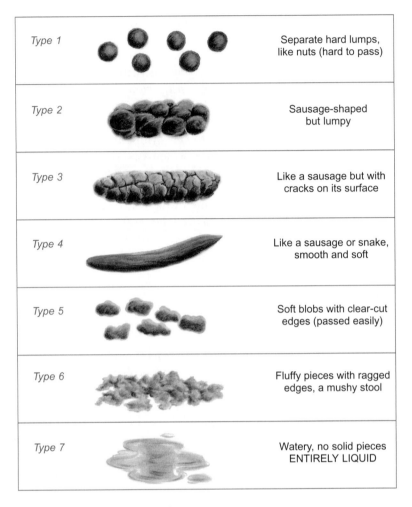

Type 1		Separate hard lumps, like nuts (hard to pass)
Type 2		Sausage-shaped but lumpy
Type 3		Like a sausage but with cracks on its surface
Type 4		Like a sausage or snake, smooth and soft
Type 5		Soft blobs with clear-cut edges (passed easily)
Type 6		Fluffy pieces with ragged edges, a mushy stool
Type 7		Watery, no solid pieces ENTIRELY LIQUID

Figure 6.3 The Bristol Stool Form Scale.

perineal or perianal area should be observed such as rectal prolapse, haemorrhoids or faecal soiling. The normal state of the rectum is empty; therefore a lack of faecal matter on DRE does not necessarily signify the absence of constipation.

Faecal impaction

Faecal impaction describes the condition when constipation has become so severe that a large mass of faeces cannot be passed. Faeces then accumulate in the rectum and may back up in the sigmoid colon and even as far as the transverse and ascending colon. Occasionally, impaction of the rectum may be due to soft poorly formed faeces as a consequence of too much osmotic laxative. In an attempt to soften hard impacted faeces the bowel produces mucus and this can result in faecal impaction with overflow, known as spurious diarrhoea.

Treatment and management of bowel problems

Constipation

The severity of constipation may vary from the slight, causing no disruption to life, to the severe, impacting upon an individual's physical, psychological and social well-being. Therefore, treatment plans will also vary from relatively simple dietary, exercise and lifestyle advice to planned evacuations employing medicines management. The aim of an individualised, planned programme is to reduce constipation without causing FI. The planned programme is tailored to the individual's needs, taking into consideration ability to toilet, carer requirement and daily plan. A predictable bowel habit means that constipation and FI can be avoided and daily activities can be organised with greater confidence (Wiesel & Bell 2004).

Correct positioning and optimum timing

Patients can be encouraged to take advantage of the morning gastro-colic reflex by having a hot drink soon after waking and sitting on the toilet around twenty minutes later. As well as encouraging mobility and appropriate dietary and fluid intake, it is helpful to ensure patients are sitting correctly on the lavatory in order to raise their intra-abdominal pressure during defecation. Some patients may need support to adopt and maintain this position. The addition of a foot-rest can help those who use raised lavatory seats or who are wheeled on a commode over the lavatory to sit in the correct position. If a patient has no sitting balance and a bed pan is the only option it is preferable for the patient to be hoisted into a sitting position above the pan rather than lying flat. It is very important to promote privacy and dignity and if the patient is able to sit on a commode they should be wheeled into a toilet on the commode rather than being left behind closed curtains which do not disguise sounds and smells.

Laxatives

Laxatives are the most commonly prescribed pharmacological intervention for the management of constipation and it is important to understand their mode of action. Treatment decisions need to take into consideration whether the constipation is acute or chronic and whether there is impaction of faeces. There are four main types of laxative:

- Bulk forming
- Stimulant
- Osmotic
- Softeners

Bulk-forming laxatives can be thought of as a method of supplementing the fibre content of the diet. They must be taken with a fluid as they work by absorbing liquid and swelling. The resultant increase in bulk increases peristalsis, in turn decreasing the transit time through the colon. The reduction in time that the faeces are in contact with the colon also reduces the amount of fluid absorbed from the faeces, thereby helping to keep the stool softer. However, these laxatives are not the best option for stroke patients who are dysphagic or who require altered consistency fluids. Brand names include ispaghula (Fybogel, Regulan, Konsyl and Isogel), methylcellulose (Celevac) and sterculia (Normacol).

Stimulant laxatives work by stimulating the nerve endings in the muscular wall of the colon. They increase peristalsis and secretion of fluid into the colon, helping to soften and lubricate the stool. They usually work within 6–12 hours and should be used short term only, when bulk-forming laxatives have proven ineffective. It should be noted that these medications can cause severe stomach cramps that can be distressing, particularly in frail elderly patients. Continued use of stimulant laxatives can reduce muscle tone in the colon and can also lead to potassium depletion and dehydration. Generic name preparations include senna, bisacodyl, docusate, glycerol and picosulphate, also combined with ispaghula (as Manevac).

Osmotic laxatives act like a sponge to draw water into the colon for easier passage of stool. They need to be taken with large quantities of water and generally produce a semi-fluid stool. Continued use can lead to electrolyte imbalances and dehydration. Products include macrogols (Movicol and Idrolax), lactulose, lactitol, magnesium hydroxide, magnesium sulphate (Epsom salts), Carbalax suppositories (also a phosphate salt), micro-enemas and phosphate enema. Movicol is a common treatment of choice in stroke patients, and is effective for both acute and chronic constipation. This medication is well tolerated by patients and does not cause stomach cramps (Corazziari et al. 2000). It is the only laxative currently recommended for faecal impaction. Lactulose has been used extensively but is no longer recommended as a first choice medication (Prodigy Guidance 2004). It contains a high concentration of non-absorbable sugars (not precluded from use by diabetic patients as the sugar does not enter the bloodstream), but takes several days to work and may cause cramps. Enemas may be useful in treating impacted faeces but should not be used as a routine treatment.

Stool softeners provide moisture to the stool and prevent dehydration. They work by coating the stool with a hydrophobic layer of oil which helps retain water in the stool, keeping it soft and lubricated. Products include arachis oil which may be given as an enema to soften and aid evacuation of impacted faeces. Only docusate sodium (also classed as a stimulant laxative) is recommended for oral use (Prodigy Guidance 2004).

Conclusion

The consequences of stroke can have a direct effect on bladder and bowel function. Problems are often complex and multifactorial, including pre-existing problems, and mobility and manual dexterity problems, which compound bladder and bowel symptoms by making toileting access difficult. Other problems such as visual disturbances, dysphagia and cognition also contribute directly to continence difficulties. Incontinence should not be accepted as an unavoidable or untreatable consequence of ageing or disease. Incontinence has a major and enduring impact on all aspects of life. All nurses should be trained in basic assessment and management of bladder and bowel problems and should know where to get further advice and help.

Bladder and bowel care requires active management – this includes a written personalised plan, taking into consideration required assistance, personal needs and goals. Close involvement and cooperation of families and carers with patients and members of the multidisciplinary team are important to ensure development, implementation and evaluation of an appropriate, individually tailored, feasible and acceptable continence or incontinence management plan.

References

Barratt, JA, 2002, Bladder and bowel problems after stroke, *Reviews in Clinical Gerontology*, vol. 12, no. 3, pp. 253–267.

Bo, K, Talseth, T, & Holme, I, 1999, Single blind, randomised controlled trial of pelvic floor exercises, electrical stimulation, vaginal cones, and no treatment in management of genuine stress incontinence in women, *British Medical Journal*, vol. 318, no. 7182, pp. 487–493.

Bo, K, Kvarstein, B, & Nygaard, I, 2005, Lower urinary tract symptoms and pelvic floor muscle exercise adherence after 15 years, *Obstetrics and Gynecology*, vol. 105, no. 5 Pt 1, pp. 999–1005.

Brittain, KR, 1998, Urinary symptoms and depression in stroke survivors, *Age and Ageing*, vol. 27 Suppl 1, p. 72.

Brittain, KR, Peet, SM, Potter, JF, & Castleden, CM, 1999, Prevalence and management of urinary incontinence in stroke long-term placement survivors, *Age and Ageing*, vol. 28, no. 6, pp. 509–511.

Brown, JS, Vittinghoff, E, Wyman, JF, Stone, KL, Nevitt, MC et al., 2000, Urinary incontinence: does it increase risk for falls and fractures? Study of Osteoporotic Fractures Research Group, *Journal of the American Geriatrics Society*, vol. 48, no. 7, pp. 721–725.

Bryant, C, Dowell, C, & Fairbrother, G, 2002, Caffeine reduction education to improve urinary symptoms, *British Journal of Nursing*, vol. 11, pp. 560–565.

Colling, J, Owen, TR, McCreedy, M, & Newman, D, 2003, The effects of a continence program on frail community-dwelling elderly persons, *Urologic Nursing*, vol. 23, no. 2, pp. 117–131.

Corazziari, E, Badiali, D, Bazzocchi, G, Bassotti, G, Roselli, P et al., 2000, Long term efficacy, safety, and tolerability of low daily doses of isosmotic polyethylene glycol electrolyte balanced solution (PMF-100) in the treatment of functional chronic constipation, *Gut*, vol. 46, no. 4, pp. 522–526.

Craggs, M, & Vaizey, C, 1999, Neurophysiology of the bladder and bowel, in *Neurology of Bladder, Bowel and Sexual Dysfunction*, CJ Fowler, ed., Butterworth-Heinemann, Oxford.

Crum, RM, Anthony, JC, Bassett, SS, & Folstein, MF, 1993, Population-based norms for the Mini-Mental State Examination by age and educational level, *Journal of the American Medical Association*, vol. 269, no. 18, pp. 2386–2391.

Department of Health, 2000, *Good practice in continence services*, Department of Health, London.

Eckford, SD, Swami, KS, Jackson, SR, & Abrams, PH, 1994, Desmopressin in the treatment of nocturia and enuresis in patients with multiple sclerosis, *British Journal of Urology*, vol. 74, no. 6, pp. 733–735.

Eustice, S, & Wragg, A, 2005, Nocturia and older people, *Nursing Times*, vol. 101, no. 29, pp. 46–48.

Eustice, S, Roe, B, & Paterson, J, 2003, *Prompted voiding for the management of urinary incontinence in adults (Cochrane review)*, Oxford. The Cochrane Library 3, Art: CD002113.

Folstein, MF, Folstein, SE, & McHugh, PR, 1975, 'Mini-mental state': A practical method for grading the cognitive state of patients for the clinician, *Journal of Psychiatric Research*, vol. 12, no. 3, pp. 189–198.

Fonda, D, DuBeau, CE, Harari, D, Ouslander, JG, Palmer, M, & Roe, B, 2005, Incontinence in the frail elderly, in *Incontinence: 3rd International Consultation on Incontinence*, P Abrams et al., eds., Health Publications Ltd, pp. 1163–1239.

Gelber, DA, Good, DC, Laven, LJ, & Verhulst, SJ, 1993, Causes of urinary incontinence after acute hemispheric stroke, *Stroke*, vol. 24, no. 3, pp. 378–382.

Getliffe, KA, & Fader, M, 2007, Catheters and containment products for continence care, in *Promoting Continence: A Clinical and Research Resource*, 3rd edn, K Getliffe & M Dolman, eds., Elsevier Science, Edinburgh.

Harari, D, Coshall, C, Rudd, AG, & Wolfe, CD, 2003, New-onset fecal incontinence after stroke: prevalence, natural history, risk factors, and impact, *Stroke*, vol. 34, no. 1, pp. 144–150.

Harari, D, Norton, C, Lockwood, L, & Swift, C, 2004, Treatment of constipation and fecal incontinence in stroke patients: randomized controlled trial, *Stroke*, vol. 35, no. 11, pp. 2549–2555.

Harbarth, S, Sax, H, & Gastmeier, P, 2003, The preventable proportion of nosocomial infections: an overview of published reports, *Journal of Hospital Infection*, vol. 54, no. 4, pp. 258–266.

Heaton, KW, Radvan, J, Cripps, H, Mountford, RA, Braddon, FE et al., 1992, Defecation frequency and timing, and stool form in the general population: a prospective study, *Gut*, vol. 33, no. 6, pp. 818–824.

Higgins, PD, & Johanson, JF, 2004, Epidemiology of constipation in North America: a systematic review, *American Journal of Gastroenterology*, vol. 99, no. 4, pp. 750–759.

Ho, YH, & Goh, HS, 1995, Anorectal physiological parameters in chronic constipation of unknown aetiology (primary) and of cerebrovascular accidents – a preliminary report, *Annals of the Academy of Medicine, Singapore*, vol. 24, no. 3, pp. 376–378.

Hodkinson, HM, 1972, Evaluation of a mental test score for assessment of mental impairment in the elderly, *Age and Ageing*, vol. 1, no. 4, pp. 233–238.

Intercollegiate Stroke Working Party, 2008a, *National Clinical Guidelines for Stroke*, 3rd edn, Royal College of Physicians, London.

Intercollegiate Stroke Working Party, 2008b, *National Sentinel Audit for Stoke 2008. National and Local Results for the Process of Stroke Care Audit 2008*, Royal College of Physicians, London.

Kenefick, N, 2004, The epidemiology of faecal incontinence, in *Bowel Continence Nursing*, C. Norton & S. Chelvanayagam, eds., Beaconsfield, Bucks, UK.

Khan, Z, Starer, P, Yang, WC, & Bhola, A, 1990, Analysis of voiding disorders in patients with cerebrovascular accidents, *Urology*, vol. 35, no. 3, pp. 265–270.

Marinkovic, SP, Gillen, LM, & Stanton, SL, 2004, Managing nocturia, *British Medical Journal*, vol. 328, no. 7447, pp. 1063–1066.

National Institute for Health and Clinical Effectiveness (NICE), 2006, *Urinary incontinence: the management of urinary incontinence in women*, Royal College of Obstetricians and Gynaecologists Press, London.

Ostaszkiewicz, J, Johnston, L, & Roe, B, 2004a, *Habit retraining for the management of urinary incontinence in adults*, Issue 2: CD002801, Oxford.

Ostaszkiewicz, J, Johnston, L, & Roe, B, 2004b, *Timed voiding for the management of urinary incontinence in adults*, Issue 1: CD002802, Oxford.

Ouslander, JG, & Schnelle, JF, 1993 Assessment, treatment and management of urinary incontinence in the nursing home, in *Improving care in the nursing home; compre-*

hensive reviews of clinical research, LZ Rubenstein & D Wieland, eds., Sage, Newbury Park, pp. 131–159.

Patel, M, Coshall, C, Rudd, AG, & Wolfe, CD, 2001, Natural history and effects on 2-year outcomes of urinary incontinence after stroke, *Stroke*, vol. 32, no. 1, pp. 122–127.

Perry, S, Shaw, C, Assassa, P, Dallosso, H, Williams, K et al., 2000, An epidemiological study to establish the prevalence of urinary symptoms and felt need in the community: the Leicestershire MRC Incontinence Study. Leicestershire MRC Incontinence Study Team, *Journal of Public Health Medicine*, vol. 22, no. 3, pp. 427–434.

Prodigy Guidance, 2004, *Practical Support for Clinical Governance – Constipation.*

RCN, 2000, *Digital Rectal Examination and Manual Removal of Faeces: Guidance for Nurses*, Royal College of Nursing, London.

Resnick, NM, 1990, Initial evaluation of the incontinent patient, *Journal of the American Geriatrics Society*, vol. 38, no. 3, pp. 311–316.

Richmond, J, 2003, Prevention of constipation through risk management, *Nursing Standard*, vol. 17, no. 16, pp. 39–46.

Rigby, D, 2007, Medication for continence, in *Promoting Continence: A Clinical and Research Resource*, 3rd edn, K Getliffe & M Dolman, eds., Elsevier Science, Edinburgh.

Robain, G, Chennevelle, JM, Petit, F, & Piera, JB, 2002, Incidence of constipation after recent vascular hemiplegia: a prospective cohort of 152 patients, *Revue neurologique (Paris)*, vol. 158, no. 5 Pt 1, pp. 589–592.

Royal College of Physicians, 2002, *National Sentinel Audit of Stroke*, Royal College of Physicians, London.

Tam, CK, Wong, KK, & Yip, WM, 2006, Prevalence of incomplete bladder emptying among elderly in convalescence wards: a pilot study, *Asian Journal of Gerontology and Geriatrics*, vol. 1, no. 2, pp. 66–71.

Thomas, LH, Barrett, J, Cross, S, French, B, Leathley, M, Sutton, C, & Watkins, C, 2005, *Prevention and treatment of urinary incontinence after stroke in adults*, Cochrane Database of Systematic Reviews, Oxford, CD004462.

Thompson, WG, Longstreth, GF, Drossman, DA, Heaton, KW, Irvine, EJ et al., 1999, Functional bowel disorders and functional abdominal pain, *Gut*, vol. 45 Suppl 2, pp. II43–II47.

Tombaugh, TN, & McIntyre, NJ, 1992, The Mini-Mental State Examination: a comprehensive review, *Journal of the American Geriatrics Society*, vol. 40, no. 9, pp. 922–935.

Van Kerrebroeck, P, Abrams, P, Chaikin, D, Donovan, J, Fonda, D et al., 2002, The standardisation of terminology in nocturia: report from the Standardisation Subcommittee of the International Continence Society, *Neurourology and Urodynamics*, vol. 21, no. 2, pp. 179–183.

Wallace, SA, Roe, B, Williams, K, & Palmer, M, 2007, *Bladder training for urinary incontinence in adults*, Issue 2: CD001308, Oxford.

Wiesel, P, & Bell, S, 2004, bowel dysfunction: assessment and management in the neurological patient, in *Bowel Continence Nursing*, C Norton & S Chelvanayagam, eds., Beaconsfield Publishers Ltd, UK, pp. 181–203.

Winge, K, Rasmussen, D, & Werdelin, LM, 2003, Constipation in neurological diseases, *Journal of Neurology, Neurosurgery and Psychiatry*, vol. 74, no. 1, pp. 13–19.

Wyndaele, JJ, Castro, D, Madersbacher, H, Chartier-Kastler, E, Igawa, Y et al., 2005, *Neurologic urinary and faecal incontinence, in Incontinence*, vol. 2, P. Abrams et al., eds., Health Publications Ltd, Paris.

Yoshimura, K, Terada, N, Matsui, Y, Terai, A, Kinukawa, N et al., 2004, Prevalence of and risk factors for nocturia: analysis of a health screening program, *International Journal of Urology*, vol. 11, no. 5, pp. 282–287.

Chapter 7

Management of physical impairments post-stroke

Cherry Kilbride and Rosie Kneafsey

Key points

- Carrying out purposeful therapeutic handling within all activities of daily living can help to drive positive neuroplastic changes in the brain to promote recovery of mobility.
- Take patients out of their preferred postures and patterns of movement and introduce variety throughout the 24-hour period to minimise risk of secondary complications, e.g. contractures and development of abnormal muscle tone.
- Patients showing both low and high tone are at risk of adaptive muscle shortening and need active intervention to minimise changes.
- Prevention remains the best approach for contractures. Specific muscle strengthening and aerobic exercise are important in the restoration of movement post-stroke.
- Opportunities for practice of task-specific activities should be encouraged in formal therapy sessions and throughout the day by all members of the team and family.

I'm back to work now, and I work in London. You can imagine, it's all a fast pace, and I used to get the bus to the station or walk to the station, jump on the train, get off the train, walk, the majority of the time I used to walk, from London Bridge to Tower Bridge which is a good 20 minute walk. Then walk back, its nice in the summer doing that. No way; no chance of doing that now. I get the train, which is not the easiest thing to get on when they're packed; because I have to have a seat, so I leave really early. I get into work at half past eight so I can leave at 4.30, to get a chance of getting a seat. I don't walk any more. I did try to get the Tube, which was a nightmare, because there was a lot of stairs, which I never really realised before, so I ended up getting a taxi, which is not cheap. At the moment I'm very dependent where before I was very independent. I had my own flat, my own car; I was doing what I wanted to do when I wanted to do it. Now I have to more depend on other people; I have to go a slower pace, which in some respects is nice, but London is a very fast pace, you cannot afford to be slow. So I think I probably will have to end up changing my job. Something like this, it makes you take stock of your life.

(Jodie, 31-year-old woman, South London, six months post-stroke)

Introduction

This chapter focuses on the early management of physical impairments post-stroke and describes rehabilitation interventions to promote activity and participation. The term *mobility* is defined using the International Classification of Functioning, Disability and Health (ICF) (World Health Organisation 2001) and incorporates:

- Changing and maintaining body position
- Carrying, moving and handling objects
- Walking and moving

Losing the ability to purposefully and easily move after a stroke impinges on the individual's capacity to remain physically independent in daily activities and invariably affects quality of life. Being in control of movement can be a source of autonomy, pride and dignity; hence mobility problems can have significant psychological and emotional effects. Mobility rehabilitation is a key aspect of the overall treatment for stroke and one in which the nurse has a central role.

This chapter begins by briefly reviewing muscle tone and the role of sensation in the production of movement as a preface to sections covering moving and handling (including risk assessment), therapeutic positioning and seating, early mobilisation, falls prevention, restoration and re-education of movement, specific rehabilitation techniques and current developments in therapy. The ongoing involvement and education of the patient, family and carers is implicit in all interventions described.

Movement

Muscle tone

The term *muscle tone* describes the resistance felt when passively moving a limb. It consists of neural and non-neural components: the active muscle tension arising from the stretch reflex contraction and the passive stiffness of the joint plus inherent viscoelastic properties of surrounding connective tissue (Britton 2004). Muscle tone is integral to all posture and movement. Whilst postural tone will vary between individuals, it must be high enough for movement to take place against the force of gravity, yet not so high that it prevents an individual making tonal adaptations in response to the constantly changing demands of the environment (Edwards 2002). Moreover, the distribution of tone within the body alters as different postures are adopted: in standing, more extensor activity is seen (Brown 1994; Markham 1987); lying supine is a position of predominant extension; and supported sitting favours flexion (Edwards 2002). The clinical relevance of this for patients following stroke will be discussed in the therapeutic positioning and seating section.

Following a stroke, changes can occur in muscle tone and these are commonly divided into:

- *Positive features*, e.g. spasticity, clonus, increased tendon reflexes extensor/flexor spasms, associated reactions
- *Negative features*, e.g. muscle weakness, fatigue, loss of dexterity/coordination
- *Adaptive features*, e.g. changes in mechanical and functional properties of muscle and connective tissue (Ada & Canning 2005; Carr & Shepherd 2003; Fitzgerald & Stokes 2004)

In the clinical setting, positive features may also be referred to as high or increased tone and negative features as low or decreased tone. Hypertonia, which is defined as 'a greater than normal resistance when moving a limb passively through range' (Boyd & Ada 2001), is linked to the presence of adaptive features, i.e. contractures. How abnormalities in muscle tone contribute to movement loss and altered function is not well understood and the detrimental effect attributed to spasticity and other positive features on decreased function post-stroke may have been overestimated. The impact of negative changes, particularly weakness, and adaptive features is now more widely recognised (Ada & Canning 2005; Carr & Shepherd 2003). Indeed, spasticity can help function in some people, i.e. increased tone in lower limbs can effectively be utilised when weakness would otherwise impede transfers or walking (Barnes 2001; Thompson et al. 2005; Ward 2002).

The role of sensation in movement

> **Case example 7.1** Jodie, the 31-year-old woman quoted at the chapter start.
>
> 'A lot of people when they have strokes, can't feel anything in the side that's affected. I could feel everything, I just couldn't move it. But I could feel everything. And when I was laying there the first day, and they was touching me, I could feel everything. It was so frustrating 'cos I couldn't move.'

The execution of functional mobility involves the integration of sensory feedback from receptors in the periphery with plans or programmes of movement stored in the central nervous system (Rothwell 2004). Following a stroke, sensory functions may be impaired, which can affect a person's ability to move (see Case example 7.1). The extent of impairment is dependent on the site and size of the lesion; for example, sensory receptors in muscles and tendons provide information about body and limb position and the information is conveyed via the dorsal column tract to be processed in the somatosensory area located in the post-central gyrus of the parietal lobe of the brain (Lindsay & Bone 2004; Marieb & Hoehn 2007). Thus following a middle cerebral artery infarct, resultant cell death can alter the brain's ability to accurately process and interpret sensory information sent from the body to the brain. This results in a loss of or diminished ability to move. Movement without sensation is possible but it lacks accuracy and exhibits increasing clumsiness in the absence of sensory feedback to update the instructions coming from the brain (Rothwell 2004). It is therefore important to be aware of the effect of sensory involvement in the rehabilitation of mobility.

Moving and handling people with stroke

As described in Chapter 2, the neuroplastic properties of the brain are influenced by sensory inputs received and motor outputs requested (Lawes 2004). Therapeutic interactions with patients post-stroke therefore have the potential to drive positive neuroplastic change for recovery of mobility. It follows that it is essential that the moving and handling of people who have experienced stroke is not treated as a routine or ritualistic task. New nurses are often socialised into a culture that is preoccupied with speed; *'getting through the work'* can become the norm of behaviour and it is well documented that patients are frequently mishandled, putting both patient and nurse at risk (Hignett 2005; Jootun & MacInnes 2005). Whilst lack of suitable moving and handling equipment may constrain nurses' practice, it is also possible that nurses do not always employ the right solving and assessment skills in relation to patient handling, leading to missed opportunities for rehabilitation and potentially the continued use of outdated patient handling approaches.

Patient handling carried out by nurses should be viewed as an important therapeutic component of rehabilitation, not simply a means of getting the individual from A to B. Each time nursing help is given with positioning, transfers or walking, it should be viewed as an opportunity to coach the patient and build aspects of treatment, initiated during formal therapy sessions, into nursing care. In this way, the nurses' 'therapy integration' and 'therapy carry on' roles (Long et al. 2002) can maximise the value of time-limited therapist–client interactions; a recent study showed patients in a stroke unit were only with therapists 5.2% of the observed day (8 am to 5 pm) (Bernhardt et al. 2007). For example, helping a patient to get to the toilet on a regular basis can form a core component of daily therapy. It is essential that continence issues are effectively managed but this can also be part of effective rehabilitation for movement or mobility. Benefits can work both ways, with regular movement helping to promote normal bowel habits.

It is generally agreed that helping patients to regain the ability to move is more successful if a consistent approach to moving and handling is adopted. This may include teaching patients new ways to move or adapt to their reduced abilities with an emphasis on maximising activities and participation. Moving and handling of rehabilitation patients has been identified as an area of specialist nursing, requiring skills above and beyond those possessed by the 'average' nurse (Gibbon 1993; Waters 1991; Waters & Luker 1996). Moreover, this advanced practical skill must also be combined with an ability to connect and communicate effectively with patients, along with the aptitude to assess the patient's progress towards rehabilitation goals (Kneafsey 2007). Nonetheless it typically remains the ward-based qualified nurse and nursing support worker that help patients with movement and mobility on a day-to-day basis (Brown-Wilson 2002; St Pierre 1998). However, since the publication of the Manual Handling Operations Regulations (MHOR) (Health and Safety Executive 1992), there has been ongoing uncertainty about how the requirements of the MHOR in the UK and processes of mobility rehabilitation may be reconciled. This is explored next.

Rehabilitation handling and the Manual Handling Operations Regulations

In the UK the MHOR legally require employers to undertake specific assessments of all manual handling operations such as patient handling, to identify potential risks of injury to patients or staff. Where risks are identified, actions must be taken to eliminate these dangers or reduce them as far as is practical (Health and Safety Executive 1992). As a result, many hospitals and community services have introduced 'no-lifting policies' to which staff are expected to adhere. However, many practitioners believe that these policies have misinterpreted the legislation and place unnecessary constraints on rehabilitation practice and patient care by demanding that all manual handling of patients that incurs risk must be eliminated (Health and Safety Executive 1992). Within the literature, there has been some exploration of how patient handling in rehabilitation settings has been managed. For example, the Chartered Society of Physiotherapy (2008) has recently published comprehensive guidance on manual handling in physiotherapy and the draft *Framework for Rehabilitation Handling* (Royal College of Nursing Rehabilitation and Intermediate Care Nurses' Forum 2002) provides nurses with guidance on rehabilitative patient handling, which complies with the 1992 UK Manual Handling Operations Regulations. The framework itself identifies three components of rehabilitation moving and handling (care, treatment and rehabilitation handling), recognising that at different times and circumstances, any of these approaches to movement might be required. Whilst the Framework is a valuable resource, it is unclear what specific nursing activities, skills and knowledge might relate to each type of handling or how nurse, physiotherapist (PT) and occupational therapist (OT) contributions overlap and blur. A useful document has also been published by the Royal College of Nursing Rehabilitation and Intermediate Care Nurses' Forum (2002), which seeks to foster evidence-based, safe, rehabilitation patient handling. It argues that assistive devices can and should be used to promote rehabilitation despite nurses' concerns that over-use of devices could affect patients' functional independence (Canadian Taskforce on Safe Patient Handling 2005; Mutch 2004).

Risk assessments

Completion of effective risk assessments is a core component of successful patient handling and in preventing accidents. Johnson (2005) provides a comprehensive overview of this process and identifies that the first step in a risk assessment is the ability to 'notice' and recognise risk factors related to patient handling. The acronym TILE is often used as a framework to assist in the comprehensive risk assessment of load handling activities and refers to an assessment of the *Task*, *Individual* capability, *Load* and *Environment*. It is vital that appropriate action is then taken, using the risk assessment to minimise the effect of identified risks. It may be that the initial risk assessment identifies that a more detailed analysis of the task is needed to help identify the best course of action. The Chartered Society of Physiotherapy (2008) and Johnson (2005) provide summaries of a number of risk assessment tools and discuss strategies for risk reduction and the ongoing monitoring of risk. Inherent within this is that practitioners have to recognise their own individual level of skill and any limitations.

Whilst all members of the multidisciplinary team (MDT) may contribute to rehabilitation handling, therapists may be more adept at rehabilitation techniques and patient assessment than those who have learnt specialist skills through observation and practical experience alone. It may be that during therapy sessions a patient practises walking and transfers with only manual assistance from a qualified physiotherapist. On the ward setting, however, it may initially be safer for both patient and nurse for the patient to be assisted using standing aids or hoists. Patients may initially need to be helped in and out of bed and with movement from place to place using a mechanical device, until a point is reached when the risk to handler and patient has reduced. As the patient progresses, however, transfers may be accomplished with only manual support from nursing staff similar to that practised by the patient with the physiotherapist in the gym, and other mobilisation activities described in this chapter can commence. Additional guidance on therapeutic handling is given in later sections of the chapter.

Therapeutic positioning and seating in the acute phase

Positioning is one of the cornerstones of stroke rehabilitation. The underlying premise is that provision of external support enables the patient to cope better with effects of gravity and to maintain postural alignment without using undue muscular activity (Pope 2006).

Therapeutic positioning whether in bed or sitting out in a chair is essential to:

- Limit sustained postures
- Maximise function
- Maintain skin integrity and prevent pressure sores
- Maintain soft-tissue length and prevent contractures

- Reduce noxious stimuli and decrease discomfort
- Promote socialisation (Thornton & Kilbride 2004)

Research demonstrates that patients on stroke units are more likely to be better positioned than patients on conventional wards, have more therapeutic contact with staff, spend less time lying down and more time sitting out of bed and standing (Lincoln et al. 1996). This arguably suggests an understanding of the need for therapeutic positioning by specialist stroke nurses. However, the relationship between positioning and outcome has yet to be confirmed and evidence remains largely based on clinical experience (Chatterton et al. 2001; Rowat 2001). A postal survey of 674 UK physiotherapists undertaken to explore patient positioning post-stroke found three main reasons underpinning choice of position: modulation (alteration) of muscle tone, prevention of damage to affected limbs and support to body segments (Chatterton et al. 2001). Sitting in an armchair, side lying on the non-hemiplegic and hemiplegic side were cited as the most frequently used positions. Findings from another study in which 150 nurses and 25 therapists in a Scottish teaching hospital were surveyed reported sitting out in a chair as the preferred position for conscious patients following stroke, and side lying on the non-hemiplegic side for those still unconscious. There was less agreement about the use of supine, high side lying and lying on the hemiplegic side (Rowat 2001). Therefore, there is no one correct position. Varying the patient's posture during the day and night, using T-rolls, pillows and wedges to achieve this in supine, prone, side lying and sitting out, has been advocated (Thornton & Kilbride 2004). Thus changing and rotating positions rather than sustaining any one posture is key.

A well-positioned patient demonstrates good biomechanical alignment of different parts of the body in relation to each other, which ultimately affects the efficiency of movement (Shumway-Cook & Woollacott 2007). Altered body alignment may be indicative of weakness or changes in muscle tone and may adversely affect the subsequent recruitment of muscle activity (Bennett & Karnes 1998; Kilbride & McDonnell 2000). For example, a patient sitting in a flexed position and weight bearing through their sacrum, rather than ischium, thighs and feet, is not only at increased risk of pressure sores, but must use excessive muscle activity elsewhere, for example, head, upper limbs, trunk or hips to remain upright. As a result, patients will use their arms to help 'fix' themselves in sitting. Poorly designed chairs, soft mattresses and lack of specialist equipment can present challenges to therapeutic positioning and may require creative use of foot blocks, pillows or folded blankets to help provide external support and attain 90 degrees° at hips, knees and ankles. Aspects of positioning identified by physiotherapists as being the most important are:

- Head alignment (neutral, midline and supported on pillow)
- Scapular protraction
- Equal weight bearing between right and left buttocks
- Hip and trunk alignment, i.e. hips are 90 degrees
- Support of distal components i.e. hands and feet (Chatterton et al. 2001)

Observational analysis of the influence of altered tone on patient postures in common positions can be made by viewing the relative alignment of the head, trunk, shoulder and pelvic girdles and associated limbs. The inter-relationship of these body parts can affect the overall influence of extension or flexion on a specified position, with this assumption based on the neurophysiological rationale that putting patients in certain positions can alter the distribution of muscle tone (Bobath 1990; Shumway-Cook & Woollacott 2007). Photographs (taken with informed consent) of the patient are increasingly seen in the clinical setting as a way of individualising information for specific patient needs, and standard positioning charts can also be individualised by drawing on additional pillows to help postural alignment.

Positioning in the early stages of acute stroke is also carried out as part of respiratory care for optimal oxygen saturation. In a systematic review of four studies including a total of 183 stroke patients, there was strong evidence that body position did not affect oxygen saturation in acute stroke patients without relevant (respiratory) co-morbidities, with limited evidence that sitting in a chair had a beneficial effect and lying positions had a deleterious effect on oxygen saturation in those patients with respiratory co-morbidities (Tyson & Nightingale 2004). Refer to Chapter 4 for more detail of positioning in the hyperacute stage.

In addition, the orientation and position of the patient within their immediate surroundings can provide valuable stimulation when visual and perceptual problems are evident. However, in the early stages it may be necessary with a patient who has marked visual and perceptual deficits, to address them in midline, i.e. straight on and within their visual field. As remediation occurs, stimulation can be provided from the affected side (Baer & Durward 2004). Special consideration is required for the small number of patients who present with the *contraversive pushing syndrome* where they lean towards the hemiplegic side, strongly resisting any attempts to passively correct posture towards or across midline as they already perceive themselves to be upright (Karnath et al. 2000; Karnath & Broetz 2003). Karnath and Broetz (2003) describe an intervention plan to address this impairment that includes helping the patient to recognise the altered perception of erect body position and the use of visual aids, i.e. the upright of a door frame, to check their own verticality.

In summary, therapeutic positioning and seating can maximise function, limit secondary complications, enhance perceptual awareness, communication, swallow function and social interaction and is therefore an essential part of rehabilitation (Clark et al. 2004; Pope 2006). Readers are referred to Pope (2006) for a comprehensive review of posture and seating.

Promoting early mobilisation

National Clinical Guidelines for Stroke recommend that people with acute stroke should be mobilised as soon as their clinical condition permits (Pope 2006). The promotion of early mobility is a key aspect in acute stroke care and can help to reduce common physiological complications associated with immobility, in particular: chest infections, pressure sores, deep vein thrombosis, constipation and urinary tract infections. Other problems associated with immobility include hypoalbuminaemia, which can lead to widespread oedema. Even short periods of immobility will lead to muscle atrophy, loss of subcutaneous fat, contractures, decreased range of movement and activity intolerance. Respiratory difficulties are also common when mobility is limited and the patient may become dyspnoeic with chest crackles and wheezes and an increased respiratory rate. Some patients may also experience cardiovascular disruption associated with immobility including orthostatic hypotension, increased heart rate and peripheral oedema (Adams et al. 2003; Bernhardt et al. 2008; Indredavik et al. 1999). Complications that may be a consequence of, or related to, immobility are detailed in Table 7.1.

To prevent such complications from occurring, it is important that patients begin to move and mobilise early after their initial stroke. Little is known about what constitutes early mobilisation. There is little agreement about what the term means, and little guidance on the required intensity, duration, frequency, and the risks and benefits of early mobilisation (Arias & Smith 2007). It is likely that local policies vary and that practice will evolve as the evidence base for stroke care develops. At the present time, a useful description of 'early mobilisation' is given by (Indredavik et al. 1999), and cited by (Arias & Smith 2007) and includes:

Table 7.1 Complications that may be related to immobility. Reproduced with permission from the STEP team, Royal Free NHS Trust, Hampstead, London.

System	Abnormal findings
Metabolic	Slowed wound healing Muscle atrophy Decreased amount of subcutaneous fat Stasis oedema
Respiratory	Decreased chest wall and diaphragmatic movement Limited alveolar ventilation, may result in dyspnoea Noisy breathing (wheeze, crackles, crepitation), increased respiratory rate
Cardiovascular	Orthostatic hypotension Deconditioning, leading to increased heart rate Weak peripheral pulses, cold extremities Peripheral oedema
Musculoskeletal	DVT: erythema, increased diameter in calf or thigh; discomfort/pain Decreased range of movement Joint contracture Loss of activity tolerance Muscle atrophy
Skin	Damage to skin integrity; pressure ulcer development
Elimination	Difficulty with micturition; scanty, cloudy or concentrated urine Decreased frequency of bowel movements; constipation Abdominal distension Decreased or increased bowel sounds

- Sitting out of bed within 24 hours
- Mobilisation is independent of whether the stroke is ischaemic or haemor-rhagic type
- Patient is assessed by a physiotherapist between 8 and 24 hours of the stroke occurring
- Training in transfers, sitting and walking begins at between 24 and 72 hours
- Mobilisation undertaken by nurses trained by a dedicated stroke unit phys-iotherapist or a neurological physiotherapist

Results from an ongoing phase III randomised controlled trial 'AVERT', *A Very Early Rehabilitation Trial*, which is investigating very early mobilisation post-stroke, i.e. sitting out of bed, standing and walking within 24 hours and no later than 48 hours, will inform this increasingly important clinical area of stroke care (Bernhardt et al. 2008).

For some nurses working in acute settings, encouraging patients to walk and change position may be a low priority compared with the demands of meeting patients' other needs. Results from a recent study showed that only 27% of 118 patients actually 'walked' whilst an inpatient and those that did walk, only did so for a mean time of 5.5 minutes. It is therefore of utmost importance that nurses, as the MDT members who are consistently present, promote this area of rehabilitation (Callen et al. 2004).

Once the decision has been taken for the patient to start rehabilitation a number of parameters should be considered to assess how well the patient is tolerating the intervention. Stiller & Phillips (2003) provide a useful overview of the safety aspects associated with mobilising acutely ill patients. For example, acute care contraindications to mobilising patients include acute infections, unstable angina, acute pulmonary embolus or infarction. Patients with a diag-nosed DVT in the lower leg will be prescribed anticoagulation. Mobilisation may be delayed until therapeutic anticoagulation has been achieved or not commenced if it is known that the patient has been over-coagulated because this may increase the risk of bleeding. If it becomes apparent that a patient's level of oxygenation is deteriorating during mobilisation, the intensity of the activity should be reduced or even ceased initially and oxygen saturation levels measured. Further guidance on oxygen saturation levels and the need for sup-plementary oxygen can be found in the British Thorax Society National Guide-lines (O'Driscoll et al. 2008). Patients with type 1 diabetes may be vulnerable to unstable blood glucose levels after a stroke and their blood glucose levels should be monitored for hyper- or hypoglycaemia in relation to mobilisation activities because these have the potential to reduce glycaemic control. Other patients may have developed hyperglycaemia in response to the stroke and the same precautions must be taken. As well as the parameters discussed, the patient should be monitored for any subjective signs of distress during mobili-sation activities. These might include signs of pain or discomfort, level of perceived exertion, shortness of breath, fatigue, anxiety, skin colour, sweatiness and clamminess. Evidence such as this will assist in ascertaining how well the patient is coping with the activity.

When the MDT has agreed a patient is medically stable, a programme of sitting–standing for antigravity extensor muscle activity and maintenance of soft tissue length can be commenced (Bernhardt et al. 2008; Carr & Shepherd 1998; Indredavik et al. 1999), alongside other aspects of mobility rehabilitation. In addition, patients must have sufficient energy to actively participate in mobility rehabilitation; nutrition and hydration needs must be met (see Chapter 5) and healthy sleep and rest patterns similarly promoted. Likewise stroke patients suffering from poorly treated pain may become reluctant to move and actively engage in rehabilitation.

Sitting out of bed

While patients should be sat out of bed within 24 hours (Bernhardt et al. 2008; Indredavik et al. 1999), it is important initially not to sit the patient out for too long because it can become very tiring and may lead to unwanted excessive muscle activity to achieve the goal, for example overuse of the head to try to remain upright. Depending on the assessment of individual needs, the patient may be sat out for approximately 15–20 minutes. Ideally, a range of wheelchairs should be available for use (e.g. tilt in space specialist seating) but invariably ward chairs are adapted (often with pillows, rolled up towels and folded blankets) to achieve optimum postures to maintain length, protect vulnerable joints such as the glenohumeral joint, help respiration and aid communication and social interaction (Clark et al. 2004; Pope 2006). Support should be provided for the head, trunk and hemiplegic upper limb as required, and be sufficient to maintain a good posture and thus help with carry-over of treatment (Chui 1995). If patients have severe prolonged difficulties with seating they may require referral to a specialist seating service.

Standing

Standing is a key component of early mobilisation and should be commenced as soon as the patient's cardiovascular system has stabilised, ideally within 24 hours (Bernhardt et al. 2008; Carr & Shepherd 2003). Encouraging patients to stand and undertake periods of weight bearing is a good way to maintain length in muscles, modulate tonal change and promote extensor muscle activity to counter the predominance of flexion incurred from prolonged periods of sitting (Carr & Shepherd 1998, 2003; Massion 1994). With the exception of standing hoists, the increasing use of mechanical lifting aids as a means to transfer people has arguably reduced the opportunities for patients to take weight through their lower limbs. Regular standing through the day can help maintain tone levels, decrease frequency of spasms, assist maintenance of joint range (Bohannon 1993) and help activate extensor muscles, which does not happen when lying in bed (Brown 1994; Markham 1987; Massion 1994). If a patient has no or only minimal movement, a tilt table can be used (Chang et al. 2004); if the patient shows more extensor activity in the trunk and lower limb, then other standing devices such as a motorised standing frame can be introduced to the patient's routine (Thornton & Kilbride 2004). It may be that periods as short as only five minutes can be tolerated initially; mechanical ventilation does not preclude standing or sitting but close monitoring of oxygen saturation and vital signs is required, particularly if autonomic disturbances are exhibited (Carter & Edwards 2002). As the patient progresses, the amount of support can be reduced and the patient can practise standing with the help of one or two team members or within parallel bars if available.

Walking

Depending on the degree of hemiparesis, walking may not be possible in the early stages post-stroke or it may require the assistance of additional equipment; the MDT should take the lead from the physiotherapist as to the best way to help the patient mobilise. For example, diminished movement in the upper limb means the use of a walking frame is often precluded, or a lack of dorsiflexion in the ankle region may require the provision of temporary ankle–foot orthoses (Olney 2005) or orthotics (Edwards & Charlton 2002). Selective functional electrical stimulation (FES) has been used successfully for foot drop (Burridge et al. 1997; Popovic et al. 2002). In recent years, partial body weight support treadmill training has offered the possibility for active and task specific gait re-education, even for stroke patients with low levels of activity because the harness system provides added security (Hesse et al. 2003; Smith & Thompson 2008; Tuckey & Greenwood 2004). However, these specialist treadmills are relatively expensive and require considerable space and tend to be confined to larger physiotherapy departments or rehabilitation units. Indeed, a recent review looking at the rehabilitation of walking speed post-stroke showed that simple low technology and conventional exercise was as effective as treadmill and robot-based interventions (Dickstein 2008).

Falls prevention

Falls are extremely common after a stroke (see Case example 7.2). A study found that of 311 inpatients, 25% suffered from a fall after their stroke (Langhorne et al. 2000). There are a number of reasons why a person may fall, as detailed in Box 7.1. Whilst it is not possible to prevent all falls from occurring, even when a patient is in hospital, it is possible to reduce the likelihood of a fall. Many hospital and community services produce useful information leaflets for patients and relatives about how to do this. It is important to try to prevent falls because handling falling or fallen people presents risks of injury to patient, carer or staff member. In particular, it is inadvisable to try to catch someone falling despite the ethical dilemma this poses.

Guidance relating to falls assessment has been published (Oliver, Daly, Martin & McMurdo, 2004); all patients who have had a fall or have gait or balance abnormalities should be offered a multifactorial falls risk assessment

---

Box 7.1 Possible causes of falls.

- Reduced strength and balance, poor gait and physical weakness
- Foot problems and footwear
- Sensory deficits, e.g. visual problems, poor hearing
- Cognitive and perceptual problems, e.g. neglect, altered judgement etc.
- Medical conditions, e.g. acute illness, stroke, cognitive decline, postural hypotension
- Fear of falling
- History of falls
- Hurrying, altered environment, space and furniture layout, poor lighting

---

Case example 7.2 Betty, 82 years old, living alone six months post-stroke.

'I was getting the breakfast stuff tidied up again, and I came in here and I went down. I knew I was going down, and I hit against this thing (coffee table). I was bleeding and all. I got as far as the door and I fell again and I couldn't get up.'

(Langhorne et al. 2000). This includes exploring the history of falls and an assessment of gait, balance, mobility, muscle weakness, osteoporosis risk, functional ability, older persons' fear of falling, visual impairment, cognitive impairment, urinary incontinence, home hazards, neurological and cardiovascular examination, and a medication review. A falls prevention intervention can then be offered if needed. This could involve modification of risk factors, strength and balance training, changes within the home, referral and improving vision and modifying medication. On the rehabilitation ward, safety measures might include using a wheelchair to take the patient to the toilet if there is an urgent need, and walking back. Alternatively, the falls risk assessment might suggest the need to position a walking aid or chair half way between bedside and toilet (Betts & Mowbray 2005).

Restoration and re-education of movement

As described earlier, the loss of movement after stroke results from the combined effect of positive (i.e. spasticity), negative (i.e. weakness) and adaptive (i.e. contractures) features. There is direct evidence to demonstrate alteration of sensory input from the periphery, i.e. moving the hemiplegic limb can affect the resultant motor output (Hamdy et al. 2000; Johansson 2000). Interventions described in this section assist with restoration and maintenance of movement post-stroke and are in addition to those already covered in previous sections.

Decreased range of movement and contractures

Altered muscle tone is often implicated in the development of contractures and without intervention the affected parts of the body tend to remain in shortened positions for prolonged periods leading to soft tissue changes and loss in range of movement (Goldspink & Williams 1990). A recent longitudinal study in Australia demonstrated for the first time that spasticity can cause contracture in the first four months after stroke but thereafter findings implicated muscle weakness as the main contributor in activity limitations (Ada et al. 2006). Tonal changes and the inability to move lead to the emergence of habitual postures, which contribute to soft tissue shortening and biomechanical changes in muscle (see earlier section on therapeutic positioning and seating). These peripheral changes play a part in muscle imbalance that compound any central motor dysfunction from the stroke itself and thus lead to more movement difficulties (Fitzgerald & Stokes 2004; Singer et al. 2001).

Patients thought to be at most risk of developing contractures are those that are:

- Unconscious
- Immobile and have altered muscle tone
- Exhibit shortening with current intervention
- Have fractures and/or pressure sores
- Have a low score on the Glasgow Coma Scale (less than nine)
- Are medically unstable and unable to be stood (Thornton & Kilbride 2004)

In addition, patients who show no functional recovery in muscle activity two to four weeks post-stroke are also highlighted as being at higher risk of contracture (Pandyan et al. 2003). Decreased range of movement and adaptive muscle changes, including contracture, are most commonly seen post-stroke in the following areas and in muscles that cross two joints:

- Hip and knee flexors
- Hip adductors
- Calf muscles and Achilles tendon affecting both the ankle and foot
- Shoulder elevators, adductor and medial rotators
- Elbow flexors and forearm muscles
- Wrist and finger flexors

Furthermore, patients with loss of movement in the limbs are likely to have loss of range of movement in the trunk, pelvis and shoulder girdles (Carter & Edwards 2002). The long-term negative effect of contractures is a loss of potential function and thus represents an important area of intervention for all team members; methods for intervention are considered next.

Stretching, assisted and passive movements

Whilst contractures are best treated by prevention, at times, despite best efforts, this is not possible. Loss of movement post-stroke and consequent enforced inactivity leads to decreased joint range motion and interventions are required to maintain the movement in all large and small joints of the body including the jaw (Carter & Edwards 2002; Davies 1994). National stroke guidelines recommend any patient whose range of movement at a joint is reduced or at risk of becoming reduced should have a programme of passive stretching of all affected joints on a daily basis and that the programme should be taught to patient and/or carers (Carter & Edwards 2002). Movements to help maintain range can be carried out in a variety of ways:

- Active – performed solely by the patient
- Active assisted – patient helped by someone else
- Passive – movements carried out solely by the therapist, nurse or carer and not the patient

While movements carried out independently by the patient do result in larger cortical sensorimotor changes (Lotze et al. 2003), passive movements have been shown to stimulate brain activity and thus may be involved in reorganisation of sensory and motor systems in the brain (Nelles et al. 1999). Therefore, in the absence of voluntary muscle action, passive movements should be carried out as part of the overall rehabilitation process.

Handling techniques that may be used for patients with differing presentations of altered tone have been described (Thornton & Kilbride 2004). Movement should be carried out at different speeds and utilising compression, traction, stretch and rotational movements, but should never be vigorous or forced due to the risk of heterotrophic ossification (the laying down of bone in muscle). Whilst taking patients out of their preferred postures, particular attention should be paid to muscles that cross two joints and to patterns of movement. The length and frequency with which sustained muscle stretch should be applied continues to be the subject of debate and varies from six hours per day (Tardieu et al. 1988) to 15–20 minutes (Carr & Shepherd 2003). A recent systematic review of stretching in spasticity recognised the complexity of the concept and recommended further research into the area (Bovend'Eerdt et al. 2008). An alternative to applying therapeutic stretch to muscles is to utilise splints or casts.

Splinting

If positioning and regular movements are ineffective in preventing adaptive feature of contractures, splinting the affected body part may become necessary (Edwards & Charlton 2002). The mechanism behind splinting remains the subject of debate but is thought to have both neural and musculoskeletal effects (Stoeckmann 2001). Casting, which encloses a limb in a cylinder (such as that used with a bone fracture), may decrease input to tactile, proprioceptive and temperature receptors and give total contact, even pressure and warmth: this is thought to lessen the excitability of neuronal output (Childers et al. 1999; Robichaud & Agostinucci 1996; see Case example 7.3). Findings from a systematic review undertaken to look at the evidence for casting in neurological patients in order to maintain or increase passive range of motion, manage hypertonia and improve function, concluded that there is evidence to support the use of casting for improving range of movement but that further research is required into the other two areas (Mortensen & Eng 2003).

Case example 7.3 Ray, 56 years old, five months post-stroke.

'I've got no control over that hand at all. It's very numb down that side still, and this, the fingers on this hand are constantly moving, I can't stop them getting into peculiar positions, because I don't feel them doing anything. The therapist fixed that up for me [a splint for the hand and arm], I wasn't sleeping because my hand exercises constantly, and it would wake me up in the night. Anyway I wear this and I get a good night's sleep.'

Splinting carries considerable risk of pressure sores and skin damage so great care is required and nursing input is vital to monitor the condition of the skin. Three main forms of splinting with the neurological patient have been described (Thornton & Kilbride 2004):

- Prophylactic (preventative) – as the name suggests, prophylactic splinting aims to prevent any loss in range of movement and includes, e.g. the use of 'plaster' boots or pressure splints (Johnstone 1995).
- Corrective – this type of splinting is used to increase range of movement in the presence of contracture. For example, cylindrical plasters (such as plaster boots as described above), drop out splints and hinged cast braces can be used for gaining activity whilst preventing movement (Edwards & Charlton 2002).
- Dynamic – this aims to facilitate recovery and assist stability for function; examples include ankle–foot orthoses, which can be hinged or fixed (Tyson & Thornton 2001), and the use of orthotic insoles (Edwards & Charlton 2002). Strapping provides an alternative short-term approach, which can be applied to most joints, the ankle and shoulder in particular (Thornton & Kilbride 2004) (also see later section on hemiplegic shoulder pain), although the evidence for efficacy is limited.

The use of botulinum toxin, which is produced by *Clostridium botulinum* and acts on the neuromuscular junction to help reduce muscle activity, may be used in conjunction with splinting when the tone is high (Thompson et al. 2005; Thornton & Kilbride 2004). However, this is unlikely to be needed except in extreme cases in the acute stroke patient.

Targeted strengthening and exercise

Muscle weakness is now recognised as a cardinal feature post-stroke with more regard given to weakness as a primary factor limiting recovery of physical function (Cramp et al. 2006). Difficulties are noted in areas such as generating force, timing and sequencing force production and sustaining force for functional activity; however, muscle weakness is modifiable through strength training of appropriate intensity (Carr & Shepherd 2003). Recent systematic reviews of exercise post-stroke (Saunders et al. 2004) and strength training (Morris et al. 2004) indicate the positive nature of both these approaches to stroke rehabilitation and support earlier research. Muscle strength and function were found to be improved by strength training, which did not increase abnormal muscle activation (Ng & Shepherd 2000). As muscle weakness post-stroke is a feature of a more general motor control impairment, it has been recommended that strength training should be task-specific or at least oriented towards characteristics of the task to be learned (Carr & Shepherd 2003). For example, repeating the task of sit to stand helps to strengthen the muscles involved in the functional activity whilst practising the action, thus addressing skills to be gained and targeting weak muscles. The task can be varied by executing the task through full, mid or inner range of the movement, changing speed, or adding resistance by changing the height of the starting position (Ada & Canning 2005). In addition, there may be a role for *specific* strengthening of muscles in preventing contractures and loss of range of movement (Shortland et al. 2002).

Along with weakness, individuals can also show signs of cardiovascular deconditioning with low levels of fitness from the enforced inactivity post-stroke (Hass & Jones 2004). As with any individual planning to undertake a new exercise regime, a risk assessment for cardiorespiratory training should be carried out (Hass & Jones 2004; Kilbreath & Davis 2005). These researchers recommend following procedures from the American College of Sports Medicine (Hass & Jones 2004), which include termination of activity with the onset of angina or angina-like symptoms, signs of poor perfusion such as light-headedness, confusion or cold and clammy skin, and failure of testing or monitoring equipment. Many types of exercise can be used depending on the individual requirements, including brisk walking (*free* walking or treadmill), stepping, static cycles, arm and leg cycle ergometers (Hass & Jones 2004; Kilbreath & Davis 2005). Indeed, people with residual moderate disability post-stroke have been shown to be capable of exercising for 30 minutes up to 90 minutes in fitness programmes incorporating aerobic and strength components (Duncan et al. 2003).

Management of the upper limb

> *My right arm, I find combing my hair, taking any weight on the arm, rather – well, trying. But I just get on with it.*
>
>   (Bill, 72 years old, five months post-stroke)

The most common cause of stroke is from an occlusion of the middle cerebral artery, which is associated with weakness and sensory loss that affects the arm and face more than the leg (Shelton & Reding 2001). Figures stated in the literature on the recovery of the upper limb post-stroke are varied, with numbers ranging from 5% to 52% (Dean & Mackey 1992; Gowland et al. 1992). When these figures are compared with the numbers regaining the ability to walk, estimated to be between 70 and 80% of patients (Rodgers et al. 2003), the size of the challenge of rehabilitation in this area becomes evident. Whilst it is generally accepted that most recovery happens in the first three months post-stroke (Wade et al. 1985), substantial recovery can happen at more than one year (Taub et al. 1993). A study followed up 54 patients with first-ever stroke for four years, assessing upper limb recovery (Broeks et al. 1999); although most of the improvement occurred during the first 16 weeks after stroke, it continued after 16 weeks in 10 patients and indeed with 13 of the patients, recovery of arm function only started after 16 weeks. At four years, loss of arm function was still perceived to be a major problem by 36 participants. Reasons for poor recovery of the upper limb are multiple and range from learnt disuse (Taub et al. 1993), corticospinal tract damage (Bourbonnais & Vanden 1989; Shelton & Reding 2001), reduced coordination of motor control (Diedrichsen et al. 2007) and the complexity of movement required for activities in the arm and hand when compared with the lower limb (Carr & Shepherd 2003). Furthermore, it has also been suggested that other functions are treated and practised at the expense of the upper limb (Lang et al. 2007; Rodgers et al. 2003). Task-specific practice and intensity of treatment, and other novel approaches are likewise relevant to restoration of movement in the upper limb.

Managing shoulder joint subluxation

Shoulder pain post-stroke is common and complicates the recovery of purposeful movement in the arm (Gamble et al. 2002). Changes in muscle tone, weakness and loss of range of movement can affect normal shoulder posture and soft tissue changes (Turner-Stokes & Jackson 2002). Subluxation is a commonly seen manifestation of the loss of tone in muscles supporting the shoulder joint because stability is reliant on muscle activity and not ligaments (Bobath 1990). However, it need not be a cause of pain if managed correctly with appropriate upper limb support (see Edwards & Charlton 2002 for an overview). A recent study in Australia looked at interventions for subluxation of the shoulder and found the collar and cuff sling was the most common approach but with low-level evidence. They found the use of a wheelchair or wheelchair attachments were most useful, with stronger supporting evidence (Foongchomcheay et al. 2005). Taping around the shoulder joint is sometimes used to help decrease inappropriate alignment, reduce subluxation and increase proprioceptive input but the mechanisms of this adjunct to treatment are still being debated and require further investigation (Alexander et al. 2003; Peters & Lee 2003). Education of staff and family, as with all areas of stroke care, is a central aspect of treatment (Intercollegiate Stroke Working Party 2008).

Hemiplegic shoulder pain

Prevention of hemiplegic shoulder pain is of prime concern to health professionals, and it is estimated to be present in 30% of patients with stroke (Intercollegiate Stroke Working Party 2008). Pain persisted in 47% of a study cohort

Stroke patients with shoulder weakness are at high risk of developing:
i)   **Shoulder subluxation**
ii)   **Painful shoulder**
iii) **Reduced shoulder mobility**
The following guide has been developed to minimise these complications:

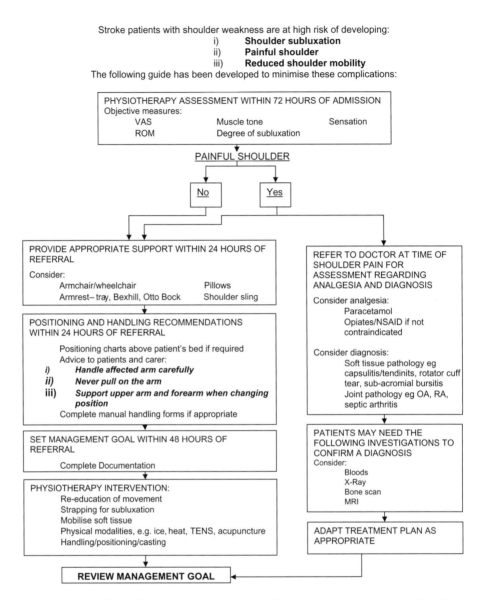

Figure 7.1 A guide for the management of the shoulder in a stroke patient. Reproduced with thanks to the STEP team, Royal Free NHS Trust, Hampstead, London.

of 297 people, with sleep being disturbed in 58%, and 40% requiring rest to relieve the pain when present. Steps to reduce the risk of trauma, provide limb support, and maintain range of movement can be structured within an integrated care pathway. A comprehensive example from a specialist rehabilitation unit is described (Jackson et al. 2003). Figure 7.1 illustrates a simpler example from an acute stroke unit. Both examples help to promote timely and coordinated intervention from the MDT. Use of overhead arm slings that encourage uncontrolled abduction should be avoided (Intercollegiate Stroke Working Party 2008; Kumar et al. 1990).

Further rehabilitation strategies and novel developments

This section looks at additional strategies that can be used in the rehabilitation of motor control post-stroke and more novel therapeutic developments that are not yet mainstream but may represent useful treatment possibilities in the future.

Task-specific training and practice opportunities

The key principle underpinning *task-specific training* is that restoration of movement should be specific to the task to be mastered or at least orientated to the characteristics of the task to be performed, because to a large degree how one action is carried out is dependent on the preceding components (Carr & Shepherd 2003; Shumway-Cook & Woollacott 2007). Furthermore, rehabilitation post-stroke can be carried out as a *whole task training*, i.e. walking practice or as *part or modified training* (Shumway-Cook & Woollacott 2007). For example, with walking it may be necessary to target a specific impairment such as weakness in the ankle dorsiflexors and practise this aspect to address overall improvement in mobility. Equally, with other tasks such as washing and dressing it may be necessary to break the task down into component parts in the progression towards functional independence. It is therefore important that opportunities are given to practise tasks. The effectiveness of motor skill learning is enhanced if the activity is goal directed (Pomeroy & Tallis 2002) and the individual is given some control over practice conditions because this is thought to lead to more active involvement in the learning process (Wulf 2007).

Intensity of activity

Practice is an essential element of rehabilitation and thus it is important that patients are given the opportunity to practise (Carr & Shepherd 2003). There is a direct relationship between practice and learning, with more intensive practice being more beneficial (Kwakkel et al. 2004; Kwakkel 2006; Winstein et al. 2004). However, traditional neurorehabilitation interventions have limited effectiveness in promoting motor recovery within the dosing parameters typically used (Wolf et al. 2008). Looking at the dose–response relationship, it was found that augmentation of routine therapy input produced additional benefits, with results of a systematic review indicating augmentation of current routine practice by a minimum of 16 hours in the first six months after stroke (Kwakkel et al. 2004). It is therefore important that all members of the MDT are involved in providing opportunities for patients to practise tasks. Patients can also be set up with self-monitored practice outside of formal treatment sessions. However, it is essential that the patient can do the exercise and that the exercises are challenging but achievable. A timetable along with written instructions, diagrams, photographs or audiotapes can be helpful depending on the individual needs of the patient. It is also important that the movements which should be avoided are clearly stated.

Constraint-induced movement therapy (CIMT)

Following stroke, patients with mild to moderate impairment of upper limb can exhibit learned disuse, meaning that despite having some return of movement in the arm they tend to favour and use the less affected side (Taub et al. 1993). In CIMT, unaffected arms are restricted during 90% of waking hours over a two-week period whilst engaging in a six-hour activity programme using affected arms (Taub et al. 1993; Wolf et al. 2008). Some active wrist and finger movement is necessary to participate in CIMT and so it is not suitable for all patients. Indeed it is estimated that four out of five patients are excluded from CIMT because of poor baseline movement (Grotta et al. 2004). Results from the recent EXCITE trial, (a single-blind randomised multicentre trial with 222 patients who had a minimum 10 degree wrist extension, 10 degree thumb adduction, and a 10 degree extension of at least two fingers) three to nine months post-stroke showed statistically significant and clinically relevant improvements in arm motor function that persisted for a year (Wolf et al. 2008).

Modified constraint-induced movement therapy (mCIMT)

Many patients find the intensity of the previously described constraint-induced movement therapy (CIMT) too difficult to comply with, and therapists often do not have the resources to administer th e approach, which led to the development of a shorter protocol that has become known as modified constraint-induced movement therapy (mCIMT) (Page et al. 2005). An mCIMT study looked at four patients one year post-stroke who initially exhibited minimal movement in affected hands (Page & Levine 2007); patients received a structured 30-minute therapy session that focused on involving the affected arms in activities valued by the participants, three times per week for 10 weeks. Less affected arms were restrained five days per week for five hours per day during the 10-week period. All participants demonstrated improvement in the use of affected arms and in the quality of that movement. Thus mCIMT may offer a programme of targeted intensity of practice that is more acceptable and achievable for both patients and therapists. The combination of mCIMT and Wii technology holds promise.

Motor imagery practice (MIP)

Brain imaging of the mental (cognitive) rehearsal of a specific motor action without actual body movement occurring shows that regions of the brain activated during mental practice are the same as when physically doing the task (Dickstein & Deutsch 2007; Sharma et al. 2006). MIP has been described as the 'backdoor' to the motor system following stroke and could be used to bridge the gap, because unlike CIMT or mCIMT, it is not dependent upon the person's ability to move (Sharma et al. 2006). It can be a way that patients in the early stages and those with enduring motor impairment can be actively involved in self practice.

Combination therapy

This approach to treatment looks at the use of electromyography-triggered muscle stimulation (ETMS) combined with mCIMT in chronic stroke. Findings from a small study of six patients with upper limb hemiparesis within one year of the stroke indicated favourable initial changes. Study participants received 35 minutes of ETMS twice every weekday for eight weeks, followed by mCIMT three times a week for ten weeks (Page & Levine 2006). Results indicated that ETMS alone did not lead to functional change but is thought to have assisted with gaining more wrist and finger extension, allowing subsequent participation in a programme of mCIMT, which demonstrated functional gains. The authors suggest that combination therapy could provide a bridge for lower functioning patients but acknowledge that further work is required. The use of EMG-triggered functional electrical stimulation (FES) in the rehabilitation of wrist and finger extensors in chronic stroke has also been reported to lead to significant improvements in grasping small objects and sustaining extensor muscle activity (Cauraugh et al. 2000; Hara et al. 2006). This approach has also been used in the acute stroke patient 15 days post-stroke, to good effect (Chae et al. 1998; Francisco et al. 1998).

Peripheral nerve stimulation (PNS)

The use of direct peripheral nerve stimulation (PNS) has been described as a form of somatosensory stimulation to enhance functional hand training in patients with chronic stroke (Celnik et al. 2007). Results from this single-blinded randomised crossover study of nine stroke patients who had two nerves (ulnar and median) in their affected upper limb stimulated as a precursor to practising motor skills showed that PNS as an adjunct positively augmented upper limb retraining.

Biofeedback

Evidence regarding the use of biofeedback as an adjunct to stroke rehabilitation is equivocal. A meta-analysis of eight published randomised controlled trials concluded the efficacy of biofeedback in stroke is yet to be established, although the effect of small study sizes was acknowledged (Glanz et al. 1995). Conversely, EMG biofeedback was reported to have had a large effect on improving function in the impaired arm following stroke (Hiraoka 2001). Other authors have found this a useful adjunct to treatment in providing feedback to patients on their performance of specific activities, for example balance retraining (Nichols 1997; Sackley & Lincoln 1996), weight transference (Cheng et al. 2004) and improving the strength of ankle dorsiflexors (Moreland et al. 1998).

Repetitive transcranial magnetic stimulation (rTMS)

Transcranial magnetic stimulation is a non-invasive, relatively painless method of mapping the cortex of the brain using a magnetic coil to induce a focused weak electrical current in brain tissue, causing stimulation of local neurons (Barker et al. 1985). Transcranial direct current stimulation (tDCS) is another recent development in the use of TMS in rehabilitation; it is able to painlessly modulate cortical activity, is undetectable and valuable in research through enabling true placebo controls (Hummel et al. 2005). Both rTMS and tDCS have demonstrated beneficial effects on the function of hemiplegic hands and early results are promising. Most recently it has been shown that a five-day course of low frequency rTMS applied over the unaffected hemisphere for 20 minutes in patients with chronic stroke who had mild to moderate impairment led to improvements in affected hand function that lasted two weeks (Fregni et al. 2006). These authors hypothesised that rTMS combined with motor training might further enhance motor recovery after stroke.

Robotic assisted movement

Robotic therapy is carried out by a robot manipulator, which applies forces to the affected arm that is held within a movable external support. Robotic therapy assists impaired upper limbs to repetitively practise movements in passive and active modes. The National Clinical Guidelines for Stroke (Intercollegiate Stroke Working Party 2008) recommend this intervention as an adjunct to conventional therapy; it should be considered in patients with deficits in arm function who are at least six months post-stroke (Lum et al. 2002; Volpe et al. 2000).

Patients' perspective on mobility rehabilitation

Patients' experiences of their rehabilitation may not always be positive. Several areas of unmet need for rehabilitation patients have been uncovered, such as a lack of information and involvement in their own rehabilitation, too little therapy and poor pain control within the context of physical care provision. Boredom and isolation were also cited as particular sources of distress (Long et al. 2001).

Whilst there is a great deal of literature discussing ways to ensure that patient handling does not result in injuries to health and social care personnel (e.g. (Billin 1998; Brown-Wilson 2002; Hignett 2003), less has been written about patients' views about being 'handled'. Patients may not like being assisted, particularly if this assistance involves a mechanical device. For example, older people may view mobility aids as a source of stigma and a threat to dignity and pride (Rush & Ouellet 1997). Client discomfort and fear have been cited by nurses as reasons for not using mechanical aids (McGuire et al. 1996).

Rehabilitation patients may want the nurse to 'do for' or 'care for' them, rather than promote their independence (Kneafsey & Long 2002). For rehabilitation staff, it may therefore be difficult to negotiate a balance between listening to patients' wishes and implementing care known to be beneficial for them. However, it is important that patients do consent to their treatment and care and are willing participants in their own rehabilitation. The way in which health care staff plan to assist patients with movement and mobility is a key part of this process. A survey of staff views about the early mobilisation of stroke patients identified that many health care professionals (including nurses, doctors and physiotherapists) believe that early mobilisation could begin irrespective of whether or not the patient wanted to get up (Arias & Smith 2007). However, it is important that health care professionals attempt to incorporate patients' wishes and opinions into rehabilitation care. For example, when discussing home care provision, UK Health and Safety Executive guidance (Health and Safety Executive 2001) suggests that 'no-lifting' policies have been misinterpreted in the past, with hoists routinely prescribed for all moves and transfers irrespective of the patients' wishes and sometimes needs. Clearly, this is unfair to patients and detrimental to the rehabilitation process. It is therefore important that patients' goals and wishes are respected (see Case example 7.4) and that decisions about patient handling and the provision of assistance with mobility and movement are made with consultation and agreement from the patient.

Conclusion

This chapter has demonstrated the importance of early and proactive management and treatment of physical impairments post-stroke as an integral part of the overall recovery of mobility. Nurses, in collaboration with the MDT, have a central role to play in this process by combining nursing care with rehabilitation principles and integrating therapeutic activity into everyday function. This chapter has reviewed familiar areas of practice like positioning and seating, falls prevention, and the complexity of assessing risk in moving and handing in rehabilitation alongside an exploration of more novel therapeutic developments in the treatment of stroke. It is only through the ongoing continual professional development of all team members and engagement with service users that rehabilitation will continue to keep up to date with new developments and research, enabling subsequent changes in this challenging but rewarding area of clinical practice.

Case example 7.4 Jodie, the 31-year-old woman quoted at the chapter start.

'I want to be able to walk down the road arm-in-arm with me boyfriend and not have people look at me because I'm limping. And some people say that's bad, you should not worry about what people think. But I think it's good that I worry about what other people think. Because if I didn't, if I didn't give a damn, and thought well it doesn't matter if I limp – come and see me 10 years later, I'd still be limping.'

References

Ada, L, & Canning, C, 2005, Changing the way we view the contribution of motor impairments to physical disability after stroke, in *Science-Based Rehabilitation: Theories into Practice*, L Ada & E Ellis, eds., Elsevier, Edinburgh, pp. 87–106.

Ada, L, O'Dwyer, N, & O'Neill, E, 2006, Relation between spasticity, weakness and contracture of the elbow flexors and upper limb activity after stroke: an observational study, *Disability and Rehabilitation*, vol. 28, no. 13–14, pp. 891–897.

Adams, HP, Jr, Adams, RJ, Brott, T, del Zoppo, GJ, Furlan, A et al., 2003, Guidelines for the early management of patients with ischemic stroke: a scientific statement from the Stroke Council of the American Stroke Association, *Stroke*, vol. 34, no. 4, pp. 1056–1083.

Alexander, CM, Stynes, S, Thomas, A, Lewis, J, & Harrison, PJ, 2003, Does tape facilitate or inhibit the lower fibres of trapezius? *Manual Therapy*, vol. 8, no. 1, pp. 37–41.

Arias, M, & Smith, LN, 2007, Early mobilization of acute stroke patients, *Journal of Clinical Nursing*, vol. 16, no. 2, pp. 282–288.

Baer, G, Durward, B, 2004, Stroke, in *Physical Management in Neurological Rehabilitation*, 2nd edn, M Stokes, ed., Elsevier, Edinburgh, pp. 75–101.

Barker, AT, Jalinous, R, & Freeston, IL, 1985, Non-invasive magnetic stimulation of human motor cortex, *Lancet*, vol. 1, no. 8437, pp. 1106–1107.

Barnes, MP, 2001, Medical management of spasticity in stroke, *Age and Ageing*, vol. 30 Suppl 1, pp. 13–16.

Bennett, SE, & Karnes, JL, 1998, *Neurological Disabilities: Assessment and Treatment*, Lippincott, Philadelphia.

Bernhardt, J, Chan, J, Nicola, I, & Collier, JM, 2007, Little therapy, little physical activity: rehabilitation within the first 14 days of organized stroke unit care, *Journal of Rehabilitation Medicine*, vol. 39, no. 1, pp. 43–48.

Bernhardt, J, Dewey, H, Donnan, G, Thrift, A, Lindley, R et al., 2008, A very early rehabilitation trial (AVERT): phase III, *Lancet.Com* (http://www.thelancet.com/journals/lancet/misc/protocol/06PRT-5424).

Betts, M, & Mowbray, C, 2005, The falling and fallen person and emergency handling, in *The Guide to the Handling of Patients*, 5th edn, J Smith, ed., Backcare in collaboration with the Royal College of Nursing and National Back Exchange.

Billin, SL, 1998, Moving and handling practice in neuro-disability nursing, *British Journal of Nursing*, vol. 7, no. 10, pp. 571–574, 576.

Bobath, B, 1990, *Adult Hemiplegia Evaluation and Treatment*, Heinemann Medical Books, Oxford.

Bohannon, RW, 1993, Tilt table standing for reducing spasticity after spinal cord injury, *Archives of Physical Medicine and Rehabilitation*, vol. 74, no. 10, pp. 1121–1122.

Bourbonnais, D, & Vanden, NS, 1989, Weakness in patients with hemiparesis, *American Journal of Occupational Therapy*, vol. 43, no. 5, pp. 313–319.

Bovend'Eerdt, TJ, Newman, M, Barker, K, Dawes, H, Minelli, C et al., 2008, The effects of stretching in spasticity: a systematic review, *Archives of Physical Medicine and Rehabilitation*, vol. 89, no. 7, pp. 1395–1406.

Boyd, RN, & Ada, L, 2001, Physiotherapy management of spasticity, in *Upper Motor Neurone Syndrome and Spasticity: Clinical Management and Neurophysiology*, MP Barnes & GR Johnson, eds., Cambridge University Press, Cambridge, pp. 96–121.

Britton, T, 2004, Abnormalities of muscle tone and movement, in *Physical Management in Neurological Rehabilitation*, 2nd edn, M Stokes, ed., Elsevier, Edinburgh, pp. 47–56.

Broeks, JG, Lankhorst, GJ, Rumping, K, & Prevo, AJ, 1999, The long-term outcome of arm function after stroke: results of a follow-up study, *Disability and Rehabilitation*, vol. 21, no. 8, pp. 357–364.

Brown, P, 1994, Pathophysiology of spasticity, *Journal of Neurology, Neurosurgery and Psychiatry*, vol. 57, no. 7, pp. 773–777.

Brown-Wilson, C, 2002, Safer handling practice: influence of staff education on older people, *British Journal of Nursing*, vol. 11, no. 20, pp. 1332–1339.

Burridge, JH, Taylor, PN, Hagan, SA, Wood, DE, & Swain, ID, 1997, The effects of common peroneal stimulation on the effort and speed of walking: a randomized controlled trial with chronic hemiplegic patients, *Clinical Rehabilitation*, vol. 11, no. 3, pp. 201–210.

Callen, BL, Mahoney, JE, Grieves, CB, Wells, TJ, & Enloe, M, 2004, Frequency of hallway ambulation by hospitalized older adults on medical units of an academic hospital, *Geriatric Nursing*, vol. 25, no. 4, pp. 212–217.

Canadian Taskforce on Safe Patient Handling, 2005, Strategies to improve patient and healthcare provider safety in patient handling and movement tasks, *Rehabilitation Nursing*, vol. 30, no. 3, pp. 80–83.

Carr, J, & Shepherd, R, 1998, *Neurological Rehabilitation Optimising Motor Performance*, Butterworth Heinemann, Oxford.

Carr, J, & Shepherd, R, 2003, *Stroke Rehabilitation: Guidelines for Exercise and Training to Optimise Motor Skill*, Butterworth Heinemann, Oxford.

Carter, P, & Edwards, S, 2002, General principles of treatment, in *Neurological Physiotherapy: a problem solving approach*, 2nd edn, S Edwards, ed., Churchill Livingstone, Edinburgh, pp. 121–153.

Cauraugh, J, Light, K, Kim, S, Thigpen, M, & Behrman, A, 2000, Chronic motor dysfunction after stroke: recovering wrist and finger extension by electromyography-triggered neuromuscular stimulation, *Stroke*, vol. 31, no. 6, pp. 1360–1364.

Celnik, P, Hummel, F, Harris-Love, M, Wolk, R, & Cohen, LG, 2007, Somatosensory stimulation enhances the effects of training functional hand tasks in patients with chronic stroke, *Archives of Physical Medicine and Rehabilitation*, vol. 88, no. 11, pp. 1369–1376.

Chae, J, Bethoux, F, Bohine, T, Dobos, L, Davis, T et al., 1998, Neuromuscular stimulation for upper extremity motor and functional recovery in acute hemiplegia, *Stroke*, vol. 29, no. 5, pp. 975–979.

Chang, AT, Boots, R, Hodges, PW, & Paratz, J, 2004, Standing with assistance of a tilt table in intensive care: a survey of Australian physiotherapy practice, *Australian Journal of Physiotherapy*, vol. 50, no. 1, pp. 51–54.

Chartered Society of Physiotherapy, 2008, *Guidance on Manual Handling in Physiotherapy*, 3rd edn, Chartered Society of Physiotherapy, London.

Chatterton, HJ, Pomeroy, VM, & Gratton, J, 2001, Positioning for stroke patients: a survey of physiotherapists' aims and practices, *Disability and Rehabilitation*, vol. 23, no. 10, pp. 413–421.

Cheng, PT, Wang, CM, Chung, CY, & Chen, CL, 2004, Effects of visual feedback rhythmic weight-shift training on hemiplegic stroke patients, *Clinical Rehabilitation*, vol. 18, no. 7, pp. 747–753.

Childers, MK, Biswas, SS, Petroski, G, & Merveille, O, 1999, Inhibitory casting decreases a vibratory inhibition index of the H-reflex in the spastic upper limb, *Archives of Physical Medicine and Rehabilitation*, vol. 80, no. 6, pp. 714–716.

Chui, ML, 1995, Wheelchair seating and positioning, in *Physical Therapy for Traumatic Brain Injury*, J Montgomery, ed., Churchill Livingstone, New York, pp. 117–136.

Clark, J, Morrow, M, & Michael, S, 2004, Wheelchair postural support for young people with progressive neuromuscular disorders, *International Journal of Therapy and Rehabilitation*, vol. 11, no. 8, pp. 365–373.

Cramp, MC, Greenwood, RJ, Gill, M, Rothwell, JC, & Scott, OM, 2006, Low intensity strength training for ambulatory stroke patients, *Disability and Rehabilitation*, vol. 28, no. 13–14, pp. 883–889.

Davies, PM, 1994, *Starting Again: Early Rehabilitation After Traumatic Brain Injury or Other Severe Brain Lesions*, Springer-Verlag, Berlin.

Dean, CM, & Mackey, FH, 1992, Motor assessment scale scores as a measure of rehabilitation outcome following stroke, *Australian Journal of Physiotherapy*, vol. 38, no. 1, pp. 31–35.

Dickstein, R, 2008, Rehabilitation of gait speed after stroke: a critical review of intervention approaches, *Neurorehabilitation and Neural Repair*, vol. 22, no. 6, pp. 649–660.

Dickstein, R, & Deutsch, JE, 2007, Motor imagery in physical therapist practice, *Physical Therapy*, vol. 87, no. 7, pp. 942–953.

Diedrichsen, J, Criscimagna-Hemminger, SE, & Shadmehr, R, 2007, Dissociating timing and coordination as functions of the cerebellum, *Journal of Neuroscience*, vol. 27, no. 23, pp. 6291–6301.

Duncan, P, Studenski, S, Richards, L, Gollub, S, Lai, SM et al., 2003, Randomized clinical trial of therapeutic exercise in subacute stroke, *Stroke*, vol. 34, no. 9, pp. 2173–2180.

Edwards, S, 2002, An analysis of normal movement as the basis for the development of treatment techniques, in *Neurological Physiotherapy: A Problem Solving Approach*, 2nd edn, S. Edwards, ed., Churchill Livingstone, Edinburgh, pp. 35–67.

Edwards, S, & Charlton, PT, 2002, Splinting and the use of orthoses in the management of patients with neurological disorders, in *Neurological Physiotherapy: A Problem Solving Approach*, 2nd edn, S. Edwards, ed., Churchill Livingstone, Edinburgh, pp. 219–253.

Fitzgerald, D, & Stokes, M, 2004, Muscle imbalance in neurological conditions, in *Physical Management in Neurological Rehabilitation*, 2nd edn, M. Stokes, ed., Elsevier, Edinburgh, pp. 501–516.

Foongchomcheay, A, Ada, L, & Canning, CG, 2005, Use of devices to prevent subluxation of the shoulder after stroke, *Physiotherapy Research International*, vol. 10, no. 3, pp. 134–145.

Francisco, G, Chae, J, Chawla, H, Kirshblum, S, Zorowitz, R et al., 1998, Electromyogram-triggered neuromuscular stimulation for improving the arm function of acute stroke survivors: a randomized pilot study, *Archives of Physical Medicine and Rehabilitation*, vol. 79, no. 5, pp. 570–575.

Fregni, F, Boggio, PS, Valle, AC, Rocha, RR, Duarte, J et al., 2006, A sham-controlled trial of a 5-day course of repetitive transcranial magnetic stimulation of the unaffected hemisphere in stroke patients, *Stroke*, vol. 37, no. 8, pp. 2115–2122.

Gamble, GE, Barberan, E, Laasch, HU, Bowsher, D, Tyrrell, PJ et al., 2002, Poststroke shoulder pain: a prospective study of the association and risk factors in 152 patients from a consecutive cohort of 205 patients presenting with stroke, *European Journal of Pain*, vol. 6, no. 6, pp. 467–474.

Gibbon, B, 1993, Implications for nurses in approaches to the management of stroke rehabilitation: a review of the literature, *International Journal of Nursing Studies*, vol. 30, no. 2, pp. 133–141.

Glanz, M, Klawansky, S, Stason, W, Berkey, C, Shah, N et al., 1995, Biofeedback therapy in poststroke rehabilitation: a meta-analysis of the randomized controlled trials, *Archives of Physical Medicine and Rehabilitation*, vol. 76, no. 6, pp. 508–515.

Goldspink, G, & Williams, PE, 1990, Muscle fibre and connective tissue changes associated with use and disuse, in *Foundations for Practice: Topics in Neurological Physiotherapy*, L Ada & C Canning, eds., Heinemann, London, pp. 197–218.

Gowland, C, deBruin, H, Basmajian, JV, Plews, N, & Burcea, I, 1992, Agonist and antagonist activity during voluntary upper-limb movement in patients with stroke, *Physical Therapy*, vol. 72, no. 9, pp. 624–633.

Grotta, JC, Noser, EA, Ro, T, Boake, C, Levin, H et al., 2004, Constraint-induced movement therapy, *Stroke*, vol. 35, no. 11 Suppl 1, pp. 2699–2701.

Hamdy, S, Rothwell, JC, Aziz, Q, & Thompson, DG, 2000, Organization and reorganization of human swallowing motor cortex: implications for recovery after stroke, *Clinical Science (London)*, vol. 99, no. 2, pp. 151–157.

Hara, Y, Ogawa, S, & Muraoka, Y, 2006, Hybrid power-assisted functional electrical stimulation to improve hemiparetic upper-extremity function, *American Journal of Physical Medicine and Rehabilitation*, vol. 85, no. 12, pp. 977–985.

Hass, BM, & Jones, F, 2004, Physical activity and exercise in neurological rehabilitation, in *Physical Management in Neurological Rehabilitation*, 2nd edn, M Stokes, ed., Elsevier, Edinburgh, pp. 489–499.

Health and Safety Executive, 1992, *Manual Handling: Manual Handling Operations Regulations 1992: Guidance on the Regulations*, Health and Safety Executive, Sudbury.

Health and Safety Executive, 2001, *Handling Homecare*, Health and Safety Executive, London.

Hesse, S, Werner, C, von Frankenberg, S, & Bardeleben, A, 2003, Treadmill training with partial body weight support after stroke, *Physical Medicine Rehabilitation Clinics of North America*, vol. 14, no. 1 Suppl, pp. S111–S123.

Hignett, S, 2003, Systematic review of patient handling activities starting in lying, sitting and standing positions, *Journal of Advanced Nursing*, vol. 41, no. 6, pp. 545–552.

Hignett, S, 2005, *Measuring the effectiveness of competency based education and training programmes in changing the manual handling behaviour of health care staff*, Health and Safety Executive, London. Research Report 315.

Hiraoka, K, 2001, Rehabilitation effort to improve upper limb extremity function in post-stroke patients: a meta-analysis, *Journal of Physical Therapy Science*, vol. 13, no. 1, pp. 5–9.

Hummel, F, Celnik, P, Giraux, P, Floel, A, Wu, WH et al., 2005, Effects of non-invasive cortical stimulation on skilled motor function in chronic stroke, *Brain*, vol. 128, no. 3, pp. 490–499.

Indredavik, B, Bakke, F, Slordahl, SA, Rokseth, R, & Haheim, LL, 1999, Treatment in a combined acute and rehabilitation stroke unit: which aspects are most important? *Stroke*, vol. 30, no. 5, pp. 917–923.

Intercollegiate Stroke Working Party, 2008, *National Clinical Guidelines for Stroke*, 3rd edn, Royal College of Physicians, London.

Jackson, D, Turner-Stokes, L, Williams, H, & Das-Gupta, R, 2003, Use of an integrated care pathway: a third round audit of the management of shoulder pain in neurological conditions, *Journal of Rehabilitation Medicine*, vol. 35, no. 6, pp. 265–270.

Johansson, BB, 2000, Brain plasticity and stroke rehabilitation: the Willis lecture, *Stroke*, vol. 31, no. 1, pp. 223–230.

Johnson, C, 2005, Manual handling risk assessment – theory and practice, in *The Guide to the Handling of Patients*, 5th edn, J Smith, ed., Collaboration with the Royal College of Nursing and the National Back Exchange, Middlesex.

Johnstone, M, 1995, *Restoration of Normal Movement after Stroke*, Churchill Livingstone, Edinburgh.

Jootun, D, & MacInnes, A, 2005, Examining how well students use correct handling procedures, *Nursing Times*, vol. 101, no. 4, pp. 38–40.

Karnath, HO, & Broetz, D, 2003, Understanding and treating 'pusher syndrome', *Physical Therapy*, vol. 83, no. 12, pp. 1119–1125.

Karnath, HO, Ferber, S, & Dichgans, J, 2000, The origin of contraversive pushing: evidence for a second graviceptive system in humans, *Neurology*, vol. 55, no. 9, pp. 1298–1304.

Kilbreath, S, & Davis, G, 2005, Cardiorespiratory fitness after stroke, in *Science Based Rehabilitation: Theories into Practice*, L Ada & E Ellis, eds., Elsevier, Edinburgh, pp. 131–158.

Kilbride, C, & McDonnell, A, 2000, Spasticity: the role of physiotherapy, *British Journal of Therapy and Rehabilitation*, vol. 7, no. 2, pp. 61–64.

Kneafsey, R, 2007, Nursing contributions to mobility rehabilitation: a systematic review examining the quality and content of the evidence, *Journal of Nursing and Healthcare of Chronic Illness, in association with Journal of Clinical Nursing*, vol. 16, no. 11C, pp. 325–340.

Kneafsey, R, & Long, A, 2002, Multi-disciplinary rehabilitation teams: the nurses' role, *British Journal of Therapy and Rehabilitation*, vol. 9, no. 1, pp. 24–29.

Kumar, R, Metter, EJ, Mehta, AJ, & Chew, T, 1990, Shoulder pain in hemiplegia. the role of exercise, *American Journal of Physical Medicine and Rehabilitation*, vol. 69, no. 4, pp. 205–208.

Kwakkel, G, 2006, Impact of intensity of practice after stroke: issues for consideration, *Disability and Rehabilitation*, vol. 28, no. 13/14, pp. 823–830.

Kwakkel, G, van, PR, Wagenaar, RC, Wood, DS, Richards, C et al., 2004, Effects of augmented exercise therapy time after stroke: a meta-analysis, *Stroke*, vol. 35, no. 11, pp. 2529–2539.

Lang, CE, MacDonald, JR, & Gnip, C, 2007, Counting repetitions: an observational study of outpatient therapy for people with hemiparesis post-stroke, *Journal of Neurologic Physical Therapy*, vol. 31, no. 1, pp. 3–10.

Langhorne, P, Stott, DJ, Robertson, L, MacDonald, J, Jones, L et al., 2000, Medical complications after stroke: a multicenter study, *Stroke*, vol. 31, no. 6, pp. 1223–1229.

Lawes, N, 2004, Neuroplasticity, in *Physical Management in Neurological Rehabilitation*, 2nd edn, M Stokes, ed., Elsevier, Edinburgh, pp. 57–72.

Lincoln, NB, Willis, D, Philips, SA, Juby, LC, & Berman, P, 1996, Comparison of rehabilitation practice on hospital wards for stroke patients, *Stroke*, vol. 27, no. 1, pp. 18–23.

Lindsay, KW, & Bone, I, 2004, *Neurology and Neurosurgery*, 4th edn, Churchill Livingstone, Edinburgh.

Long, AF, Kneafsey, R, Ryan, J, Berry, J, & Howard, R, 2001, *Teamworking in rehabilitation: exploring the role of the nurse*, English National Board for Nursing, Health Visiting and Midwifery, London. Researching Professional Education, Research Reports Series Number 19.

Long, AF, Kneafsey, R, Ryan, J, & Berry, J, 2002, The role of the nurse within the multi-professional rehabilitation team, *Journal of Advanced Nursing*, vol. 37, no. 1, pp. 70–78.

Lotze, M, Braun, C, Birbaumer, N, Anders, S, & Cohen, LG, 2003, Motor learning elicited by voluntary drive, *Brain*, vol. 126, no. 4, pp. 866–872.

Lum, PS, Burgar, CG, Shor, PC, Majmundar, M, & Van der Loos, M, 2002, Robot-assisted movement training compared with conventional therapy techniques for the rehabilitation of upper-limb motor function after stroke, *Archives of Physical Medicine and Rehabilitation*, vol. 83, no. 7, pp. 952–959.

Marieb, E, & Hoehn, K, 2007, *Human Anatomy and Physiology*, 7th edn, Pearson, San Francisco.

Markham, CH, 1987, Vestibular control of muscular tone and posture, *Journal of Canadian Science and Neurology*, vol. 14, no. 3 Suppl, pp. 493–496.

Massion, J, 1994, Postural control system, *Current Opinion in Neurobiology*, vol. 4, no. 6, pp. 877–887.

McGuire, T, Moody, J, & Hanson, M, 1996, An evaluation of mechanical aids used within the NHS, *Nursing Standards*, vol. 11, no. 6, pp. 33–38.

Moreland, JD, Thomson, MA, & Fuoco, AR, 1998, Electromyographic biofeedback to improve lower extremity function after stroke: a meta-analysis, *Archives of Physical Medicine and Rehabilitation*, vol. 79, no. 2, pp. 134–140.

Morris, SL, Dodd, KJ, & Morris, ME, 2004, Outcomes of progressive resistance strength training following stroke: a systematic review, *Clinical Rehabilitation*, vol. 18, no. 1, pp. 27–39.

Mortensen, PA, & Eng, JJ, 2003, The use of casts in the management of joint mobility and hypertonia following brain injury in adults: a systematic review, *Physical Therapy*, vol. 83, pp. 648–658.

Mutch, K, 2004, Changing manual-handling practice in a stroke rehabilitation unit, *Professional Nurse*, vol. 19, no. 7, pp. 374–378.

Nelles, G, Spiekermann, G, Jueptner, M, Leonhardt, G, Muller, S et al., 1999, Reorganization of sensory and motor systems in hemiplegic stroke patients. A positron emission tomography study, *Stroke*, vol. 30, no. 8, pp. 1510–1516.

Ng, SS, & Shepherd, RB, 2000, Weakness in patients with stroke: implications for strength training in neurorehabilitation, *Physical Therapy Reviews*, vol. 5, pp. 227–238.

Nichols, DS, 1997, Balance retraining after stroke using force platform biofeedback, *Physical Therapy*, vol. 77, no. 5, pp. 553–558.

O'Driscoll, BR, Howard, LS, & Davison, AG, 2008, BTS guideline for emergency oxygen use in adult patients, *Thorax*, vol. 63 Suppl 6, pp. vi1–68.

Oliver, D, Daly, F, Martin, FC, McMurdo, MET, 2004, Risk factors and risk assessment tools for falls in hospital in-patients: a systematic review. *Age and Ageing*, vol. 33, pp. 122–130.

Olney, S, 2005, Training gait after stroke: a biomechanical perspective, in *Science Based Rehabilitation: Theories into Practice*, K Refshauge, L Ada, & E Ellis, eds., Elsevier, Edinburgh, pp. 159–184.

Page, SJ, & Levine, P, 2006, Back from the brink: electromyography-triggered stimulation combined with modified constraint-induced movement therapy in chronic stroke, *Archives of Physical Medicine and Rehabilitation*, vol. 87, no. 1, pp. 27–31.

Page, SJ, & Levine, P, 2007, Modified constraint-induced therapy in patients with chronic stroke exhibiting minimal movement ability in the affected arm, *Physical Therapy*, vol. 87, no. 7, pp. 872–878.

Page, SJ, Levine, P, & Leonard, AC, 2005, Modified constraint-induced therapy in acute stroke: a randomized controlled pilot study, *Neurorehabilitation and Neural Repair*, vol. 19, no. 1, pp. 27–32.

Pandyan, AD, Cameron, M, Powell, J, Stott, DJ, & Granat, MH, 2003, Contractures in the post-stroke wrist: a pilot study of its time course of development and its association with upper limb recovery, *Clinical Rehabilitation*, vol. 17, no. 1, pp. 88–95.

Peters, SB, & Lee, GP, 2003, Functional impact of shoulder taping in the hemiplegic upper extremity, *Occupational Therapy in Health Care*, vol. 17, no. 2, pp. 35–46.

Pomeroy, VM, & Tallis, RC, 2002, Restoring movement and functional ability after stroke: Now and the future, *Physiotherapy*, vol. 88, no. 1, pp. 3–17.

Pope, P, 2006, *Severe and Complex Neurological Disability: Management of the Physical Condition*, Butterworth-Heinemann, Edinburgh.

Popovic, MB, Popovic, DB, Sinkjaer, T, Stefanovic, A, & Schwirtlich, L, 2002, Restitution of reaching and grasping promoted by functional electrical therapy, *Artificial Organs*, vol. 26, no. 3, pp. 271–275.

Robichaud, JA, & Agostinucci, J, 1996, Air-splint pressure effect on soleus muscle alpha motoneuron reflex excitability in subjects with spinal cord injury, *Archives of Physical Medicine and Rehabilitation*, vol. 77, no. 8, pp. 778–782.

Rodgers, H, Mackintosh, J, Price, C, Wood, R, McNamee, P et al., 2003, Does an early increased-intensity interdisciplinary upper limb therapy programme following acute stroke improve outcome? *Clinical Rehabilitation*, vol. 17, no. 6, pp. 579–589.

Rothwell, JC, 2004, Motor control, in *Physical Management in Neurological Rehabilitation*, 2nd edn, M Stokes, ed., Elsevier, Edinburgh, pp. 3–19.

Rowat, AM, 2001, What do nurses and therapists think about the positioning of stroke patients? *Journal of Advanced Nursing*, vol. 34, no. 6, pp. 795–803.

Royal College of Nursing Rehabilitation and Intermediate Care Nurses' Forum, 2002, *Framework for Rehabilitation Handling*.

Rush, KL, & Ouellet, LL, 1997, Mobility aids and the elderly client, *Journal of Gerontological Nursing*, vol. 23, no. 1, pp. 7–15.

Sackley, CM, & Lincoln, NB, 1996, Physiotherapy treatment for stroke patients: a survey of current practice, *Physiotherapy Theory and Practice*, vol. 12, no. 2, pp. 87–96.

Saunders, DH, Greig, CA, Young, A, & Mead, GE, 2004, *Physical Fitness Training for Stroke Patients (Cochrane Review)*, John Wiley and Sons, Chichester, UK. Issue 3.

Sharma, N, Pomeroy, VM, & Baron, JC, 2006, Motor imagery: a backdoor to the motor system after stroke? *Stroke*, vol. 37, no. 7, pp. 1941–1952.

Shelton, FN, & Reding, MJ, 2001, Effect of lesion location on upper limb motor recovery after stroke, *Stroke*, vol. 32, no. 1, pp. 107–112.

Shortland, AP, Harris, CA, Gough, M, & Robinson, RO, 2002, Architecture of the medial gastrocnemius in children with spastic diplegia, *Developmental Medicine and Child Neurology*, vol. 44, no. 3, pp. 158–163.

Shumway-Cook, A, & Woollacott, M, 2007, *Motor Control: Translating Research into Clinical Practice*, 3rd edn, Lippincott Williams and Wilkins, Philadelphia.

Singer, B, Dunne, J, & Allison, G, 2001, Clinical evaluation of hypertonia in the triceps surae muscles, *Physical Therapy Review*, vol. 6, no. 1, pp. 71–80.

Smith, PS, & Thompson, M, 2008, Treadmill training post stroke: are there any secondary benefits? A pilot study, *Clinical Rehabilitation*, vol. 22, no. 10–11, pp. 997–1002.

St Pierre, J, 1998, Functional decline in hospitalized elders: preventive nursing measures, *AACN Clinical Issues*, vol. 9, no. 1, pp. 109–118.

Stiller, K, & Phillips, A, 2003, Safety aspects of mobilising acutely ill inpatients, *Physiotherapy Theory and Practice*, vol. 19, no. 4, pp. 239–257.

Stoeckmann, T, 2001, Casting for the person with spasticity, *Topics in Stroke Rehabilitation*, vol. 8, no. 1, pp. 27–35.

Tardieu, C, Lespargot, A, Tabary, C, & Bret, MD, 1988, For how long must the soleus muscle be stretched each day to prevent contracture? *Developmental Medicine and Child Neurology*, vol. 30, no. 1, pp. 3–10.

Taub, E, Miller, NE, Novack, TA, Cook, EW, III, Fleming, WC et al., 1993, Technique to improve chronic motor deficit after stroke, *Archives of Physical Medicine and Rehabilitation*, vol. 74, no. 4, pp. 347–354.

Thompson, AJ, Jarrett, L, Lockley, L, Marsden, J, & Stevenson, VL, 2005, Clinical management of spasticity, *Journal of Neurology, Neurosurgery and Psychiatry*, vol. 76, no. 4, pp. 459–463.

Thornton, H, & Kilbride, C, 2004, Physical management of abnormal tone and movement, in *Physical Management in Neurological Rehabilitation*, 2nd edn, M Stokes, ed., Elsevier, Edinburgh, pp. 431–450.

Tuckey, J, & Greenwood, R, 2004, Rehabilitation after severe Guillain-Barre syndrome: the use of partial body weight support, *Physiotherapy Research International*, vol. 9, no. 2, pp. 96–103.

Turner-Stokes, L, & Jackson, D, 2002, Shoulder pain after stroke: a review of the evidence base to inform the development of an integrated care pathway, *Clinical Rehabilitation*, vol. 16, no. 3, pp. 276–298.

Tyson, SF, & Nightingale, P, 2004, The effects of position on oxygen saturation in acute stroke: a systematic review, *Clinical Rehabilitation*, vol. 18, no. 8, pp. 863–871.

Tyson, SF, & Thornton, HA, 2001, The effect of a hinged ankle foot orthosis on hemiplegic gait: objective measures and users' opinions, *Clinical Rehabilitation*, vol. 15, no. 1, pp. 53–58.

Volpe, BT, Krebs, HI, Hogan, N, Edelstein, OL, Diels, C et al., 2000, A novel approach to stroke rehabilitation: robot-aided sensorimotor stimulation, *Neurology*, vol. 54, no. 10, pp. 1938–1944.

Wade, DT, Wood, VA, & Hewer, RL, 1985, Recovery after stroke – the first 3 months, *Journal of Neurology, Neurosurgery and Psychiatry*, vol. 48, no. 1, pp. 7–13.

Ward, AB, 2002, A summary of spasticity management – a treatment algorithm, *European Journal of Neurology*, vol. 9 Suppl 1, pp. 48–52.

Waters, KR, 1991, *The role of the nurse in the rehabilitation of elderly people in hospital*, Unpublished PhD, *University of* Manchester.

Waters, KR, & Luker, KA, 1996, Staff perspectives on the role of the nurse in rehabilitation wards for elderly people, *Journal of Clinical Nursing*, vol. 5, no. 2, pp. 105–114.

Winstein, CJ, Rose, DK, Tan, SM, Lewthwaite, R, Chui, HC et al., 2004, A randomized controlled comparison of upper-extremity rehabilitation strategies in acute stroke: a pilot study of immediate and long-term outcomes, *Archives of Physical Medicine and Rehabilitation*, vol. 85, no. 4, pp. 620–628.

Wolf, SL, Winstein, CJ, Miller, JP, Thompson, PA, Taub, E et al., 2008, Retention of upper limb function in stroke survivors who have received constraint-induced movement therapy: the EXCITE randomised trial, *Lancet Neurology*, vol. 7, no. 1, pp. 33–40.

World Health Organisation, 2001, *International Classification of Functioning, Disability and Health (ICF)*, World Health Organisation, Geneva.

Wulf, G, 2007, Self-controlled practice enhances motor learning: implications for physiotherapy, *Physiotherapy*, vol. 93, no. 2, pp. 96–101.

Chapter 8

Communication

Jane Marshall, Katerina Hilari and Madeline Cruice

Key points

- Communication difficulties are common after a stroke.
- Stroke patients can experience a wide variety of communication difficulties, not all of which are immediately obvious.
- It is important to understand the range of problems which individual stroke patients can demonstrate in order to make best use of remaining communication abilities.
- Particular care needs to be taken when evaluating communication abilities of people from language minority groups and those who have more than one language, to ensure a full and detailed picture is obtained.
- Communication difficulties can significantly affect quality of life, and cause distress and frustration for families, friends and staff as well as stroke survivors.
- Staff should be able to support patients in not only expressing their basic wants and needs but also participating in higher level activities requiring communication; these activities might include understanding their condition, the treatment required and decision-making, as well as normal social interaction.

R   *How have things been since you left hospital? Any health problems?*
S1   *No ... (pause) no new problems.*
R   *What would you say is the most important effect of the stroke in your life?*
S1   *Well, altogether, I am, mix up with speech. And ... I ...*
S2   *Go on.*
S1   *I well, uh,*
S2   *I think what Martha feels is: it's the speech more than anything else – which obviously has been affected – which is the biggest problem. Apart*

*from the physical side, with the hand, it is the speech and getting the
words right. Because she tends, she mixes it up –*

S1 *Yeah.*

S2 *Not all the time.*

R *Are you still seeing speech therapists?*

S1 *Yes, uh, I have to phone, and he, somebody else – I don't know.*

R *So you're going to make a phone call ...?*

S1 *Yes.*

S2 *We're still waiting for, what was it, the speech therapist. She's due out
here this month. As a follow-up.*

S1 *Yes.*

R *So your speech, is your speech making a difference to your life?*

S1 *Yes, it has, it has. In a way. If I'm completely alone with one person,
and it's just me and that person that is speaking. Please beg my pardon
if Danesland come into because – I don't know sometimes.*

(R: Researcher. S1: Danish stroke survivor. S2: stroke survivor's husband.
Interview at six months post-stroke, South London, UK)

Introduction

Communication is important for all aspects of stroke care. This chapter
describes the communication impairments caused by stroke with some examples, and suggests strategies that nurses and other members of the stroke team
can use to facilitate communication. Special considerations in relation to people
from language minority groups are flagged. The role of the speech and language
therapist (SLT, or speech pathologist) for communication is discussed, as is the
impact of communication difficulties in relation to psychosocial issues and
quality of life.

Communication in the acute stroke care context

A variety of factors can make communication in hospital difficult for any
patient, such as anxiety, pain, sleep deprivation, the noisy and unfamiliar environment, and lack of privacy. Staff communication styles and attitudes can also
be unhelpful and create difficulties (McCooey et al. 2000). After a stroke,
problems are often confounded by speech and language impairments. Graham,
who was unable to speak after his stroke, gives this example:

> *[I] attracted the nurses' attention in hospital by throwing things at their
> office, as [I] was unable to call them ... [they] thought I was delirious.*
>
> (Jordan & Kaiser 1996)

Such problems can be made worse by the misconceptions of others. For
example, Elsie's inability to speak was misconstrued as unwillingness, and
Dorothy's as a cause for exclusion:

When you first came into hospital you were a poor little thing. You sat in the corner and wouldn't say a thing. (Hospital porter commenting to Elsie)

(Jordan & Kaiser 1996, p.16)

Initially, as people realised that Dorothy couldn't take part in the conversation, they would talk to me. Perhaps Dorothy would be sat between the two of us and they would talk about her, over her and through her to me. And Dorothy would be sat, as though she was attending a tennis match, looking from one to the other, but nobody was really talking to her … it made her very angry.

(Jordan & Kaiser 1996, p.16)

Research shows that good communication between ward staff and patients has many advantages. It leads to more accurate diagnoses, more effective treatment, better patient compliance and higher patient satisfaction (McCooey et al. 2000). It is also crucial that patients are able to make their needs known to staff and participate in decision-making about their care. Whilst the SLT can play a particular role in creating a positive communication environment, this is the responsibility of all members of the stroke team. Perhaps most importantly, staff need to ensure that their communication behaviours do not add to the barriers faced by stroke patients. This chapter will suggest techniques and strategies that can prevent staff communication behaviours from becoming a barrier, particularly when nursing patients who have communication problems following stroke.

Communication impairments caused by stroke

Aphasia

In the early stages of stroke, just under one-third of patients have aphasia (Enderby & Davies 1989). This is an acquired language disorder arising from brain injury, with stroke being the most common cause. It affects all aspects of language, i.e. speaking, listening, reading and writing, and can even impair non-verbal devices like gestures. Almost everyone with aphasia has left hemisphere damage, as the left brain plays the primary role in processing language. Below are some examples of how people with aphasia define the condition (Parr et al. 1997, pp.104–106):

> 'It's taken my voice'
> 'My brain is just buzzing about and me lips is a different kettle of fish'
> 'It was just as if my brain was a cake and a piece was cut out'
> 'I know the right word, but the wrong word comes out'

One of the most obvious signs of aphasia is a loss of speech. This affects content rather than simply pronunciation. For some people the loss is total. Others, like Karl in Case example 8.1, can produce isolated words or phrases. Repetitive utterances are also fairly common. Unfortunately these are often swear words and cannot be inhibited (Code 1982).

Case example 8.1 Karl, a patient with aphasia.

Karl is a 49-year-old car salesman, admitted to hospital one week ago following a left hemisphere middle cerebral artery stroke causing right-sided hemiplegia and severe aphasia.

Karl grew up in India and spoke Hindi and English fluently before his stroke. Now he is only able to say one repetitive phrase: 'I've got it' and occasional single words, such as 'arm' and 'coffee'. Ward staff are not sure whether these words are accurate. For example, Karl was pointing to his leg when he said 'arm'. His wife has tried speaking to him in Hindi, but says that he was not able to reply. Karl is cooperative with the nurses and follows instructions. For example, if a nurse wants to check his blood pressure he will hold out his arm. Karl is also resourceful. On one occasion a student nurse wanted to take Karl for a bath. He said 'no' which initially surprised the nurse. Then Karl found his calendar of appointments and indicated that he was expecting his physiotherapy.

Karl sometimes becomes very agitated and distressed. These episodes have recently become more frequent. Karl is due to be discharged from hospital in a couple of days.

Case example 8.2 Examples of fluent aphasia.

RG describing Interflora:

'There's a stage of firms that arrange the ... nation of children er er want to insert them in the area where the person that is expected to receive the flowers is going to be so he hasn't got to buy the flowers and wait a hell of a distance for them to come there.' (Marshall et al. 1996)

GF saying how she has been over the weekend:

'I was quite ... erm ... that's why I can't get wayerdkeep erm makes me very erm here up here makes him all ... all setoytaid but these come and I can't it might be because I had another mingsing.' (Robson et al. 1998)

Aphasia is often described as 'non-fluent' or 'fluent'. Karl has non-fluent aphasia, since his speech is hesitant and fragmented. This is also termed Broca's aphasia, after the 19th century neurologist who first described the condition. People with this problem cannot produce grammatical sentences. So they might say 'Saturday ... shops' instead of 'on Saturday I went shopping'. Usually there are problems with word-finding and often dyspraxia (see below). Broca's aphasia typically arises from lesions to the left frontal lobe.

The stroke survivors speaking in Case example 8.2 have fluent aphasia, since the quantity and rate of their speech is normal. However, they are difficult to understand because they make a lot of errors, including nonsense words and neologisms. Puzzlingly, some fluent aphasic speakers seem unaware that their speech is disordered (Marshall et al. 1998). As a result they are surprised and even angry when care staff fail to understand them, and may refuse rehabilitation. Such speakers are sometimes described as having jargon aphasia or Wernicke's aphasia (again after a 19th century scientist). They typically have more posterior lesions than those with Broca's aphasia.

The problems of aphasia extend beyond speech. In most cases there are also difficulties with comprehension. These may be subtle, for example only affecting the understanding of complex language, or profound, where even single words are affected. Typically, comprehension difficulties are most evident in Wernicke's aphasia, although there are exceptions to this.

In the example of Karl (Case example 8.1), he seemed to understand speech. He followed instructions and, when asked if he wanted a bath, responded appropriately. However, we need to be cautious. Karl may have picked up clues from the environment that helped him understand what was being said. For example, the student nurse may have (helpfully) pointed to the bathroom when asking about the bath. We therefore need to test comprehension when no such clues are available before drawing firm conclusions.

Reading and writing are usually impaired in aphasia. Not being able to read in the acute care environment can be particularly disorientating for the patient. For example, the person may not be able to read basic signs such as 'toilet', 'dining room', and 'call bell', or recognise their name. It will also be difficult to select options from a menu card. Writing varies across individuals. Some people are completely unable to write, while others achieve occasional written words, or even sentences. Importantly, we often see dissociations between writing and speech. So someone who has no meaningful speech may be able to write a few words (and vice versa). As with speech, people with aphasia often make errors in writing. So they might write MOTHER when they meant to write 'wife' or make a spelling error, such as WITE. Also many people with aphasia have to write with their non-preferred hand, because they have a right hemiplegia. This will add to their difficulties by making writing slow and effortful. Writing problems can be very distressing, possibly because of the negative impact on the person's self-esteem.

Research has produced conflicting findings about prognosis in aphasia. For example, some studies find that younger patients achieve better outcomes than older patients, (e.g. Holland et al. 1989), whereas others do not (Wertz & Dronkers 1990). Less disputed is the relationship between initial severity and recovery. So, people with low initial scores on language tests also have the poorest final scores (Basso 1992; De Riesthal & Wertz 2004). Despite this, most people with aphasia improve to some extent, providing there are no further neurological events. Progress is most rapid in the period immediately following the stroke, but may continue throughout the first year and even beyond. We also know that recovery may be assisted by speech and language therapy, particularly when two or more hours per week are provided (Robey 1998; Bhogal, Teasell & Speechley 2003).

Identifying aphasia

The SLT plays the key role in diagnosing aphasia. However, most patients are referred to SLT by nurses, doctors and other rehabilitation staff. It is therefore important to pick up the signs of aphasia that might prompt a referral (see Table 8.1).

In some cases there may be obvious communication problems, but it may be less obvious whether these are due to aphasia. For example, relatives may hint

Table 8.1 Signs of aphasia.

Modality	Possible signs
Speech	Limited output with long pauses
	Obvious word-finding difficulties
	Word selection or production errors, such as calling a carrot a 'potato' or a 'karrik'
	Fluent but incomprehensible speech that may contain non-words
	Grammatical errors or a lack of grammar
Comprehension	Failure to follow instructions
	Errors in following instructions, such as looking down when asked to look up
	Helped by repetition, simplified speech, pointing and gesture
Reading and writing	Refuses books and newspapers, or only chooses texts with pictures
	Fails to complete menu card or makes obviously incorrect selections
	Not able to clarify information when given a pen and paper
	Distress when asked to write
	Obvious discrepancy between pre-morbid writing and current abilities
	Word selection or spelling errors in writing; only parts of words achieved

at a dementia that pre-dated the stroke. In these instances a referral should still be made to the SLT as they can help clarify the diagnosis. Aphasia can also be difficult to identify in patients who speak little or no English. Again a referral should be made, so that a language assessment can be conducted through an interpreter or bilingual co-worker (see below).

The SLT will be able to confirm whether or not aphasia is present, often by using a screening test. This may take the form of a quick to administer language measure (e.g. the Frenchay Aphasia Screening Test; Enderby et al. 1987), or a structured interview (e.g. the Inpatient Functional Communication Interview – IFCI; McCooey et al. 2004). The therapist will also be interested in nurses' observations about the patient. Indeed the IFCI includes a Staff Questionnaire, which asks nurses (or other staff) to indicate how patients communicate on the ward.

Strategies to use when nursing patients with aphasia

Communication problems that arise from aphasia make nursing difficult. However, there are a number of strategies that can be applied, Karl's use of his calendar being a good example.

For a start, everyone should think carefully about the language they use. For example, most people with aphasia struggle if sentences are long or complex; they understand concrete words better than abstract ones. Concrete words refer to things that can be seen and touched, examples being banana and drum. Abstract words refer to concepts that cannot be experienced by the senses,

Table 8.2 Adapting language for the patient with aphasia.

Message	Aphasia friendly version
After I have taken your blood pressure I need to give you your cardiac medication	I am going to take your blood pressure (the nurse shows the patient the equipment and carries out the test). Now I need to give you your pills (the nurse shows the patient the medication). They are for your heart (the nurse gestures to his/her own heart)
After you have been discharged tomorrow you will receive correspondence from us about your review appointment	Tomorrow you are going home. The doctor will write to you. She will ask you to come back to the hospital so we can find out how you are getting on

examples being democracy and idea. Therefore, short simple speech, constructed mainly from concrete words, is easier. Many people with aphasia are helped by slowed speech, although it is important that this does not sound patronising. Table 8.2 gives examples of how to make speech 'aphasia friendly'.

Clues about what is being said can also accompany speech. So, if a nurse wants to tell a man with aphasia that they are going to give him an injection, it would be a good idea to show him the syringe, or make a simple gesture. Many people with aphasia find written words and pictures helpful. So, if the patient is being taken for a scan, it would be a good idea to show him the written sign and a picture of the equipment. It can be difficult to know whether a person with aphasia has understood. In some cases they may even repeat what you say, but without comprehension. Therefore, important information should be conveyed several times, with the support of pictures, written words and symbols.

Other things can also help a person with aphasia get their message across. Firstly, give them plenty of time and do not be afraid of silences. Remind the person to use alternatives to speech. For example, if the person has a pain, they can be asked to point to where it hurts. Some people with aphasia make very effective use of gesture or drawing, either spontaneously or in response to therapy (Rose 2006; Sacchett et al. 1999). It is also worth exploring whether writing is better than speech, for example by giving the person a pen and paper when they are trying to convey something. If the person is able to produce some speech, remember that it may contain errors: important information should be checked for accuracy. This is an example of a nurse doing this:

Nurse   Do you take any pills or medicine?
Patient   Yes ... er espro
Nurse   Is that aspirin (writes 'aspirin')?
Patient   Yes
Nurse   How many do you take each day?
Patient   er ... four
Nurse   (Writes 4 and holds up four fingers) You take four. Is that right?
Patient   No ... er one
Nurse   (Writes 1 and holds up one finger) You take one. Is that right?
Patient   Yes.

Some people with aphasia are helped by cues when they are stuck for a word. For example, providing them with the first sound of a word, or information about its meaning may help them to say it (Nickels 1997). However, this is rather unnatural and only works if the nurse knows the target word. So, an alternative is to provide people who have aphasia with props to assist with communication. Karl had a written weekly calendar of his rehabilitation appointments that was kept by his bed. By using this, he could show the student nurse that it was not a good time for his bath. Other props include communication charts, with symbols for everyday basic needs, maps, family photographs and pictures. There are also special resources to assist communication with people with aphasia, like 'Stroke Talk' (Cottrell & Davies 2006), which has been designed to help with commonly encountered tests and treatments during a hospital stay after stroke (for example, see http://www.ukconnect.org/upload/StrokeTalksamplepages.pdf).

Dysarthria and dyspraxia

Dysarthria and dyspraxia are problems of speech production, rather than language. So, assuming there are no other deficits, the person will be able to read, write and comprehend what other people say. Their own speech, however, will be difficult, if not impossible, to understand.

Annette (Case example 8.3) has dysarthria, a condition affecting at least 20% of stroke patients (Warlow et al. 2000). In dysarthria the neurological control of the muscles involved in speech is disrupted. These are the muscles of the chest, used for breathing, the muscles of the larynx, used for voice production, and the muscles of the face, tongue, lips and throat, used for articulation (making different speech sounds). There are different types of dysarthria, depending on the nature of the neurological damage (see Table 8.3). Flaccid, spastic and ataxic are the most common *single* types of dysarthria following

---

Case example 8.3 Annette, a patient with dysarthria.

Annette is 43 years old and has a thriving life coaching business. She has a moderate hearing loss in her left ear, for which she uses a hearing aid. Annette was admitted to hospital five hours ago with slurred speech and difficulties swallowing. The CT scan suggests that Annette has suffered a brainstem stroke, in the area where both the left and right upper motor neuron pathways run together (causing bilateral damage). She is finding it extremely difficult to communicate with nursing staff, and is very distressed by her uncontrollable crying (a pseudobulbar effect) and the way she looks (drooling onto her blouse). Her hearing aid has been lost en route to the hospital, making it hard for her to hear other people's and her own speech. Annette's speech is slow and it takes a lot of effort for her to talk. Despite this, she is still difficult to understand. She sounds monotone and her voice has a strained-strangled quality. The SLT has already assessed Annette's swallow. Later when Annette had rested for a couple of hours, the SLT returns to determine what parts of Annette's speech are affected by her stroke. Her symptoms suggest a spastic dysarthria.

Table 8.3 The six different types of dysarthria (Murdoch 1990).

Type of dysarthria	Signs and symptoms
Flaccid	Nasal sounding speech with air escaping down the nose, breathy voice, audible breathing, imprecise consonants, flat speech with no variation of pitch, harsh voice quality, short phrases and no variation in loudness; particular speech characteristics depend on which nerves are damaged
Spastic	Spasticity, weakness, limited range of movement, slowness of movement; slow, effortful speech
Hypokinetic	Reduction in the amplitude (size) of voluntary movements, slowness of movement, initiation difficulties, muscular rigidity, loss of automatic movements, tremor at rest, no variation in pitch, reduced stress (or speech emphasis), no variation in loudness; common in patients with Parkinson's disease
Hyperkinetic	Abnormal involuntary movements, which disturb the rhythm and rate of speech; there are quick and slow forms of hyperkinesiac movements
Ataxic	Arises from damage to the cerebellum; characterised by inaccurate articulation, abnormal stress and intonation (affecting lilt and emphasis), and quiet/weak voice
Mixed	Commonly caused by amyotrophic lateral sclerosis (ALS), multiple sclerosis and Wilson's disease. Quite different presentations can result

stroke, with spastic being the most prevalent (Duffy 1995). Dysarthria is often accompanied by dysphagia and both are particularly common after brainstem strokes (Teasell et al. 2002). It can also co-occur with aphasia, although less frequently.

The role of the SLT in managing dysarthria

In the very acute stage, the assessment and management of dysphagia are typically a greater priority than speech (see Chapter 5). Assessment of communication aims to determine the patient's level of intelligibility, or the degree to which speech can be understood, and why this is breaking down. A commonly used test is the Frenchay Dysarthria Assessment (FDA) (Enderby 1983). This explores each aspect of speech, such as breathing, volume, pitch and rate. It also examines the movements of the tongue and the lips and measures the patient's intelligibility with single words and sentences. Such systematic assessment helps to identify which aspects of speech are impaired or intact, so helps to pinpoint appropriate aims for therapy. Results on the FDA are recorded on a graph and this is often included in the patient's notes.

As time progresses, the SLT will involve the patient and family more in discussing their perception of the patient's speech. This is important as therapy for dysarthria typically requires the patient to monitor and exert more control over their speech. Other aspects of therapy include speech exercises, and training in compensatory strategies, such as slowed speech, gesture and writing (for examples of therapy see Mackenzie & Lowit 2007). In some cases, particularly where there is no accompanying aphasia, technological aids may be recommended, such as keyboard-activated speech synthesisers.

Dysarthria can be caused by a number of conditions aside from stroke, such as Parkinson's disease and motor neuron disease. Patients with dysarthria from stroke often have a good prognosis for recovery. A recent study found that 40% of patients had normal speech at six months post-stroke, and most of the others had only mild impairments (Urban et al. 2006).

Dyspraxia

A variety of dyspraxias can occur after stroke, for example affecting limb movements or dressing. This condition can also disrupt the coordination and sequencing of speech movements. This happens whenever speech is planned, i.e. when the person wants to say something or is asked to talk. Surprisingly, automatic speech may still be possible; so the person may be able to recite the days of the week or count. Dyspraxia is marked by hesitant, imprecise speech, with errors on the sounds of words. Often there are signs of struggle during speech, as the person tries to control the movements of their tongue and lips. In severe cases, all speech is impossible. Although dyspraxia may occur in isolation it often coexists with aphasia. It typically arises from left hemisphere damage. Both aphasia and dyspraxia are more commonly associated with stroke than dysarthria (Yorkston et al. 1987).

Strategies to use when nursing a patient with dysarthria or dyspraxia

Dysarthria makes it difficult for the patient to communicate their needs and concerns (Box 8.1). Often problems are worse with fatigue, so it is best to hold important conversations in the morning or after a period of rest. They are also affected by posture, so it is important that the patient is in an upright sitting

---

Box 8.1   Communication strategies for supporting the patient with dysarthria (adapted from American Speech-Language-Hearing Association (ASHA) 2007).

Try to speak to the patient in a quiet environment with no distractions:
- Hold important conversations in the morning when the patient is most rested
- Make sure the patient is in a good sitting position
- If relevant, make sure the patient has their hearing aid and glasses
- Pay careful attention to the patient and watch them as they talk
- Be honest and let the patient know if you do not understand them; do not pretend to understand
- Repeat the part of the message that you understood so that the patient does not have to repeat the entire message
- If you cannot understand the message after repeated attempts, ask yes/no questions and/or encourage the patient to write

Things to suggest to the patient:
- Encourage them to indicate the topic with a word or a short phrase, before they attempt a full sentence
- Encourage them to speak slowly and loudly, and pause frequently
- Encourage them to use other methods as well as speech, such as pointing, gesturing, or writing key words
- Finally, if the patient gets frustrated, encourage them to take a rest, and come back later to try communicating again

position. Talking during concurrent activities, especially eating, is no longer possible, so distractions need to be removed. It is important that communication is made as easy as possible, so, for example, ensure that the patient can hear properly (remember Annette's hearing aid). Depending on the nature of the damage, patients with dysarthria often have unimpaired language and cognition, so can make good use of strategies and easily follow spoken or written instructions.

Lesions in the right hemisphere

Lesions in the right hemisphere (RHD) can cause a range of problems (see Chapter 9). These include left-side neglect; visual agnosias, including occasionally prosopagnosia (face-blindness); constructional apraxia (inability to assemble parts correctly to make a meaningful whole, e.g. being unable to copy a two- or three-sided design); and disorientation in space. There may be anosognosia, that is, a lack of awareness of illness or disability; and problems of attention, memory, organisation and problem solving. Some individuals lose the perception of sounds, making it difficult for them to appreciate music. Many of these problems have consequences for communication (Cherney & Halper 1999), and are distressing for the person and their family. Face-blindness, for example, can result in the patient not recognising his own wife or children.

In the 1960s it was recognised that RHD may affect language (Eisenson 1962). Eisenson (1962) found that people with RHD often failed 'difficult' language tests, for example where they had to finish a sentence with an abstract word. He concluded that the right hemisphere might be involved in high-level and abstract language processing. Overall, up to 50% of people with RHD show language difficulties, with about 20% having a marked impairment (Benton & Bryan 1996). Problems include:

- Difficulties interpreting the context of a conversation or the speaker's intentions. These are called pragmatic difficulties. A person with RHD may have no problems understanding the words they hear but they may have difficulty interpreting non-verbal signs or the overall meaning of a conversation. For example, they may want to ask a passing nurse a question, while missing signs that the nurse is dealing with something else and is in a hurry. Pragmatic difficulties are often evident in non-verbal behaviours, such as reduced eye contact, reduced facial expression and reduced use of gesture. There may be difficulties with intonation and stress; the person's own speech may sound flat and they may not be able to interpret other people's intonation, for example, to detect anger or amusement.
- Difficulties with non-literal uses of language. These include difficulties with jokes, metaphors and with making inferences.
- Difficulties with conversation, such as verbosity (wordiness) and poor turn-taking. The person may be poor at keeping to the topic of a conversation, or may stick inappropriately on the same topic.

> **Case example 8.4** James, a patient with right hemisphere damage. In his initial assessment, the SLT noticed that James had a blank facial expression and his speech lacked intonation. He talked a lot but had a tendency to take everything literally and veer off the topic in conversation.
>
> James is an 83-year-old retired judge. He lives with his wife who has disabling visual and hearing problems and is her main carer. James was admitted to hospital with left-sided weakness and slurred speech. A CT scan confirmed a small area of haemorrhage in the right parietal lobe. Other left-sided signs included facial weakness, neglect, absent reflexes and reduced sensation.
>
> James was referred to SLT for his speech and swallowing problems. Sarah, his nurse, said he followed instructions and although his speech was quiet and somewhat slurred (James has dysarthria), she could understand what he was saying. However, James's daughter reported difficulties conversing with her father. Sarah could not understand why this was, although she noticed that James missed light-hearted comments, did not smile or engage much with the other patients. Betty, the person in the bed next to his, complained that he ignored her and described him as 'odd'. Also, James seemed forgetful and anxious. He asked the same questions again and again, e.g. who was looking after his wife while he was in hospital.

- Reading and writing deficits. These may arise from visuo-spatial disturbances or from the pragmatic and cognitive deficits. People with the latter will not follow the plot of a story and will misinterpret humour, irony and metaphor. As a result, reading for pleasure will be lost. Visuo-spatial impairments make it difficult to cope with page layouts. There may be left neglect dyslexia (failure to read information in the left visual field) causing errors with the beginning of words or sentences. There may be comparable problems in writing (the person may only write on the right side of a page and may make spelling errors on the left of words, e.g. writing 'Lenny' instead of 'Penny').

Taking all this into account, it is easier to understand James's problems (Case example 8.4). James's RHD took away his sense of humour. It caused him to take things literally and miss the person's intention to make a joke. His daughter often commented on how she missed his witty sense of humour. In conversations, James's facial expression was flat and he would often pick on a minor detail and talk about it at length. His problems with inference affected his interactions with Betty. For example, once Betty wanted to borrow James's newspaper. She hinted at this by saying 'I wonder what's in the news today'. James completely missed her intention and simply said 'I don't know', which upset her.

Strategies to use when nursing a person with RHD

Right hemisphere communication deficit does not present the same challenges as aphasia, in that these individuals can usually follow simple instructions and make their basic needs known. As we have seen, however, their subtle pragmatic problems will affect communication on the ward. In addition, difficulties in laying down new memories will affect their ability to cope with the changes

Table 8.4 Strategies to help the patient with RHD.

Modality	Sign	Strategy
Comprehension	Takes expressions like 'the physio will be up in a minute' literally and gets anxious when the physio is 'late'	Be literal, e.g., say 'the physio will be up soon'
	Has difficulty drawing inferences	Be clear and check understanding
		If appropriate, alert other patients to the nature of RHD communication difficulties
	Has difficulty recognising the speaker's intention	Make your intention obvious; e.g. if you are being funny say: 'I am only joking'
Memory	Gets disorientated; asks the same questions again and again	Have a daily routine. Discuss the routine, e.g. at the beginning of the day and after lunch
	Forgets appointments	Have a diary of events and frequently remind the patient to use it
	Does not practise exercises	
Reading	Has difficulty reading menu cards, TV guide due to left side neglect	Have something of different texture and colour under reading material, and track the left edge with finger before starting reading
		Write key words vertically

caused by stroke and can make them appear obsessively worried, for example, because they ask the same questions over and over again. Alternatively, awareness and memory disorders can make them seem indifferent to their problems and to the efforts of the stroke team. Above all it is worth remembering that people with RHD have problems with social communication. This will affect their relationships with other patients and, potentially, with staff. Being aware of these difficulties is essential to ensure their well-being on the ward. Table 8.4 summarises some ways to help.

Language minorities

It is very important that aphasia and other communication impairments are not missed in stroke patients from minority language groups (for evidence that this can happen, see Marshall et al. 2003). For example, we should not assume that communication problems following stroke simply reflect limited premorbid English. Ideally, the patient should be assessed by a speech and language therapist from his or her language community. If this is not possible, the therapist will assess through interpreters or bilingual co-workers. It is preferable not to use family members and friends as interpreters, as this can disrupt family relationships and yield unreliable data (Roberts 2001). Relatives can, however, provide invaluable insights, for example about what happens when the person tries to speak in their home language(s).

If the person is bi- or multilingual it is important that all their languages are assessed. In our case example of aphasia (see Case example 8.1), Karl's Hindi and English were both affected. Karl's case is typical, in that aphasia rarely leaves one language unscathed. However, the profile of impairments may vary, with one language being stronger than another: see examples in Fabbro (1999). Typically the language that was learnt earlier in life, or which was used most commonly by the individual, is most resistant to damage. However, occasionally the person's second language is less impaired following stroke. Discrepancies like this call for careful assessment to uncover whatever language resources remain to the individual.

The role of the speech and language therapist in acute stroke care

The SLT has four main responsibilities, which are to:

- Assess the patient's communication and swallowing impairments and their impact on the patient's life
- Help the patient communicate on the ward
- Advise the patient, family members and care staff about communication and swallowing
- Provide therapy to reduce the communication and swallowing problems

Assessment

SLT assessment aims to find out the nature and severity of the communication impairment, its effect on communication activities and the role played by environmental factors. Assessment may additionally explore broader issues such as social participation and quality of life (Hilari et al. 2003b). A further purpose is to provide a baseline against which recovery can be compared. Therapists draw upon the views of the patient and family during assessment. For example, they will ask how they perceive the difficulties and elicit their priorities for intervention (Pound et al. 2000). Therapists also consult with the nursing and rehabilitation staff to determine how the patient is communicating with them during activities of the day, for example at mealtimes or ward rounds.

Therapists have a number of measures for exploring these issues, such as formal speech and language tests and interview protocols (i.e. for the patient and/or family members). They will often record and analyse samples of the patient's language and carry out informal observation, for example to find out how the person responds to conversation or copes with situations on the ward.

Supporting communication on the ward

Hospital patients have important communication needs. For example, they need to understand their medical diagnosis and its implications. They probably want to ask questions about their care and the various procedures they are undergoing. At the most basic level, they need to be able to call for a nurse. These functions can be hard if there are communication impairments following a stroke. Through observation and discussion with ward staff, the SLT can help to pinpoint the particular communication needs of each patient, and help them meet those needs during the hospital stay. This is likely to involve the implementation of strategies such as providing pictures or symbols in place of words for important signs. Often the therapist will offer short training sessions for ward staff on how to make communication easier, both with all stroke patients and in specific cases.

Advice

Most people know very little about the communication impairments arising from stroke (Code et al. 2001; Elman et al. 2000). Patients and family members are therefore in great need of information, for example about the nature of the problem and how to help (see below). Advice may be provided individually, or through relatives' support groups and training programmes. Such provision makes a positive impact on family interaction (Turner & Whitworth 2006).

Therapy

Results from assessment will help direct therapy. In many cases, therapy is provided by the community team after the patient returns home. However, it may begin in hospital. Therapy methods are diverse and include language exercises, group work and work on strategic compensation, such as gesture or drawing. Often therapy will involve family members, friends and staff, for example to give them skills in communicating with the person who has aphasia. Case example 8.5 provides an example of therapy.

Case example 8.5 Rachael, an example of speech and language therapy.

Rachael was 75 years old when she had a left hemisphere stroke causing severe aphasia and a right hemiplegia. Her speech was fluent but incomprehensible, with almost no recognisable words. Her writing was also affected, although she could occasionally write part of a word. Rachael could still understand spoken and written words, but not complex sentences. Rachael was a retired academic who lived alone in a first floor flat. She had two loyal friends who visited regularly. Communication about Rachael's nursing and care needs resulted in frequent misunderstandings. For example, Rachael often refused to be taken to physiotherapy, particularly if the therapist was unfamiliar. She also found it very difficult to make requests, e.g. if she needed her glasses or the lavatory.

The first communication aim, therefore, was to alleviate these difficulties. The SLT produced a *chart of strategies* to use when communicating with Rachael. This was discussed with Rachael, and given to all staff and her friends. With Rachael, the SLT developed *a simple booklet of her main rehabilitation and care needs*. On one page she wrote 'physiotherapy' alongside a photo of the gym. This booklet was then used consistently by all members of the team. The therapist practised using the booklet with Rachael, for example to help her make requests.

The therapist also employed *writing therapy*. The aim was for Rachael to write ten words that related to her immediate needs, examples being the names of clothing, the names of her friends, and object names like 'toothbrush'. Rachael practised these words in tasks that progressed from copying, copying after a delay, filling in a missing letter and finally writing the name from a picture. Once Rachael could make a recognisable attempt at all these words, they were incorporated into communication activities. For example, the therapist might ask Rachael 'who is visiting this afternoon?' as a cue for her to write her friend's name. Therapy was also stepped up by introducing new words.

It was clear that Rachael would have long-term mobility, daily living and communication needs. It was important that this was discussed with Rachael and that she was fully involved in *decisions about her future*. However, her severe language impairments made this hard. Working with Rachael's friends, the SLT and occupational therapist instituted a programme of consultation. They used photographs of Rachael's flat to identify the obstacles that she would face (such as the stairs). They also mapped out a typical day (with pictures) and thought about the help that she would need (e.g. with dressing). The therapists then provided Rachael with labels and images of the different care options. For example, they outlined how Rachael might be supported at home, with images of a stair lift, visiting care staff, meals on wheels, bath hoist and a panic button. They also showed her brochures from local residential homes, with simplified financial information about the fees. Rachael was able to use these images to indicate her preference, which was for residential care. This was followed up with a visit to a care home and a successful trial stay.

Psychosocial issues and quality of life

Onset and acute care

The onset of stroke with acquisition of a speech or language impairment is a crisis point in a person's life. To date, much of our evidence about this comes from people with aphasia. For example, they report feelings of shock, anger, frustration, anxiety (particularly about the toilet), aggression, shame, guilt, grief, loss and embarrassment (Lafond et al. 1993; Parr et al. 1997). It is also important to recognise that stroke can isolate patients from one another, as illustrated by Betty and James earlier in this chapter, and by Jean's comment here:

> *When I had a stroke I found nobody talk to me and that other patients you know walk by the bed and look and um let's [never] say a word because they knew I couldn't speak. (Jean, Personal Insights audiotape, Dysphasia Matters package)*

(Davies & Woolf 1997)

Family members may also be overwhelmed by negative feelings. A recent study stressed their need for support and information in the acute stages of stroke (Avent et al. 2005). Families wanted answers to questions like: what is stroke? What is aphasia? What are the coexisting problems? Where can we get more information? A particular need was for honest but hopeful information about the prognosis. For example, one participant stated:

when I was talking to the therapist, I was like, I have heard all the bad.
How about the positive?

(Avent et al. 2005, p. 359)

It is essential to provide accessible information for people with aphasia and their families and the SLT can help with this. This is important, as many existing leaflets are too difficult for people with aphasia to read and understand. Useful resources are: *The Stroke and Aphasia Handbook* (Parr et al. 2004) and the *Stroke Talk* manual (Cottrell & Davies 2006), both available from Connect (http://www.ukconnect.org).

Discharge

Discharge from hospital, although eagerly anticipated, can be a time of particular stress for both the patient and family. There may be uncertainty about the future and worries about coping with the mobility and communication problems at home (see (Parr et al. 1997). Karl (Case example 8.1) showed increased signs of distress as discharge approached. A big concern is safety, including communication safety. For example, it is essential that the person has a method of summoning help in an emergency.

It is important to ensure that when patients are discharged, they have accurate information and strategies in place to assist communication. Research emphasises the importance of information and support at this time. For example, the participants in the Avent et al. (2005) study felt it was crucial to leave hospital armed with information about support groups and other resources in the community. It is also critical that care plans are put in place, and that these are effective:

You leave with this great package and are told you will be getting all this back-up. You think great there will be all this back-up then nothing materialises for six weeks. You get home and think great, physio is going to come and this person is going to come and nobody comes at all and then six weeks later they come. Once it happens it's alright, but when you first get home nothing, it's really awful.

(Anderson 1992)

The needs of stroke patients and their family persist after discharge. Wiles et al. (1998) found that families still needed information about recovery and prognosis well past discharge, together with advice about practical tasks and social activities.

Long term

Communication disability has a long-term negative impact on recovery after stroke (Tilling et al. 2001). It significantly affects quality of life, even when other variables, such as emotional state and social support, are factored out (Cruice et al. 2003; Hilari et al. 2003a). The long-term social consequences of stroke and aphasia include loss of work and consequent drop in income, a need to give up driving, restrictions in social life, and falling away of friends (Cruice et al. 2006; Hilari & Northcott 2006; Parr et al. 1997). There may be lasting emotional effects such as volatility, irritability, loss of confidence and fear of another stroke. Fatigue is often a profound and persistent problem.

However, the long-term picture for people with communication difficulties after stroke is not all negative. Some individuals report positive changes that include: freedom from previous restrictions including work; having more time; a slower, more relaxed lifestyle; closer family relationships; and an enhanced sense of the value of life (Parr in Jordan & Kaiser 1996). There are personal accounts in the literature of individuals with long-term aphasia who have achieved new and satisfying lives (see Hinckley (2006) and Aphasia Now website: http://www.aphasianow.org). Positive experiences of care in the acute phase can be the first step towards attaining this goal.

Conclusion

Whilst communication problems are common, many and various after stroke, and can negatively affect all aspects of recovery, rehabilitation, well-being and quality of life for the stroke survivor as well as family and friends, the picture is not all bleak. Some degree of spontaneous recovery occurs with some impairments, and therapies are available with demonstrated effectiveness. A wide range of strategies can support communication with affected stroke survivors. Education, explanation and teaching for families, next of kin and carers are also priorities, not just in preparation for discharge from hospital or transfer of care, but to help maintain normal social communication and relationships.

Whilst speech and language therapists have a key role in this, it is essential that nurses, with their 24-hour, seven days per week contact with stroke patients in hospital and during rehabilitation have a good understanding of this topic. Ultimately, however, all members of the multidisciplinary stroke team require expertise and skills in supporting communication with communication-impaired stroke survivors, and it is important that all who work with stroke patients incorporate these within their daily practice.

Acknowledgements

The authors thank Elina Tripoliti for her helpful comments on the Dysarthria section of this chapter.

References

American Speech-Language-Hearing Association (ASHA), 2007, *Dysarthria*, http://www.asha.org/public/speech/disorders/dysarthria.htm 20/11/2009.

Anderson, R, 1992, *The Aftermath of Stroke: The Experience of Patients and Their Families*, Cambridge University Press, Cambridge.

Avent, J, Glista, S, Wallace, S, Jackson, J, Nishioka, J et al., 2005, Family information needs about aphasia, *Aphasiology*, vol. 19, no. 3–5, pp. 365–375.

Basso, A, 1992, Prognostic factors in aphasia, *Aphasiology*, vol. 6, pp. 337–348.

Benton, E, & Bryan, K, 1996, Right cerebral hemisphere damage: incidence of language problems, *International Journal of Rehabilitation Research*, vol. 19, no. 1, pp. 47–54.

Bhogal, SK, Teasell, R, Speechley, M, 2003, Intensity of Aphasia Therapy, Impact on Recovery. Stroke vol 34 pp. 987–993

Cochrane Stroke Review Group at http://www.dcn.ed.ac.uk/csrg/

Cherney, LR, & Halper, AS, 1999, Group treatment for patients with right hemisphere damage, in *Group Treatment of Neurogenic Communication Disorders: The Expert Clinician's Approach*, R Elman, ed., Butterworth Heinemann, Boston, MA.

Code, C, 1982, Neurolinguistic analysis of recurrent utterance in aphasia, *Cortex*, vol. 18, no. 1, pp. 141–152.

Code, C, Mackie, NS, Armstrong, E, Stiegler, L, Armstrong, J et al., 2001, The public awareness of aphasia: an international survey, *International Journal of Language and Communication Disorders*, vol. 36 Suppl, pp. 1–6.

Cottrell, S, & Davies, A, 2006, *Stroke Talk: Patient Communication Kit*, Connect Press, London.

Cruice, M, Worrall, L, Hickson, L, & Murison, R, 2003, Finding a focus for quality of life with aphasia: social and emotional health, and psychological well-being, *Aphasiology*, vol. 17, no. 4, pp. 333–353.

Cruice, M, Worrall, L, & Hickson, L, 2006, Quantifying aphasic people's social lives in the context of non-aphasic peers, *Aphasiology*, vol. 20, no. 12, pp. 1210–1225.

Davies, P, & Woolf, C, 1997, *Dysphasia Matters: A Training Package for Medical Professionals*, Creative Film Productions.

De Riesthal, M, & Wertz, R, 2004, Prognosis for aphasia: relationship between selected biographical variables and outcome improvement, *Aphasiology*, vol. 18, no. 10, pp. 899–915.

Duffy, J, 1995, *Motor Speech Disorders: Substrates, Differential Diagnosis, and Management*, Mosby, St Louis.

Eisenson, J, 1962, Language and intellectual modifications associated with right cerebral damage, *Language and Speech*, vol. 5, pp. 49–53.

Elman, R, Ogar, J, & Elman, S, 2000, Aphasia: awareness, advocacy and activism, *Aphasiology*, vol. 14, pp. 455–459.

Enderby, P, 1983, *Frenchay Dysarthria Assessment*, Pro-Ed, Austin, Texas.

Enderby, P, & Davies, P, 1989, Communication disorders: planning a service to meet the needs, *British Journal of Disorders of Communication*, vol. 24, no. 3, pp. 301–331.

Enderby, P, Wood, V, & Wade, D, 1987, *Frenchay Aphasia Screening Test*, NFER-Nelson, Windsor.

Fabbro, F, 1999, *The Neurolinguistics of Bilingualism*, Psychology Press, Hove.

Hilari, K, & Northcott, S, 2006, Social support in people with chronic aphasia, *Aphasiology*, vol. 20, no. 1, pp. 17–36.

Hilari, K, Wiggins, RD, Roy, P, Byng, S, & Smith, SC, 2003a, Predictors of health-related quality of life (HRQL) in people with chronic aphasia, *Aphasiology*, vol. 17, no. 4, pp. 365–381.

Hilari, K, Byng, S, Lamping, DL, & Smith, SC, 2003b, Stroke and Aphasia Quality of Life Scale-39 (SAQOL-39): evaluation of acceptability, reliability, and validity, *Stroke*, vol. 34, no. 8, pp. 1944–1950.

Hinckley, JJ, 2006, Finding messages in bottles: living successfully with stroke and aphasia, *Topics in Stroke Rehabilitation*, vol. 13, no. 1, pp. 25–36.

Holland, AL, Greenhouse, JB, Fromm, D, & Swindell, CS, 1989, Predictors of language restitution following stroke: a multivariate analysis, *Journal of Speech and Hearing Research*, vol. 32, no. 2, pp. 232–238.

Jordan, L, & Kaiser, W, 1996, *Aphasia: A Social Approach*, Chapman Hall, London.

Lafond, D, Joanette, Y, Ponzio, J, Degiovani, R, & Taylor Sarno, M, 1993, *Living with Aphasia: Psychosocial Issues*, Singular Publishing Group Inc, California.

Mackenzie, C, & Lowit, A, 2007, Behavioural intervention effects in dysarthria following stroke: communication effectiveness, intelligibility and dysarthria impact, *International Journal of Language and Communication Disorders*, vol. 42, no. 2, pp. 131–153.

Marshall, J, Pring, T, Chiat, S, & Robson, J, 1996, Calling a salad a federation: an investigation of semantic jargon, Paper 1, Nouns, *Journal of Neurolinguistics*, vol. 9, no. 4, pp. 237–250.

Marshall, J, Robson, J, Pring, T, & Chiat, S, 1998, Why does monitoring fail in jargon aphasia? comprehension, judgment, and therapy evidence, *Brain and Language*, vol. 63, no. 1, pp. 79–107.

Marshall, J, Atkinson, J, Thacker, A, & Woll, B, 2003, Is speech and language therapy meeting the needs of language minorities? The case of deaf people with neurological impairments, *International Journal of Language and Communication Disorders*, vol. 38, no. 1, pp. 85–94.

McCooey, R, Toffolo, D, & Code, C, 2000, A socioenvironmental approach to functional communication in hospital in-patients, in *Neurogenic Communication Disorders: A Functional Approach*, L Worrall & C Frattali, eds., Thieme, New York.

McCooey, R, Worrall, L, Toffolo, D, Code, C, & Hickson, L, 2004, *Inpatient Functional Communication Interview*, Singular Publishing.

Murdoch, B, 1990, *Acquired Speech and Language Disorders: A Neuroanatomical and Functional Neurological Approach*, Chapman and Hall, London.

Nickels, L, 1997, *Spoken Word Production and its Breakdown in Aphasia*, Psychology Press, Hove.

Parr, S, Byng, S, & Gilpin, S, 1997, *Talking about Aphasia: Living with Loss of Language After Stroke*, Open University Press, Milton Keynes.

Parr, S, Pound, C, Byng, S, & Long, B, 2004, *The Stroke and Aphasia Handbook*, Connect Press, London.

Pound, C, Parr, S, Lindsay, J, & Woolf, C, 2000, *Beyond Aphasia: Therapy for Living with Communication Disability*, Speechmark, Bicester.

Roberts, P, 2001, Aphasia assessment and treatment for bilingual and culturally diverse patients, in *Language Intervention Strategies in Aphasia and Related Neurogenic Communication Disorders*, 4th edn, R Chapey, ed., Lippincott Williams and Wilkins, Baltimore.

Robey, P, 1998, A meta-analysis of clinical outcomes in the treatment of aphasia, *Journal of Speech, Language and Hearing Research*, vol. 41, pp. 171–187.

Robson, J, Marshall, J, Pring, T, & Chiat, S, 1998, Phonological naming therapy in jargon aphasia: positive but paradoxical effects, *Journal of the International Neuropsychological Society*, vol. 4, pp. 675–686.

Rose, ML, 2006, The utility of arm and hand gestures in the treatment of aphasia, *Advances in Speech Language Pathology*, vol. 8, no. 2, pp. 92–109.

Sacchett, C, Byng, S, Marshall, J, & Pound, C, 1999, Drawing together: evaluation of a therapy programme for severe aphasia, *International Journal of Language and Communication Disorders*, vol. 34, no. 3, pp. 265–290.

Teasell, R, Foley, N, Doherty, T, & Finestone, H, 2002, Clinical characteristics of patients with brainstem strokes admitted to a rehabilitation unit, *Archives of Physical Medicine and Rehabilitation*, vol. 83, no. 7, pp. 1013–1016.

Tilling, K, Sterne, JA, Rudd, AG, Glass, TA, Wityk, RJ et al., 2001, A new method for predicting recovery after stroke, *Stroke*, vol. 32, no. 12, pp. 2867–2873.

Turner, S, & Whitworth, A, 2006, Conversation partner training programmes in aphasia: a review of key themes and participants' roles, *Aphasiology*, vol. 20, no. 6, pp. 483–510.

Urban, PP, Rolke, R, Wicht, S, Keilmann, A, Stoeter, P et al., 2006, Left-hemispheric dominance for articulation: a prospective study on acute ischaemic dysarthria at different localizations, *Brain*, vol. 129, no. 3, pp. 767–777.

Warlow, C, Dennis, M, Van Gijn, J, Hankey, G, Sandercock, P, Bamford, J, & Wardlaw, J, 2000, *Stroke: A Practical Guide to Management*, Blackwell Scientific, Oxford.

Wertz, R, & Dronkers, N, 1990, *Effects of Age on Aphasia*, American Speech-Language Hearing Association, Rockville, MD.

Wiles, R, Pain, H, Buckland, S, & McLellan, L, 1998, Providing appropriate information to patients and carers following a stroke, *Journal of Advanced Nursing*, vol. 28, no. 4, pp. 794–801.

Yorkston, K, Beukelman, D, & Bell, K, 1987, *Clinical Management of Dysarthria Speakers*, Taylor and Francis, London.

Chapter 9

Mood and behavioural changes

Peter Knapp

Key points

- Mood and behavioural changes following a stroke are common.
- Changes are distressing for patients, families and friends.
- If unrecognised and untreated, these changes will have a negative impact on the patient's recovery.
- Early recognition, assessment and onward referral to an appropriate clinician is key.

I just feel I might as well be dead. The only thing is I don't want to die alone, you see, its different when you've got loved ones, nice to have them there when it does happen, but when you're on your own it easy could happen, couldn't it? Any time. What I find the most terrible, it's a day, a day's long, every day when you're on your own. If I could get out it would be better, what people don't understand, there's no pleasure in giving yourself a lot of pain, just to go out … It all goes back to this, you see. I can't help it, I just think, all day. I can't help it, my children say, come on Dad, you've got to cheer up, eat your food, that would be similar advice I would give to someone in my position, but it's not so easy carried out. You can sit and say, and really think you're giving good advice but, and you'd like to think you could do what they say, I know they mean it with all their love, all sincerity, eat your food or you'll be bad, but unless you're a marvellous man I don't think you could do it.

Richard, 72 years old, 6 months post-stroke, South London

Introduction

Stroke can result in many different effects on the patient's mood and behaviour. Many of these changes can be distressing – both for the patient and for their close relatives – and it is common for such changes to have an impact on other outcomes in stroke, such as physical recovery, the return to normal social activities, and longer-term health. Thankfully, many patients find that changes to their mood and behaviour are short-lasting, and there are interventions that can assist in the recovery from changes that are more long-lasting.

There have been a number of significant changes in the way that health professionals care for stroke patients over the past 20 years or so. The care provided to patients with mood and behavioural changes has altered dramatically, largely as a result of an increased recognition of the prevalence of mood disorders. Importantly, there has also been a shift away from the sense that mood disorder after stroke is inevitable (and therefore not responsive to intervention) to a view that most people have some psychological reaction to the onset of stroke, and that mood disorder is a pathological response. A look at general nursing textbooks published in the 1980s reveals that mood disorder, behavioural changes and cognitive impairment are largely ignored in the sections on stroke care.

The increased recognition of these impairments and their effects on patients has resulted in the development of new interventions, some growth in the numbers of professionals skilled to intervene, and an increased quantity of research evidence on the effectiveness of the interventions. However, as will become obvious when reading this chapter, the care provided to patients with mood and cognitive impairments after stroke remains sub-optimal. Disorder and distress continue to be under-recognised; some disorders are incorrectly diagnosed and treated; and the relative lack of a research base means that nurses and doctors may be treating disorders in their patients without a great deal of certainty about the outcomes (Intercollegiate Stroke Working Party 2008).

Psychological reactions to the onset of stroke

The onset of a stroke, particularly in those experiencing a first stroke, can be distressing and worrying. For many patients, the stroke comes without warning, resulting in emergency admission to hospital and an inpatient stay. If the stroke causes a loss of function, whether that is physical or communicative, then the patient is more likely to be unsettled and react emotionally (Hackett & Anderson 2005).

It is common for stroke patients to experience worry, a sense of confusion and tearfulness in the first few days after the onset of stroke. In this way stroke differs little from the onset or acute worsening of many other conditions (Hackett et al. 2005; House et al. 1991). In the first few days patients may have concerns about practical aspects of their lives, often centred on roles and responsibilities. For example, the patient may worry about how their spouse will manage alone at home, or who will run the family business while they are in hospital, or even who will look after family pets. Worries about the future can be more distressing, since, by comparison with concerns about home life, there are no easy practical solutions to take them away. The patient will understandably be concerned about how long-lasting any disability will be, and its possible effects on their ability to carry on their lives as they did before the stroke. This is sometimes seen as role crisis or role anxiety: concerns about their ability or, in this case, future ability to fulfil their normal roles (as partner, parent, worker, social club committee member, and so on).

Early emotional reactions to stroke can also include frustration (provoked by any number of factors, including physical disability, communication problems, and inpatient hospital stay), irritability and anger. Such reactions can be distressing for patients' relatives and may be difficult for staff to deal with, and are sometimes explained as being due to a 'personality change' after stroke. A much more robust explanation is that irritability, frustration, worry and anger are understandable responses to the onset of a sometimes disabling and life-threatening condition.

Coping with stroke

Psychological models of coping can help to explain patients' reactions. Coping theory (for example, see Pearlin & Schooler 1978) explains the way that people respond to threatening events – whether they are anticipated (such as a driving test or dental treatment) or unanticipated (such as being bereaved or becoming seriously ill). Coping theory suggests that people cope, i.e. manage to deal with a threatening situation, by drawing on skills and experience they have used previously. If they respond successfully to the onset of disabling illness, it is because they have successfully adapted skills they may have developed months or years earlier, for example when they became unemployed or were bereaved or dealt with a difficult family situation. That is, people cope successfully by drawing on resources to deal with the demands made by the new threatening situation (Lazarus & Folkman 1984).

However, coping theory argues that problems will arise when the demands are too great and overwhelm people's ability to cope, or when the resources they have to respond to the demand (in this case, the stroke) are insufficient or ineffective. It is in that situation that people will benefit from additional resources, and these may be financial (in the form of disability benefits), instrumental (such as help with personal or household tasks), or psychological (such as emotional support from friends or more formal input from a counsellor).

Not all coping is effective, however, and people may deal with threatening situations in a maladaptive way. Examples include an increased emotional dependence on other people, repeated reassurance seeking, and avoidant behaviours, including denying the existence of the disability or seeking comfort in alcohol or drugs. As with coping that is successful, maladaptive coping is often patterned, in that people use it because it is their conventional response to a threatening situation. So, if their response to any difficult situation is to drink heavily, they are likely to drink heavily after a stroke. Such coping responses are unlikely to be successful, particularly in response to a stroke, which may require weeks or months of concentrated effort on the part of the patient to achieve recovery.

Depression

The emotional outcome most often associated with stroke is depression (or depressed mood), and the frequency with which it is noted after stroke has led some commentators to suggest that post-stroke depression (or PSD) is a distinct type (Robinson 2003). This view holds that depressed mood is in some way physiological in origin, caused by the neurological damage from the stroke. From this viewpoint, lesions located in some areas of the brain are more likely to lead to depressed mood than those located in other areas. However, a systematic review of the studies that have assessed the link between the location of the lesion and mood after stroke showed that it was not strong (Carson et al. 2000). That is, there is no robust evidence that depressed mood after stroke is caused by a lesion in a particular area, or on a particular side of the brain.

Clinical depression is a syndrome, that is, a cluster of symptoms or signs. The symptoms include lowered mood (or affect) lasting for at least a month, which causes distress to the patient. Diagnostic signs also include change in sleep pattern and/or appetite, a lack of pleasure in activities, a pattern of negative thinking (including about one's self-worth) and a lack of energy. That is, clinical depression is a significant pattern of disordered mood and associated symptoms, and is more than a feeling of sadness or consistent tearfulness, distressing though these behaviours can be to the patient and relatives (World Health Organisation 2003).

But is there something about having stroke that leads to depression? Certainly it is true that depression occurs frequently after stroke. Depressed mood is more common in people who have recently had a stroke than people of a similar age without stroke. However, this effect is probably not specific to stroke: higher rates of depression are also seen in people with other disabling conditions, when compared to similar aged people without disability.

There have been so many studies that have looked at the rate of depression after stroke that (Hackett et al. 2005) conducted a systematic review, in an attempt to combine the data from them to produce an overall numerical summary. The review included more than 50 studies and overall they found that depression occurred in about 33% of patients when assessed within a month of stroke. It is important to note that the rates did vary according to the way that depression had been assessed, what sort of stroke patients were included in the study, and how long after the stroke the assessment had been made.

What the studies do show is that not all depression after stroke occurs straight away. Some can occur for the first time many months after stroke (Andersen et al. 1994; House et al. 1991); indeed there is a suggestion (based on anecdote only) that depression is often provoked by the return home after hospital. This onset might be explained by the patient desiring to go home and holding that as a target during the long weeks of inpatient rehabilitation. The return home might be anti-climactic and, perhaps, the difficulty of living at home with a disability becomes a depressing reality. The studies also suggest that depressed mood can be relatively short-lasting in many patients and that it can remit spontaneously, perhaps once the patient is able to adjust psychologically to their disability.

Depression is more likely to occur in stroke patients with significant physical disability, but there is no automatic link between the two (Hackett & Anderson 2005). There are many severely disabled stroke patients who never suffer depression, while there are some patients who become depressed after having a stroke that has caused only minor or transient disability. The relationship between depression and communication impairment is also not straightforward. It is sometimes accepted as fact that the patient who cannot speak or who has trouble speaking is more likely to suffer depression. However, the research evidence suggests that depression is not more likely to occur in patients with communication problems.

One robust predictor of depression after stroke is depression immediately before the stroke, or depression or other psychological problems earlier in life. Depression also tends to occur more often in patients who have little 'social support', that is friends and acquaintances that can be a source of help in difficult times. The absence of close, confiding relationships seems to be particularly important. Depression is also more likely in those who find it difficult to adjust to a new situation. Examples of adjustment difficulties include having expectations of recovery that are unrealistically optimistic, or adopting an overly negative and generalised attitude (so thinking that things will turn out badly).

Diagnosing depression

Depressed mood after stroke should be diagnosed by a clinical interview undertaken by a health professional with appropriate mental health training or experience (Intercollegiate Stroke Working Party 2008). Ideally this would be a psychiatrist or clinical psychologist, although in the UK it is most often undertaken by a stroke physician or general physician. Since depression occurs in about 30% of stroke patients in the first year, its presence ought to be assessed in all patients admitted to hospital after stroke. Conducting a lengthy clinical interview with all patients is unrealistic and unnecessary, and there are brief screening measures that might be used to help identify those patients at risk of depression. These include the General Health Questionnaire GHQ-12 (Goldberg & Williams 1988), the Hospital Anxiety and Depression scale HAD (Zigmond & Snaith 1983), the Geriatric Depression Scale GDS (Yesavage et al. 1982) and the Patient Health Questionnaire PHQ-9 (Kroenke & Spitzer 2002). Each of these has been shown to be valid when used to assess mood in stroke populations. There is evidence that a simple question (such as 'are you feeling depressed?') can be as effective as a questionnaire with 9 or 12 items (Watkins et al. 2007b). One significant advantage of a questionnaire is that it allows the patient's mood score to be assessed and recorded on two or more occasions, to assess change. The questionnaire will give more detail than is possible with a single item 'yes/no' measure.

Asking a patient about their mood, and whether or not they are experiencing particular emotional symptoms, is seen as awkward and uncomfortable by some nurses. However, the situation can be explained to the patient and/or their relatives, by the use of what is sometimes termed a 'permission giving' preamble, such as:

We know that many people who have had a stroke feel low or emotional. Do you mind if I ask you a few questions about how you feel?

or

Sometimes after stroke people find that they that feel as if the situation will never improve. Is that something that you have felt?

Once screening has occurred, it is important that the outcome or score is recorded in the patient's notes, even if the scores indicate that they are unlikely to have a mood disorder. If the scores suggest that that they might be at risk, then this information should be recorded in the notes and the details passed on to the doctor or nurse in charge of their care, and a referral made to the clinician responsible for assessing the patient for possible treatment. It is also important that the information is fed back to the patient, such as:

Thank you for answering those questions. I am a little concerned about your mood and I want to arrange for a doctor to come to see you to ask you some more detailed questions about it.

The use of a screening measure alone should not be enough to indicate that treatment for the depression should be started. This is because screening questionnaires tend to produce 'false positive' scores, with people who don't have depression but scoring highly on the questionnaire (Gilbody et al. 2001). This and the knowledge that much depressed mood after stroke remits without treatment suggest that mood after stroke is best assessed on two separate occasions a few weeks apart (Hill 2008). If a patient scores highly on both occasions, then they should be interviewed clinically and considered for treatment. The obvious exception to this 'double screening' rule is the patient whose depression is so severe (perhaps including suicidal thoughts) that it would be irresponsible not to start treatment after the first assessment.

Assessing for depression after stroke can be very difficult in the patient with significant cognitive or communication problems. If the patient's communication problems are limited to the expressive, then many screening questionnaires can be converted to questions with 'yes/no' response formats: research shows that they can be as effective as the conventional method with spoken responses. However, in patients with more severe cognitive or communication difficulties, question-based assessments of any type are problematic. This has led to the development of alternative methods of assessment. The 'smiley faces' scales are used by some stroke services. However, research suggests that they are not dependable as a method of assessment. Other studies have attempted to develop reliable methods of assessing mood using observation only, that is, by looking at the patient's behaviour. Measures such as the Strengths and Difficulties Questionnaire SDQ-H show some promise, but are currently some way short of being reliable measures that can be depended on (Bennett et al. 2006; Laska et al. 2007; Lee et al. 2008).

It is important that depression after stroke is recognised and treated. Not only can it be distressing for the patient, relatives and staff, but it has been shown to have effects on important outcomes of stroke. For example, patients who become depressed tend to have a longer hospital stay, make less or slower progress in physical rehabilitation, may be less likely to take their medicine as prescribed or to stop smoking, and may be at increased risk of death after stroke. A large cohort study found that patients who were depressed within one month of stroke, particularly those who expressed significant depressive thoughts, were less likely than other stroke patients to be alive one and two years later (House et al. 2001).

Treating depression

The most common treatment for depression after stroke is antidepressant medication, as is the case for older patients in general: one study reported that almost one in seven patients aged 75 and above registered at UK general practices were being prescribed an antidepressant (Petty et al. 2006). The rate of prescribing may be as high as one in three patients within one month of stroke (Ruddell et al. 2007). There is a growing groundswell of opinion that antidepressants are used too liberally and too soon in patients with low mood. After stroke, unless the depression is particularly marked or trouble-some, it may be better to wait for a few weeks and reassess the patient to see if the lowered mood has continued. In patients with mild or borderline depression, it may be useful to introduce counselling, or hobbies or exercise (if possible) or some other social activity. There is no strong evidence in studies of stroke patients that these forms of therapy are effective (Knapp et al. 2000), but they may be helpful in some patients, and should be considered as an early alternative to antidepressants. The research evidence for the effec-tiveness of antidepressants in stroke is not strong, although the studies have tended to be small and have generally not been well conducted, and so are inconclusive (Hackett et al. 2008a, 2008b). An alternative to drug treatment is structured psychological treatment or 'talking treatment'. Such treatment can be given by appropriately trained stroke nurses, and brief therapy comprising a few sessions can be effective. Trials of forms of preventive psychological treatment (problem-solving therapy and motivational interviewing) and case management have shown small but promising effects on reducing the likelihood of being depressed several months later (Watkins et al. 2007a; Williams et al. 2007).

Emotionalism

Emotionalism is a common occurrence after stroke – it is said to affect around 21% of patients six months after the stroke (House et al. 1989) – and is dis-tinctive and easily recognised (see, for example, Case example 9.1). It is some-times called emotional lability, and it is the quickly changeable nature of people's emotions that makes this condition so distinctive. Its cause is not clear, although there is some evidence that it is neurological in origin. The emotional response most often seen is crying, although sometimes people laugh (often in response to sad or upsetting situations). There is a view that the emotional

---

Case example 9.1 Sandra.

Sandra, an active 55-year-old mother of three children and eight grand-children, suffered a stroke that left her unable to walk and dress independently. Sandra was a determined woman and she worked hard in her rehabilitation sessions. She remained positive in her outlook. However, she became emotional when talking about her home and her family. When her children or grand-children visited she struggled to talk to them, such was her tearfulness and upset. Some relatives found this embarrassing and distressing, such that they preferred not to visit. Sandra's reaction was thought not to be depression – her mood remained positive – but emotionalism. Staff spent time explaining the condition to Sandra and her relatives, encouraging them not to stay away from visits. Although her mood was not depressed, treatment with an antidepressant medicine was effective. Over the next three weeks before hospital discharge, the periods of emotionalism occurred less often, such that Sandra was able to talk about her family and have visitors with only occasional tears. Two months after discharge the emotionalism was no longer present and, a few weeks later, she was able to stop the medication.

---

responses of patients with this condition are in some way emotionally 'empty' and not associated with sad thoughts. This is the view often found on the early textbook accounts of emotional lability. The account seen in more recent research is different: it suggests that people with emotionalism do tend to cry (or laugh) to appropriate provocations; that is, the crying or laughing behaviour is most often seen in response to emotionally-laden situations. Emotionalism is also more likely to occur in patients with depressed mood (Calvert et al. 1998).

Emotionalism often responds well to antidepressant treatment (House et al. 2004), adding further to the view that its cause is neurological. When patients have emotionalism, there is an important nursing role in helping the patient (and relatives) to deal with it. It can be distressing for the patient to experience it, and relatives can be upset by it and request interventions to deal with it. There is a suggestion that patients deal with it by avoiding emotionally laden situations, such as visits from grandchildren or visiting places with sentimental significance after discharge from hospital (Eccles et al. 1999). Emotionalism can be a distressing and isolating condition, particularly if it persists. The social embarrassment caused by public tearfulness can mean that patients begin to avoid socialising, particularly with close family and friends, thus adding to social isolation after stroke (House et al. 1989).

Anxiety

Anxiety after stroke occurs less frequently than depression (Burvill et al. 1995), but it is thought that it is relatively unrecognised and is consequently under-diagnosed. Its lack of recognition by clinicians is also reflected in research: compared with depression after stroke there are very few studies to guide practice.

Like depression, anxiety is a syndrome or clustering of symptoms (World Health Organisation 2003). It includes an unpleasant and uncontrollable

---

Case example 9.2 George.

George, a 70-year-old widower who lived alone, suffered a stroke that left him with weakness in both his left arm and his left leg and foot. As a result he became unsteady on his feet. During his stay in the stroke unit he accidentally fell from the toilet onto the floor while trying to take himself back to his bed. His injury was minor but the psychological effect was much greater: he became anxious about being left alone in the toilet or anywhere else on the unit. He became avoidant (e.g. by drinking less water and tea so that he had to go to the toilet less often) and he sought reassurance, repeatedly asking care staff not to leave him alone in case he fell. This presented a problem, since he was physically ready to return home, but he was anxious about being in the house by himself. Treatment involved a form of cognitive-behavioural therapy while he was on the unit, in which George's cognitions (e.g. that he would come to some harm if left alone) were challenged, such as by leaving him alone on the toilet for a short time, then a little longer, and so on. A similar process was undertaken with some home visits – leaving George in the house alone for a few minutes at first, then longer. After three weeks of this therapy he was able to return home independently.

---

emotional feeling, most commonly of fear or apprehension. People experiencing anxiety have physical symptoms, such as breathlessness, palpitations and trembling. Like depression, it can have a wide range of severity and, at worst, can be a disabling and very restricting condition.

Anxiety can be provoked by a variety of situations, although there are people with 'generalised anxiety' whose symptoms are brought on by no specific provocation. In patients with stroke and other physical disabilities, anxiety might arise due to a fear of falling (see, for example, Case example 9.2). This fear may be based on real experience – perhaps the patient fell once in hospital when transferring from wheelchair to toilet soon after stroke. The experience may have been painful, embarrassing and distressing. The mood disturbance arises when the patient then generalises from that instance to all situations, such that he then fears falling whenever he tries to use the toilet. It is not hard to see how the patient might choose to cope with his feelings of anxiety by avoiding the situation that provokes it. So he avoids having to transfer to and from the toilet by drinking less fluid and reducing the need to use the toilet.

Forms of social anxiety may also occur after stroke. Patients may become fearful of social contact with strangers, or of any social contact, and seek to avoid the anxiety by withdrawing from social situations.

Patients who have suffered stroke and other conditions with sudden unexplained onset may have a fear of recurrence – of suffering another stroke – that may cause unpleasant and disabling symptoms of anxiety. In some patients, anxiety may take the form of over-generalised thoughts about the cause of stroke, such that they have a fear of situations they associate with the stroke's onset. An exaggerated fear of recurrence can result in reassurance-seeking behaviour, such as repeatedly asking caring staff 'Am I going to be alright?' Repeated requests can be difficult for staff to deal with, but answering 'yes' to the question for the tenth occasion that day may be the easy response but is likely not to be helpful. The answer to the question does not help the patient – hearing 'yes' has no effect of reducing their fear of 'not being alright' and it may reinforce the behaviour (i.e. make it more likely that the question will be asked again).

The development of the condition of anxiety is not well understood – its cause in an individual patient is most likely complex and multifactorial. However, there are often situations or experiences that the patient may be able to recall and which may have played an important role in the development of the condition in a patient who was otherwise vulnerable. For example, as described above, the patient may recall falling from the toilet, or may have a form of social anxiety that is attributed to having been embarrassed or humiliated socially soon after stroke.

There is little strong research evidence to inform treatments for anxiety after stroke: recommendations for treatment are based on research from other settings (Gould et al. 1997; National Institute for Health and Clinical Excellence (NICE) 2004; Westen & Morrison 2001). In some patients, pharmaceutical treatment can be effective, with antidepressant medicines having a sedating effect that can be beneficial. More likely to have a longer-term beneficial effect are structured psychological therapies, such as forms of cognitive-behavioural therapy (or CBT). These need to be given by appropriately trained practitioners, such as a clinical psychologist or psychiatric nurse.

Post-traumatic stress disorder

Post-traumatic stress disorder (PTSD) is becoming increasingly recognised as a potential response to ill health. Its recognition as a sequela of stroke has yet to achieve the attention it requires, despite PTSD occurring in 5–15% of people post-stroke (Holcroft 2007; Merriman et al. 2007; Sembi et al. 1998; Weallens 1998; Wealleans et al. 2009). Identification of PTSD is important in order to inform intervention practices, which differ from those for depression (see Table 9.1). Clinicians must understand that PTSD can manifest as depression, and that only differential diagnosis and specific treatment is likely to result in improvement. Consequently, when screening for depression after stroke, clinicians and researchers must be aware that those screening positive for depression may have PTSD.

A recent study (Holcroft 2007) has confirmed the potential for a stroke to be experienced as a traumatic event, and to result in PTSD. They found that those with PTSD were more likely to be younger, more disabled, had experienced previous stressful life events, and had had previous mental health problems. The extent to which the person felt frightened at the time of stroke, and how incapacitating an individual believed a stroke could be were found to be significant factors in those with PTSD.

It is clearly important for people who have had a stroke to have a comprehensive assessment of psychological problems, and all professionals working with people post-stroke should be aware of the clinical presentation of the disorder. Teasing out the difficulties experienced by individuals following

Table 9.1 DSM-IV PTSD criteria (First et al. 2002).

Criterion A

The person has been exposed to a traumatic event in which both of the following were present
(1) person experienced, witnessed or was confronted with an event or events that involved actual or threatened death or serious injury or threat to the physical integrity of self or others
(2) the person's response involved fear, helplessness or horror

Criterion B

The traumatic event is persistently re-experienced in **one** (or more) of the following ways:
(1) recurrent/intrusive distressing recollections
(2) recurrent distressing dreaming
(3) flashbacks
(4) psychological distress at exposure to cues
(5) physiological reactivity on exposure to cues

Criterion C

Persistent avoidance of stimuli associated with the trauma and numbing of general responsiveness (not present before the trauma) as indicated by **three** (or more) of the following:
(1) efforts to avoid thoughts or feelings or talking about the event
(2) efforts to avoid activities, places or people that are reminders
(3) inability to recall an important aspect of the trauma
(4) diminished interest in activities used to enjoy
(5) feeling of detachment or estrangement from others
(6) restricted range of affect e.g. unable to feel love or happiness
(7) sense of foreshortened future

Criterion D

Persistent symptoms of increased arousal (not present before the trauma) as indicated by **two** (or more) of the following:
(1) difficulty falling or staying asleep
(2) irritability or outbursts of anger
(3) difficulty concentrating
(4) hypervigilance
(5) exaggerated startle response

Criterion E

Duration of the disturbance is more than 1 month

Criterion F

The disturbance caused clinically significant distress or impairment in social, occupational or other important aspects of functioning

Full PTSD: Criterion A, Criterion B = 1 or more, Criterion C = 3 or more, Criterion D = 2 or more, Criterion E and Criterion F.

stroke is much more complex than illustrated within the literature due an existing overwhelming focus on depression. This has implications for education and training of practitioners.

It is important to acknowledge that a primary traumatic response to stroke may present as depression. If not explored further, depression could be inappropriately pursued as the primary treatment goal to address. As advised in the NICE guidance (National Institute for Health and Clinical Excellence 2005), to focus on depression and not PTSD would be unlikely to result in positive change.

When PTSD and depression are co-morbid, the PTSD should be addressed primarily and it is expected that the depression may dissipate accordingly. Importantly, NICE guidelines also highlighted that specific screening for PTSD should be undertaken in high-risk groups including those with a history of depression and those with a significant physical illness causing disability. As can be seen, this is highly applicable to the stroke population.

Cognitive and sensory impairment

The damage caused by the stroke to the brain can result in significant impairment associated with sensory or cognitive activity. 'Cognitive' is used by researchers and clinicians to denote thinking, and so cognitive impairment often includes a reduction in the efficiency of memory or decision-making. Sensory impairment includes effects on the processing of incoming information, such as visual or auditory information. However, it also includes effects on the way that the brain perceives the world, for example the sophisticated processing work that the brain does in order to perceive, among others, three-dimensional vision, the movement of objects, smell, and the taste of food.

All patients with stroke are at risk of cognitive loss and it can occur in patients with little or no physical disability. One view is that almost all stroke patients suffer some form of cognitive impairment, albeit temporary in most patients. This emphasises the importance of being aware of potential problems. It also suggests that the need to screen for cognitive impairment in patients soon after stroke, and there are basic screening measures available that can be used quickly by the non-specialist.

Attention problems

Impairments of attention can have significant effects on the patients and their ability to live independently after stroke, since attention is needed for almost all cognitive functions. Attention relates to the unconscious activity of focusing on particular aspects of the environment. We are bombarded with many sensory stimuli, and our attentional abilities allow the brain to disregard many of them and focus on whatever needs to be attended to in order to function effectively.

Attentional deficits can impede even the most basic of functions, but in particular they have an impact on complex and demanding behaviours. For example, a patient with attentional deficits would find it very hard to drive a car. An everyday example of attention can be illustrated by audio recording conversations taking place in a large room. At the time of the conversation, the brain will focus on the one conversation being attended to, or being participated in. Playing back the recording will reveal a number of conversations happening simultaneously, all of similar volume, as well as the presence of extraneous background noise. The brain is able to attend to one conversation and filter out the potentially competing noises.

Attentional impairments require the input of neuro-psychologists, not just for the diagnosis, but also for the interventions that might improve the situation of the patient. They involve a degree of re-training of the brain to identify and focus on some stimuli, while rejecting or lowering the 'volume' of many others (Lincoln et al. 2000; Michel & Mateer 2006).

Memory impairments

Memory problems after stroke are quite common and, in contrast to some other cognitive impairments, the patient is often aware of the problem. Memory problems can respond to treatments and the patient can be taught relatively straightforward techniques to allow them to make improvements, or at least to compensate for memory loss (Hildebrandt et al. 2006; Nair & Lincoln 2007).

Memory can be assessed by standardised assessment measures. If problems are identified, it would be important to check that there is no underlying physiological cause, for example hypothyroidism. In the patient with memory problems, referral to a specialist is recommended. However, therapy sessions and the inpatient ward environment can both be adjusted to best suit the patient's impairment.

Visuo-spatial disorders

Disorders of this type include neglect (that is, the disregard of a portion of the vision of the world) and inattention (that is, taking no notice of what is going on in part of the visual field), agnosias (that is, not recognising familiar objects or people), and dyspraxia (difficulty experienced in trying to do activities). Impairments of this type are often the result of lesions on the right parietal lobe of the brain.

It is hard to give a reliable estimate of the frequency of disorders of this type, since the rates published in research studies vary so much. They may occur in around one in ten patients with left hemisphere stroke and up to half of patients with right hemisphere stroke. Recovery can be quick: the problems may go away after two to three weeks in many patients, but problems can persist. For example, Stone et al. (1992) suggest that in patients who have visuo-spatial problems as a result of the stroke, around one in ten will continue to have the problems three months later.

Visuo-spatial disorders can be disturbing for the patient and can be significantly disabling: they interfere with many routine activities and can make it difficult for the patient to live and function independently. The effects of visuo-spatial problems can cause significant problems during rehabilitation. Not surprisingly, the continuation of these problems can result in the patient having a lengthy hospital stay, a greater chance of discharge to residential care, and potential social isolation with obvious resultant psychological impact (Jehkonen et al. 2006).

The diagnosis of visuo-spatial problems may be made by clinical assessment, although there are formal tests that a neuro-psychologist might use to clarify the diagnosis. Currently, few interventions have been developed for visuo-spatial impairments (Bowen & Lincoln 2007), so the emphasis for the patient will need to be on safety and compensatory techniques.

Disorientation

An impairment of the ability to orient oneself may have an impact on the most basic functioning. Disorientation can affect knowledge of time, person or place. Disorientation is not infrequent, since many neurological conditions can cause it. For example, it occurs acutely in many situations, such as after severe infection or traumatic injury. One in seven stroke patients may experience a form of disorientation in the first few weeks after stroke (Wade et al. 1989). Most recovery from problems of this type happens soon after stroke, often within the first few weeks. Disorientation in the patient can have an impact both in hospital and after discharge home. It may affect performance during rehabilitation and the patient's discharge home, particularly to independent living, will be more risky.

Executive functioning

This aspect of cognition has been categorised relatively recently, and it refers to the ability to organise, plan and execute (i.e. carry out) tasks. Executive functioning also refers to the ability to anticipate the consequences of actions. When functioning of this type is impaired it is termed 'dysexecutive syndrome' and stroke patients who have it have difficulty in planning and organising tasks, particularly series of tasks. They may also have difficulty in monitoring their behaviour and, as a result, not adapt to changed circumstances. Problems with executive functioning are relatively rare after stroke, but are more commonly seen after subarachnoid haemorrhage.

Conclusion

It is common for patients to experience mood or behavioural changes after stroke. Many of them are relatively short-lasting and may remit spontaneously. However, their onset can be distressing for the patient and their relatives, and their presence can provide a challenge during the acute phase of stroke care.

Mood problems and cognitive impairments appear to be recognised and diagnosed more frequently than before, and there is a growing body of evidence to inform treatments. In common with other aspects of stroke care, the emphasis needs to be placed on early recognition, monitoring and referral, and ensuring that the patient understands what is happening and why.

References

Andersen, G, Vestergaard, K, Riis, J, & Lauritzen, L, 1994, Incidence of post-stroke depression during the first year in a large unselected stroke population determined using a valid standardized rating scale, *Acta Psychiatrica Scandinavica*, vol. 90, no. 3, pp. 190–195.

Bennett, HE, Thomas, SA, Austen, R, Morris, AM, & Lincoln, NB, 2006, Validation of screening measures for assessing mood in stroke patients, *British Journal of Clinical Psychology*, vol. 45, no. 3, pp. 367–376.

Bowen, A, & Lincoln, N, 2007, *Cognitive rehabilitation for spatial neglect following stroke*, Cochrane Database of Systematic Reviews, Issue 2: CD003586.

Burvill, PW, Johnson, GA, Jamrozik, KD, Anderson, CS, Stewart-Wynne, EG et al., 1995, Anxiety disorders after stroke: results from the Perth Community Stroke Study, *British Journal of Psychiatry*, vol. 166, no. 3, pp. 328–332.

Calvert, T, Knapp, P, & House, A, 1998, Psychological associations with emotionalism after stroke, *Journal of Neurology, Neurosurgery and Psychiatry*, vol. 65, no. 6, pp. 928–929.

Carson, AJ, MacHale, S, Allen, K, Lawrie, SM, Dennis, M et al., 2000, Depression after stroke and lesion location: a systematic review, *Lancet*, vol. 356, no. 9224, pp. 122–126.

Eccles, S, House, A, & Knapp, P, 1999, Psychological adjustment and self reported coping in stroke survivors with and without emotionalism, *Journal of Neurology, Neurosurgery and Psychiatry*, vol. 67, no. 1, pp. 125–126.

First, M, Frances, A, & Pincus HA, 2002, *DSM-IV-TR Handbook of Differential Diagnosis*, American Psychiatric Publishing, Arlington.

Gilbody, SM, House, AO, & Sheldon, TA, 2001, Routinely administered questionnaires for depression and anxiety: systematic review, *British Medical Journal*, vol. 322, no. 7283, pp. 406–409.

Goldberg, D, & Williams, P, 1988, *A User's Guide to the General Health Questionnaire*, NFER-Nelson, Windsor.

Gould, RA, Otto, MW, Pollack, MH, & Yap, L, 1997, Cognitive behavioural and pharmacological treatment of the transition of generalised anxiety disorder: a preliminary meta-analysis, *Behavior Therapy*, vol. 28, no. 2, pp. 285–305.

Hackett, ML, & Anderson, CS, 2005, Predictors of depression after stroke: a systematic review of observational studies, *Stroke*, vol. 36, no. 10, pp. 2296–2301.

Hackett, ML, Yapa, C, Parag, V, & Anderson, CS, 2005, Frequency of depression after stroke: a systematic review of observational studies, *Stroke*, vol. 36, no. 6, pp. 1330–1340.

Hackett, ML, Anderson, CS, House, AO, & Halteh, C, 2008a, *Interventions for preventing depression after stroke*, Cochrane Database of Systematic Reviews, Issue 3: CD003689.

Hackett, ML, Anderson, CS, House, AO, & Xia, J, 2008b, *Interventions for treating depression after stroke*, Cochrane Database of Systematic Reviews, Issue 4: CD003437.

Hildebrandt, H, Bussmann-Mork, B, & Schwendemann, G, 2006, Group therapy for memory impaired patients: a partial remediation is possible, *Journal of Neurology*, vol. 253, no. 4, pp. 512–519.

Hill, K., 2008, *Mood state after stroke and its effect on outcome: a prospective cohort study*, Presented at the UK Stroke Forum, Harrogate: http://www.ukstrokeforum.org/events/past_forum_conferences/2008_uksf_conference.html 7-5-2009

Holcroft, L, 2007, *Post-traumatic stress disorder in survivors of stroke*, University of Lancaster, DClinPsych Thesis.

House, A, Dennis, M, Molyneux, A, Warlow, C, & Hawton, K, 1989, Emotionalism after stroke, *British Medical Journal*, vol. 298, no. 6679, pp. 991–994.

House, A, Dennis, M, Mogridge, L, Warlow, C, Hawton, K et al., 1991, Mood disorders in the year after first stroke, *British Journal of Psychiatry*, vol. 158, pp. 83–92.

House, A, Knapp, P, Bamford, J, & Vail, A, 2001, Mortality at 12 and 24 months after stroke may be associated with depressive symptoms at 1 month, *Stroke*, vol. 32, no. 3, pp. 696–701.

House, AO, Hackett, ML, Anderson, CS, & Horrocks, JA, 2004, *Pharmaceutical interventions for emotionalism after stroke*, Cochrane Database of Systematic Reviews, Issue 2: CD003690, Oxford.

Intercollegiate Stroke Working Party, 2008, *National Clinical Guideline for Stroke*, 3rd edn, Royal College of Physicians, London.

Jehkonen, M, Laihosalo, M, & Kettunen, JE, 2006, Impact of neglect on functional outcome after stroke: a review of methodological issues and recent research findings, *Restorative Neurology and Neuroscience*, vol. 24, no. 4–6, pp. 209–215.

Knapp, P, Young, J, House, A, & Forster, A, 2000, Non-drug strategies to resolve psycho-social difficulties after stroke, *Age and Ageing*, vol. 29, no. 1, pp. 23–30.

Kroenke, K, & Spitzer, RL, 2002, The PHQ-9: A new depression diagnostic and severity measure the nine-item Patient Health Questionnaire depression scale is a dual-purpose instrument that can establish provisional depressive disorder diagnoses as well as grade depression severity, *Psychiatric Annals*, vol. 32, no. 9, pp. 509–521.

Laska, AC, Martensson, B, Kahan, T, von Arbin M, & Murray, V, 2007, Recognition of depression in aphasic stroke patients, *Cerebrovascular Diseases*, vol. 24, no. 1, pp. 74–79.

Lazarus, RS, & Folkman, S, 1984, *Stress, Appraisal, and Coping*, Springer Publishing, New York.

Lee, AC, Tang, SW, Yu, GK, & Cheung, RT, 2008, The smiley as a simple screening tool for depression after stroke: a preliminary study, *International Journal of Nursing Studies*, vol. 45, no. 7, pp. 1081–1089.

Lincoln, NB, Majid, M, & Weyman, N, 2000, *Cognitive rehabilitation for attention deficits following stroke*, Cochrane Database of Systematic Reviews, Issue 4: CD002842.

Merriman, C, Norman, P, & Barton, J, 2007, Psychological correlates of PTSD symptoms following stroke, *Psychology Health and Medicine*, vol. 12, no. 5, pp. 592–602.

Michel, JA, & Mateer, CA, 2006, Attention rehabilitation following stroke and traumatic brain injury. A review, *Europa Medicophysica*, vol. 42, no. 1, pp. 59–67.

Nair, R, & Lincoln, NB, 2007, *Cognitive rehabilitation for memory deficits following stroke*, Cochrane Database of Systematic Reviews, Issue 3, CD002293.

National Institute for Health and Clinical Excellence, 2004, *Anxiety: management of anxiety (panic disorder, with or without agoraphobia, and generalised anxiety disorder) in adults in primary, secondary and community care*, NICE, London.

National Institute for Health and Clinical Excellence, 2005, *Post-traumatic stress disorder (PTSD): the management of PTSD in adults and children in primary and secondary care*, Clinical Guideline 26, NICE, London.

Pearlin, LI, & Schooler, C, 1978, The structure of coping, *Journal of Health and Social Behaviour*, vol. 19, no. 1, pp. 2–21.

Petty, DR, House, A, Knapp, P, Raynor, T, & Zermansky, A, 2006, Prevalence, duration and indications for prescribing of antidepressants in primary care, *Age and Ageing*, vol. 35, no. 5, pp. 523–526.

Robinson, RG, 2003, Poststroke depression: prevalence, diagnosis, treatment, and disease progression, *Biological Psychiatry*, vol. 54, no. 3, pp. 376–387.

Ruddell, M, Spencer, A, Hill, K, & House, A, 2007, Fluoxetine vs placebo for depressive symptoms after stroke: failed randomised controlled trial, *International Journal of Geriatric Psychiatry*, vol. 22, no. 10, pp. 963–965.

Sembi, S, Tarrier, N, O'Neill, P, Burns, A, & Faragher, B, 1998, Does post-traumatic stress disorder occur after stroke: a preliminary study, *International Journal of Geriatric Psychiatry*, vol. 13, no. 5, pp. 315–322.

Stone, SP, Patel, P, Greenwood, RJ, & Halligan, PW, 1992, Measuring visual neglect in acute stroke and predicting its recovery: the visual neglect recovery index, *Journal of Neurology, Neurosurgery and Psychiatry*, vol. 55, no. 6, pp. 431–436.

Wade, DT, Skilbeck, C, & Hewer, RL, 1989, Selected cognitive losses after stroke. Frequency, recovery and prognostic importance, *International Disability Studies*, vol. 11, no. 1, pp. 34–39.

Watkins, CL, Auton, MF, Deans, CF, Dickinson, HA, Jack, CI et al., 2007a, Motivational interviewing early after acute stroke: a randomized, controlled trial, *Stroke*, vol. 38, no. 3, pp. 1004–1009.

Watkins, CL, Lightbody, CE, Sutton, CJ, Holcroft, L, Jack, CI et al., 2007b, Evaluation of a single-item screening tool for depression after stroke: a cohort study, *Clinical Rehabilitation*, vol. 21, no. 9, pp. 846–852.

Weallens, G, 1998, *Post-traumatic stress disorder in survivors of stroke*, University of Liverpool, DClinPsych Thesis.

Wealleans, G, Watkins, CL, Sharma, AK, & Daniels, L, 2009, *PTSD in survivors of stroke*, British Association of Stroke Physicians Conference, poster presentation.

Westen, D, & Morrison, K, 2001, A multidimensional meta-analysis of treatments for depression, panic, and generalized anxiety disorder: an empirical examination of the status of empirically supported therapies, *Journal of Consulting and Clinical Psychology*, vol. 69, no. 6, pp. 875–899.

Williams, LS, Kroenke, K, Bakas, T, Plue, LD, Brizendine, E et al., 2007, Care management of poststroke depression: a randomized, controlled trial, *Stroke*, vol. 38, no. 3, pp. 998–1003.

World Health Organisation, 2003, *The ICD-10 Classification of Mental and Behavioural Disorders: Diagnostic Criteria for Research*, World Health Organisation, Geneva.

Yesavage, JA, Brink, TL, Rose, TL, Lum, O, Huang, V et al., 1982, Development and validation of a geriatric depression screening scale: a preliminary report, *Journal of Psychiatric Research*, vol. 17, no. 1, pp. 37–49.

Zigmond, AS, & Snaith, RP, 1983, The hospital anxiety and depression scale, *Acta Psychiatrica Scandinavica*, vol. 67, no. 6, pp. 361–370.

Chapter 10

Minimally responsive stroke patients

Elaine Pierce and Aeron Ginnelly

> ## Key points
>
> - Irrespective of patients' level of response, their needs should be identified and appropriate health care provided.
> - Privacy, dignity, confidentiality and other basic rights should be observed.
> - Those affected (relatives and carers) should be kept informed and involved in decisions.
> - Values, beliefs and previous wishes should be respected.
> - The right to approach death should be respected.
> - Those affected should be supported emotionally.
> (Further details in National Health and Medical Research Council 2008.)

Introduction

Stroke is a disease with high levels of enduring disability and morbidity amongst survivors. A very small proportion of those who survive with severe and enduring disabilities do so in a state of minimal consciousness or minimal responsiveness: this is often referred to as post-coma unresponsiveness (PCU), vegetative state, or minimally conscious or minimally responsive state (MRS). A further tiny minority will survive in a 'locked-in' state, with cognition and the ability to communicate retained but lacking the physical functional abilities to do so. MRS and 'locked-in' syndrome are situations of high stress and distress for families and for health care staff. For the 'locked-in' syndrome at least, we have some insight into the patient's experience, depicted as traumatic, distressing, depressing and deeply frustrating by Jean-Dominique Bauby (1997), the editor of the French journal *ELLE*, who experienced this as the result of a stroke in 1995. Both MRS and 'locked-in' syndrome result in patients being totally dependent on carers for all their daily needs. It is therefore essential that stroke nurses, who may be involved with such patients and their families, have a good understanding of these conditions and what care is required. Such patients and families are highly vulnerable, given the combination of conditions that are not easy to correctly identify or make prognostic judgements about, allied with a high level of dependence upon medical and other health care services.

This chapter sets out the pathophysiology, aetiology, presentation and management of these two conditions occurring as a result of stroke. A case example of one patient, Elizabeth (not her real name), illustrates treatment and care required for one key element of her long-term rehabilitation, whilst many other chapters of the book set out other aspects of care that need to be provided (e.g. nutrition and hydration, bladder and bowel management, mobility, moving and handling).

Definitions and identification

Definitions of these states have been established (see Box 10.1), but while PCU is a clinically clearly defined condition, correctly identifying whether a patient has PCU, MRS or is in a 'locked-in' state may not be easy. Being conscious means being in a state of awareness of one's self and the environment, but other people can only recognise this through a person's behaviour. There is no definitive diagnostic test for lack of consciousness; it can only be identified through lack of behaviour that positively indicates consciousness.

The first steps in diagnosis entail establishing the cause of the condition, and excluding any persisting effect of anaesthesia, drugs or metabolic disturbance. The possibility of treatable structural causes should be excluded by brain imaging. Criteria for PCU require there is:

- No evidence of awareness of self or environment
- No response to visual, auditory, tactile or other stimuli suggesting conscious purpose
- No use of language comprehension or meaningful expression

Box 10.1 Definition of terms.

Coma: a state of presumed profound unconsciousness from which the person cannot be roused when examined. Coma is not brain death: some brain function remains, and some or all may be recoverable.

Post-coma unresponsiveness (PCU): a state or condition in which a person has emerged from coma to the extent that they are observed to have sleep–wake cycles over a period of time but no purposeful responses to stimuli. Responsiveness may gradually return in some people, leading to MRS or even better, although improvement may be very slow. Some recovery may be achievable but full recovery is highly improbable.

Minimally responsive state (MRS): may arise when a person has emerged from coma or PCU. There is a minimal level of purposeful response, with discernible but inconsistent evidence of consciousness. Cognitively mediated behaviour occurs often enough or for long enough to distinguish it from reflex behaviour, and the more complex the response, the easier it is to make this distinction. In MRS, the responses do not indicate a capacity for decision-making (National Health and Medical Research Council 2008).

'Locked-in' syndrome: is quite distinct from PCU and MRS. The patient is aware and awake, but cannot move or communicate due to complete paralysis of nearly all voluntary muscles in the body. It is the result of a brainstem lesion such as a stroke at the level of the basilar artery causing damage to the pons. The term was coined in 1966 (Plum & Posner 1966) but the condition is also referred to as cerebromedullospinal disconnection, de-efferented state, pseudocoma, and ventral pontine syndrome.

- An apparent sleep–wake cycle
- Continuing hypothalamic and brainstem function, ensuring respiration and circulation (British Medical Association 2007)

Any purposeful movement or evidence of communication or awareness indicates that the patient is not in PCU. Differentiation of PCU, MRS and 'locked-in' syndrome can take time, and repeated observations are necessary to determine whether a simple movement (e.g. finger movement, eye blink, eye movement) that is seen occasionally is reflexive, simply coincidental or is actually a response to a stimulus such as a command to move fingers. By contrast, a complex response such as an intelligible word, heard only a few times, may make it clear that the person is conscious. There may be a lag time between the stimulus and the person's response, further confusing the picture. All assessments must allow sufficient time to be sure whether or not a response was initiated. In 'locked-in' syndrome, the ability to respond is minimal, due to extensive motor paralysis. Detailed assessment is required to identify residual motor function and how best to use this residual motor function in order to achieve communication. Accuracy of assessment, management and consequently, appropriateness of care, depends on understanding and using the correct terminology and applying appropriate training and skills. This will facilitate the tailoring of care to the individual's needs through the combined efforts of the multidisciplinary team (MDT). The main focus of the MDT should be on the benefits and effects of assessment, management and care for the minimally responsive individual, their families, partners, friends and informal carers (hereafter referred to as 'carers') not only in the present, but also the longer term (Laureys et al. 2006).

Minimally responsive state

This chapter will now briefly describe the nurses' role in the assessment process for MRS – an extensive overview of all assessment, management and care involved in MRS is beyond the scope of this chapter. Nurses are involved in, and contribute to, many aspects of assessment, management and health care scenarios (Figure 10.1), including medical and therapies as well as nursing activities.

Prerequisites to assessment

Generally, with individuals who have severe and complex neuro-disability, the main reasons for undertaking an assessment are to: identify problems; collect information about what the patient can or cannot do; and identify how well they can perform a task. Additionally, assessments will show how much of a task a person can successfully achieve and the level of support needed (physical or verbal). With a person who has MRS, it is necessary to consider how and what information can be obtained (e.g. from observations, history, other health

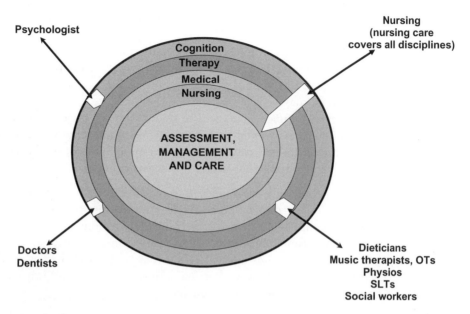

Figure 10.1 Staff involved in assessment and care of minimally conscious state individuals. OTs, occupational therapists; SLTs, speech and language therapists.

care professionals and carers) in order to prioritise, plan, implement and evaluate the provision of care. In sharing and gathering information carers should also be assessed, for example in relation to their psychological state. The medical and emotional state of carers as well as the patient is important. The level of stress experienced by carers needs to be assessed because they may require support and professional intervention. The following list describes the important aspects to take into account prior to making an assessment:

- The medical stability of the individual. For example, are they in a fit state to be assessed, due to, for example, abnormal nutritional status such as dehydration or malnourishment?
- The suitability of the environment. Noise or other distractions could lead to the assessor not receiving the patient's full attention; the temperature, if too hot or too cold, could affect how the patient responds. The assessment should be done in private.
- Attributes of the assessor, who should:
  - Have knowledge and skills in dealing with people in an MRS and their carers.
  - Be very clear in their approach. For example, the language used should be simple, the stimuli appropriate.
  - Ascertain the best position for the patient in order to obtain the relevant responses. For example, it may be better for the patient to be upright in bed or in a chair rather than lying flat. Whichever position is chosen, the patient should be comfortable.
  - Be alert to the fact that the patient may be more aware than first thought.

- Use the tool agreed by the MDT and have had the necessary training in its use.
- Be consistent and realise the limitations of themselves and the patient.
- To get the best responses from the patient, carefully choose the time when the assessment is carried out. For example, after a therapy session, the patient may be too exhausted to respond.
- Preferably, undertake the assessment after the patient has had a rest period.
- All activities should take into consideration cultural and language considerations for patients and carers, especially those of black and minority, culturally and linguistically distinctive ethnic groups.

For people with MRS referred from acute to rehabilitation or continuing care institutions, it may be necessary to do a nursing pre-assessment. Such assessment would typically cover breathing, nutrition, personal care, continence, mobility, communication, orientation, skin integrity, sleeping, medication, motivation, wounds and behaviour (day and night). It may also be important to have a pre-admission meeting with carers for purposes of introduction and orientation to the services and staff.

Assessment

The considerations listed previously are very important if the assessment is to be accurate and successful. Some or all of these considerations can also be utilised in goal setting and the delivery of care to patients. Assessments should be given priority by all members of the MDT because assessment findings are crucial for accurate diagnosis and for individual management of disability after the event (Davenport et al. 1995; Wade et al. 1985). Assessment of quality of life should also be included amongst standard assessments leading to clinical decisions (Varricchio 2006).

Initial assessments should be comprehensive (Figure 10.1). UK national stroke guidelines (Intercollegiate Stroke Working Party 2008) stipulate early (within the first 48 hours) assessment using physical and diagnostic tests for brain injury, swallow function, immediate needs in relation to positioning, mobilisation, moving and handling, bladder and bowel control, risk of developing skin pressure ulcers, capacity to understand and follow instructions, capacity to communicate needs and wishes, nutritional status, and sight and hearing. Later, assessments also address motor control and tone, sensation, pain, depression, anxiety and emotionalism, spatial and perceptual awareness. Oral health, abnormal oral reflexes and lip biting should also be assessed (Millwood et al. 2005). The purpose of these assessments is to:

- Ascertain the arousal levels of the person with MRS
- Describe their and their carers' actual and potential problems
- Together with the MDT:
  - Set achievable goals including the time frame
  - Provide a baseline by which to monitor the person with MRS for changes in condition or management, care and interventions

The frequency of assessment depends on the result of the evaluation of each goal set for the person with MRS (see Management and care section). Assessments may need to be repeated on more than one occasion: assessors should use their professional judgement as to whether an assessment is necessary and whether the person with MRS is medically stable and fit. Assessors should exercise caution to ensure that assessments do not become onerous or burdensome. Clinical assessment is a continuous process and nurses are crucial to this process, since they are in a position to observe patients continuously (e.g. for restlessness and arousal levels), and monitor changes in behaviour and response. Nurse reporting and communication processes should be standardised, and ensure findings are shared between and across all members of the MDT (Scherb et al. 1998).

Tools and measures used in assessment, management and care

Tools used should have been tried and tested, and demonstrated validity and reliability (Wade et al. 1985); they must be based on sound methods, use valid and reliable approaches and their results must be relevant for improving care and patient outcomes (Varricchio 2006). The tools and measures used in the clinical setting should be 'user friendly'; that is, understandable by all (ranging from carers and unqualified care staff through to medical staff, Registered Nurses and qualified therapists), easy to complete and interpret, not time-consuming and able to be completed within a specified time period. Multidisciplinary rehabilitation programmes utilise a wide range of measures, some of which are referred to in topic-specific chapters of this book. Many commonly used tools such as the Functional Independence Measure, Disability Rating Scale, Rancho Los Amigos Levels of Cognitive Function Scale, Barthel Index, Lowenstein Communication Scale and Wessex Head Injury Matrix include aspects of arousal, functional motor, auditory, visual and communication skills, and are useful in assessing change in responses over time (Cullen et al. 2007; Magee & Andrews 2007). A number of tools have been developed specifically for those with very severe disability or MRS. For example:

- Putney Auditory Comprehension Screening Test – PACST (Beaumont et al. 1999)
- Music therapy Assessment Tool for Patients in Low-Awareness States – MATLAS (Magee 2007)
- Sensory Modality Assessment Rehabilitation Technique – SMART (Gill-Thwaites 1997; Gill-Thwaites & Munday 1999, 2004)
- Putney Auditory Single Word Yes/No Assessment – PASWORD (Mackenzie et al. 2005)
- Multidisciplinary Evaluation of Neuro-dependency – MEND (Pierce & McLaren 2003)

The choice of tool depends on purpose: for example, an assessment tool such as the SMART might be used to assess auditory senses, followed by the MATLAS, where there is a subtle use of hearing components, to assess response and changes in arousal levels to music or music therapy (Magee & Andrews 2007).

What makes good assessments and care management?

Some assessment tools have floor and ceiling effects, which means they are not sensitive enough to detect all ranges of changes and responses (Wade et al. 1985). The choice of tools should be agreed within the MDT. The responses of someone with MRS may fluctuate and be inconsistent and so it is necessary to be cautious with initial findings and/or repeat assessments. There should be a fit between all aspects of assessment, management and care. The purpose of the assessment should dictate which tool is to be used; the result of the assessment should inform management and care; the management and care can then be evaluated against assessment outcomes.

MDT members should take account of each other's findings and adopt a team approach to management and care. A unified approach should be agreed. Barriers between professional groups, and between staff and patients, can be avoided through awareness of approach, body language, attitude, verbal language, tone and pace, whether communicating or delivering care. Something as simple as the unnecessary wearing of gloves may present a psychological barrier. This awareness is also important in relationships with carers. Previous experiences with health professionals or particular assumptions or prejudices may colour attitudes and require sensitive handling.

A key consideration in the early stages is to establish decision-making processes. Every individual has the right to make decisions about treatment and care, but people with MRS are not able to make their own decisions. This requires determination of:

- Who holds responsibility for such decisions, how such a person is appointed, and the nature and limits of that person's responsibility.
- The role of the previously expressed wishes of the person with MRS. These may have been documented in a non-specific way that guides rather than directs, documented formally and specifically, expressed informally by others to whom the person has previously made known his or her wishes, or constructed hypothetically based on what others believe the person would have wished.
- The exercise of the professional duty of care of health care professionals involved (National Health and Medical Research Council 2008).

Management and care

High-quality nursing care is needed to minimise the risks of complications, and detail of what high-quality nursing care comprises is the subject of chapters of this book. In the short term it is good medical practice to provide artificial nutrition and hydration to sustain any patient whose prognosis is uncertain. Medical treatments, including artificial nutrition and hydration, may be withdrawn later if they are considered futile (British Medical Association 2007). Futility of treatment can be demonstrated based on establishment of clear goals prior to commencement of treatment.

When planning care programmes it is important to consider the balance of benefit versus burden from all treatments and interventions. Benefits of treatment may include:

- Slowing the progress of disease
- Sustaining the person's life
- Reducing disability and improving health
- Relieving distress or discomfort (National Health and Medical Research Council 2008)

Burdens of treatment include distress and suffering to the patient and carers, and also the wider community. Treatments may be considered overly burdensome if the burden for the patient is disproportionate to the likely benefits. Burden can derive from the risky, intrusive, destructive, exhausting, painful or repugnant nature of the treatment, or from low benefit.

Management should include strategies to deal with:

- General arousal levels
- Sensory stimuli and responses – touch, taste, smell, sound (Gill-Thwaites 1997; Gill-Thwaites & Munday 1999; Wilson & Gill-Thwaites 2000)
- Attempts to speak, eye contact, visual tracking (Ansell & Keenan 1989)
- Use of assistive technology (Naude & Hughes 2005)
- Sleep disturbances (Thaxton & Myers 2002)
- Command-following (Whyte et al. 1999)
- Social behaviours (disinhibition)
- Maintenance or regaining of movement of joints – such as splinting for contractures, postural tremor, clawed toes.

An intensive rehabilitation programme for all people with MRS should be pursued and should incorporate goal setting and regular care reviews. This should involve all specialties and carers, since management and care cannot be provided in isolation. The MDT should have a leader, plan and work together to tailor care to the individual's needs. This may involve using evidence-based protocols, possibly modified to suit the individual. Management should at all times utilise the best available evidence, including expert advice, to maximise prospects for recovery. Management should include goal setting by the patient's teams and carers. This does not prevent inclusion of other disciplines that may use their own assessments, as long as this occurs within a coordinated approach and with the full cooperation of the person with MRS, carers and MDT. Chapter 11 gives more detail of the goal-setting process.

Communication is the key to good management and care. The person with MRS may not be able to hold a conversation, but that should not stop MDT team members from informing them, seeking their consent for each procedure or even obtaining their permission before entering their room. Withholding what may appear to be irrelevant information can lead to carer stress. For example, a patient's partner was observed becoming upset on finding that a change in management had been introduced since the last visit because they believed every change was for the worst. If the rationale for change is not communicated, even something as simple as a plaster over a site where blood has been taken can cause concern. Education of carers as to the patient's condition, what to observe or ways in which the carer can assist should enhance their understanding, lessen fear and stress levels, and encourage them to provide information through their observations. Carers' observations reinforce or supplement staff observations and provide information on new areas of management and care for consideration. Good communication also creates a sense of trust between the carers and the MDT.

Monitoring and evaluating care

Consciousness can only be inferred from behaviour and this can be problematic for clinicians (Katz 2001). Most people with MRS are incapable of complex behaviours. If, when asked to obey simple commands like closing their eyes, a blink follows a few seconds later, it may be unclear as to whether this is a response to the command or whether the blink was a reflex action (Whyte et al. 1999). Staff may miss or misinterpret changes in response, which despite increases in consistency, at first look random or coincidental (Childs et al. 1993). This occurs especially in those new to the specialty, who lack knowledge and skills in assessment of this patient group and/or who spend brief periods of time delivering care or evaluate only during ward rounds. It may be necessary to be inventive and use props or markers to ensure a response is consistent and reliable. For example, marking tape placed a short distance in front of the foot of a person with MRS will show that the person is making a positive response if they kick their toe beyond the tape (Whyte et al. 1999). Since responses in people with MRS can be erratic, the MDT should not dismiss reports of changes observed by carers (Childs et al. 1993). Any reported change should be followed by careful observation for consistency and managed to facilitate improvement of the patient.

It is pointless asking people with MRS to follow commands which, because of limitations such as sensory, motor or cognitive impairments (hearing, language-processing, paralysis), they are unable to perform (Whyte et al. 1999). Repeatedly asking someone to squeeze an assessor's hand, for example, may result in an intermittent random behaviour or a grasp reflex (Whyte et al. 1999). Being able to follow a command is one of the important factors in distinguishing patients in vegetative states from those with MRS, and misdiagnosis of vegetative state has been reported (Andrews et al. 1996; Gill-Thwaites 2006). Much is dependent on the nurse's assessment, implementation, monitoring and evaluation of care.

Finally, because people may emerge from MRS, long-term effects should be borne in mind (Laureys et al. 2006; Taylor et al. 2007). Good nursing care, implemented, monitored and evaluated in such as way as to avoid complications (e.g. bowel and bladder problems, pulmonary infections, electrolyte and liver function imbalance, seizures and dystonia), optimises quality of life, whatever degree of recovery and rehabilitation may be achieved (Chua et al. 2007; Pierce et al. 2001).

Long-term care

The prognosis for people with MRS is often uncertain but some survive many years. Long-term management and care may therefore need to be considered. Some may require ongoing rehabilitation because improvement may be slow but continue for years. Decisions will have to be made about the level of ongoing rehabilitation and care that is appropriate to the person's needs, as well as the setting in which this care will be delivered. Aspects of care that will likely be ongoing include: nutrition and hydration; comprehensive social care, to maintain health and well-being and prevent pressure damage; physical therapy, to prevent contractures and maintain level of function; ongoing review, for early detection of any changes; and anticipation and treatment of infections or symptoms of distress.

Ongoing care may be delivered in various settings, and decisions about the long-term accommodation of the person with MRS can be difficult and stressful. Decisions about care at home are dependent both on community support and services available, and the family's capacity to undertake care at home. Modifications to the home may be required to accommodate necessary equipment such as hoist and tube feeding supplies. Health professionals need to consider the impact of such care; very high stress levels have been reported by families who care at home for a person with severe brain damage. Respite care may also need to be considered as part of the package. A trial period may be useful before committing to care at home, as well as consideration of what support carers may need for the situation to be sustainable. Conversely, if it is decided that care should not be provided at home then carers may need support to accept this decision.

Alternative accommodation options include nursing home, specialist long-term rehabilitation hospital and community group homes. The choice will depend on local availability, individuals' needs and preferences compared with details of service provision, and resourcing. Palliative care also has a role with people with severe and enduring illness, and referral should be considered if symptoms become burdensome or withdrawal of futile treatments is being considered.

Finally, decisions about continuance or withdrawal of treatments and resuscitation options should be considered through discussion between all involved and clear plans and instructions established. Decisions should be informed by consideration of the person's best interests, including what is known about their wishes, as well as the interests of carers.

Conclusion: MRS

Nurses are central to the assessment, management and delivery of care for people with MRS. Through their round-the-clock presence on the ward, they are able to assess and monitor change and maintain continuity. Nurses are the cornerstone of communication within the MDT, keeping the team informed and updated so that care management works in the best interest of the person with MRS and their carers. Nurses are also the key link with carers, who are often invaluable in identifying and evaluating the needs, and speeding the recovery, of the person with MRS. People with MRS represent a very small proportion of the stroke survivor population, but as a patient group they present challenges for all who work with them. The 24/7 nursing role makes a unique contribution to their care.

Acknowledgement

With grateful thanks to colleagues at the Royal Hospital for Neuro-disability, Putney, London, for generously sharing their knowledge of assessment, management and care of people with MRS.

'Locked-in' syndrome

Describing the syndrome

The 'locked-in' syndrome was first defined in 1966 and redefined twenty years later as quadriplegia and anarthria with preservation of consciousness (Haig et al. 1987; Plum & Posner 1966). It is rare, and no incidence rates have been established (Smith & Delargy 2005). It is caused by trauma or disease of the ventral pons, although extensive bilateral destruction of corticobulbar and corticospinal tracts in the cerebral peduncles may also be responsible, see Table 10.1 (Smith & Delargy 2005).

Three categories are described (Bauer et al. 1979):

- *Classic* – quadriplegia and anarthria, retained consciousness and vertical eye movement

Table 10.1 Causes and mechanisms of locked-in syndrome. Reproduced from Smith, E, Delargy, M, *Locked-in syndrome*, British Medical Journal, vol. 330, no. 7488, pp. 406–409, copyright 2005 with permission from BMJ Publishing Group Ltd.

Cause	Mechanism
Ischaemic	Basilar artery occlusion, stroke, hypotensive, hypoxic events
Haemorrhage	Haemorrhage within or into the pons
Traumatic	Direct brainstem contusion, vertebrobasilar axis dissection
Tumour	Primary, or secondary metastasis
Metabolic	Central pontine myelinolysis
Demyelination	Multiple sclerosis
Infectious	Abscess, brainstem encephalitis

- *Incomplete* – the same as classic but with some additional voluntary movement
- *Total* – total immobility and inability to communicate, with full consciousness

Typically, those affected have complete paralysis of voluntary muscles in all parts of the body except for the control of eye movement. Whilst horizontal gaze palsies are usual, patients usually retain upper eyelid control and vertical eye movement because of sparing of the mid-brain tectum. Associated problems can include blurred or double vision, impaired visual accommodation, vertigo, insomnia, and emotional lability. In one series, 6 out of 44 recovering patients reported visual deficits, 39 said they cried or laughed more easily, 8 reported memory problems and 6 had attentional deficits (Leon-Carrion et al. 2002).

Mortality rates amongst these patients were estimated at 60% in 1986: mortality was higher in the first four months in patients with vascular compared to non-vascular causes, and in older people (Patterson & Grabois 1986). Recent adoption of more intensive support therapies in the acute stages may have improved survival, and earlier rehabilitation (within one month of onset) has demonstrated a mortality of only 14% at five years (Casanova et al. 2003). Although most survivors remain either in a chronic locked-in state or severely impaired, early signs of recovery can be taken advantage of by multidisciplinary rehabilitation (Smith & Delargy 2005). Early referral to specialist rehabilitation services is therefore important. There is no cure for 'locked-in' syndrome, but a wide range of therapies and assistive technologies may make significant improvements in quality of life, particularly in communication.

Initially, low technology forms of alternative and augmentative communication such as AEIOU auditory and visual scanning (see Case example) are used. However, a wide range of assistive computer interface technologies have been developed to exploit eye movements. These are used to drive a variety of communication devices, but also as a means for these people to control their environment in relation to electrical appliances, heating, lighting, and window openers. For example, an eye-gaze system has been described, based on the corneal-pupil reflection relationship technique. This is non-intrusive and calibrated by the user successively looking at nine points on the screen. On-screen, the user has a main menu from which to select one of several controlling screens whereby the user can typewrite, place a telephone call, turn appliances on or off by looking at the screen (Chapman 1991). Eye-gaze and eye tracking systems may be used to help patients communicate (Frey et al. 1990).

New direct brain interface mechanisms may provide future technological options. A brain–computer interface (BCI), also called a direct neural interface or a brain–machine interface, is a direct communication pathway between a brain and an external device. Invasive BCI research has focused on replacing damaged sight and providing new avenues of function to paralysed people. Invasive BCIs are implanted directly into the grey matter of the brain during neurosurgery. They provide the most effective communication of the BCI devices but are prone to produce scar tissue which can result in loss of signal. The first such implant was installed in a patient with 'locked-in' syndrome in

1998, allowing the recipient to learn to control a computer cursor. Partially-invasive BCIs are devices implanted inside the skull but outside the brain. They produce better signals than non-invasive BCIs where the bone of the skull deflects and deforms signals, and have a lower risk of scar-tissue formation than invasive BCIs. Non-invasive BCIs have been trialled to power muscle implants and restore partial movement but poor signal resolution makes the technology more difficult to control. Altogether, there is potential for such assistive technologies to radically enhance the lives of those living with 'locked-in' syndrome.

Case example

Elizabeth was admitted to a specialist rehabilitation centre following a haemorrhagic stroke in the brainstem region in February 2005. Prior to her stroke she worked as a full-time accountant and was a mother to her three-year-old daughter. She was 42 years old, and had a supportive mother, brother and two sisters. The referral to the rehabilitation centre offered a putative diagnosis of 'locked-in' syndrome. The following is an account of her journey through rehabilitation. Speech pathology (speech and language therapy) rehabilitation is predominantly discussed, but her full rehabilitation programme was multidimensional and multidisciplinary, essential when an individual has such significant impairments.

Airway and dysphagia management

Elizabeth arrived at the rehabilitation centre with a cuffed tracheostomy tube in situ. The tracheostomy had been performed five days after the brain haemorrhage, when it became clear that she would require longer-term support for her airway. She had been free of chest infections for three months when she was transferred to the centre, was maintained with nil orally, receiving all nutrition and hydration via a percutaneous endoscopic gastrostomy tube.

The majority of patients with 'locked-in' syndrome require tracheostomy initially at least, because:

- There is potential for damage to the respiratory control centre located in the medulla, resulting in physiological changes in breathing and subsequent need for ventilatory support
- Bulbar muscles are weakened or paralysed, with resultant risk of airway obstruction from anatomical structures, for example low toned base of tongue or vocal cord paralysis
- Paralysis of bulbar muscles is associated with risk of aspiration of food, fluid or saliva into the airway, with the potential for development of aspiration pneumonia
- Weakened respiratory musculature with resultant weak or absent cough reflex leads to inability to clear chest secretions. A tracheostomy tube provides an entry point into the airway by which secretions can be removed via suctioning

An initial role of the speech pathologist was to assess how effective Elizabeth's swallow function was for saliva, and from this to determine if it was appropriate to consider starting a tracheostomy tube weaning programme. The decision to commence a tracheostomy weaning programme is one made by the MDT; in this instance, speech pathologist in conjunction with nursing staff, doctors and physiotherapists.

Swallow assessment

Speech pathology assessment of Elizabeth's bulbar muscles revealed low tone throughout her face, lips and tongue. At the bedside there was no observable swallow initiated either to command or reflexively. Reflexive bobbing and twitching movements were observed in the laryngeal area of the neck and in Elizabeth's facial muscles. No other reflexive or volitional movements were observed. Severe drooling of her saliva (to the level of her chin and beyond) was observed due to lack of movement of her lip, tongue and throat muscles and the absent swallow reflex. Given the severity of deficits observed at the bedside, oral intake was not trialled.

The cuff on Elizabeth's tracheostomy tube was creating a barrier between the upper and lower airways, resulting in the flow of air occurring only through the tracheostomy tube to the lungs. The upper airway and larynx were bypassed. This barrier (cuff) was helping prevent aspiration of oral secretions; however, cuffs are not designed to prevent large volume aspiration, and aspiration of secretions around the cuff can occur (Dikeman & Kazandijan 1996). The presence of a cuffed tracheostomy tube may impair swallow function as there is loss of airflow in and around the larynx and laryngeal receptors, with reduced sensation (Sasaki et al. 1977). Long term, a cuffed tracheostomy tube may cause complications such as malachia, stenosis, and granulation (Law et al. 1993) although such events are less often reported with newer cuff materials.

The goal of intervention with such patients is to normalise their situation as much as possible, whilst managing any risks this might involve. With this goal in mind, the MDT decided that given Elizabeth's clear chest status, short periods of cuff deflation should be trialled despite her high risk of aspiration of oral secretions. Because cuffed tracheostomy tubes do not eliminate aspiration of secretions, it was likely that Elizabeth had been aspirating her oral secretions without detrimental impact on her respiratory health. Cuff deflation would expose Elizabeth to a more normal breathing and swallow experience and possibly reduce her risk of long-term complications associated with tracheostomy tubes.

Over one month, periods of cuff deflation were trialled and extended. By the end of the month continuous cuff deflation was tolerated. Throughout, careful monitoring and documentation of Elizabeth's chest condition and respiratory status was essential to progression of the weaning pathway. At this stage it was decided that detailed information about Elizabeth's swallow function and airway was required, and she was referred for a fibreoptic endoscopic evaluation of swallow (FEES). This is a swallow assessment that may be conducted by an appropriately trained speech pathologist, sometimes in conjunction with an Ear Nose and Throat medical officer; it involves examination of the airway and swallow physiology using an endoscope.

The FEES revealed severe dysphagia with copious amounts of saliva in the pharynx, and severe subglottic stenosis, likely as a result of prolonged endotracheal intubation. This stenosis was occluding approximately 70% of her airway. Elizabeth also had myoclonus present throughout her pharynx, larynx and base of tongue: rhythmical pulsing-type movements associated with lower motor neuron lesions, which, when severe, can compromise an individual's ability to breathe independently. Given these findings and the duration since the initial brain haemorrhage it was felt unlikely that Elizabeth would ever achieve full decannulation. Given her clear chest history, however, it was decided to continue with cuff deflation and the tracheostomy tube was changed to a cuffless tube.

Communication

Elizabeth arrived at the rehabilitation centre with no established method of communication. Given the diagnosis of a haemorrhage in the medulla it was not anticipated that Elizabeth would have significant cognitive or linguistic impairments. A joint assessment between Speech Pathology and Occupational Therapy revealed that Elizabeth had just two movements in her body under her control: she could raise her right thumb and she could move her eyes up and down. Her thumb movement was inconsistent, due to muscle fatigue rather than impaired control, but due to this inconsistency of muscle movement it was decided to utilise eye movement as a method of communication because this was a more robust and reliable movement.

The initial role of speech pathology was to determine the level of linguistic understanding. There are few assessments available for speech pathologists working with patients who have 'locked-in' syndrome. Much of the assessment therefore comprised non-standardised material and informal observations of responses over time, to allow the clinician to build up a profile of the patient's communicative strengths and weaknesses. The vertical eye movement was used as the yes/no response. Elizabeth rolled her eyes up for yes, and lowered them for no. Using these responses an assessment, using paired yes/no questions, was completed, for example, is this a bell? (The patient is shown a bell); is this money? (The patient is shown a bell). In order to score correctly the patient must answer both questions correctly. Paired questions are used with yes/no responses to assess comprehension because of the effect of chance. If non-paired questions are used, the patient has a 50% chance of a correct answer by luck for each question; pairing the questions reduces this. Biographical questions were used initially using information provided by the family, for example, do you have a daughter? (Yes); do you have a son? (No). Next, a 60-question yes/no informal assessment was carried out: Elizabeth scored 60/60 correctly, indicating intact linguistic functioning.

Next, the role of the speech pathologist was to develop a broader means of communication with Elizabeth. The idea of AEIOU auditory/visual scanning was introduced (Figure 10.2). This is a low technology form of alternative and

A	B	C	D		
E	F	G	H		
I	J	K	L	M	N
O	P	Q	R	S	T
U	V	W	X	Y	Z

Figure 10.2 The AEIOU auditory/visual scanning device.

augmentative communication. It involves the communication partner (e.g. nurse or relative) reading out letters from an alphabet board. The AEIOU row column method of scanning was designed to speed up the system, because not all of the letters of the alphabet are read out all of the time. The communication partner started by reading aloud the letters in the far left hand column (AEIOU); Elizabeth would roll her eyes up when she heard the letter at the beginning of the row containing the letter she wanted. For example, if Elizabeth wanted to spell the word GIRL, she would roll her eyes when the letter E was read out, the communication partner would then read aloud the letters contained in that row (EFGH). Elizabeth would then roll her eyes up when the letter G was spoken, indicating the target letter was G. The communication partner would make a note of this and begin scanning again from A, and so on to allow Elizabeth to complete her message.

Although initially a time-consuming and laborious method of communication (for Elizabeth as well as her communication partners – staff and family), this was an initial step. In the absence of any other method of communication, this approach can literally 'unlock' an individual and enable a high level of communication. With practice this method of communication can become fast and efficient, with short cuts introduced. Eventually it is common for both patient and communication partner not to require the board and scanning can be done from memory.

An alternative and more high technology communication aid was then introduced, aiming to support independent communication. However, after trialling the device Elizabeth chose to stay with the low tech method above, describing this as a quicker and easier way for her to communicate with people that knew the system. Extensive education was provided to Elizabeth's family, friends and carers on use of the communication technique and a video was made with Elizabeth in preparation for her discharge to a long-term care facility, demonstrating her method of communication.

Conclusion

MRS and 'locked-in' syndrome are rare outcomes of stroke, but when they occur they are devastating for patients, carers and staff. Nurses and their care for these patients make significant contributions at all stages of the patient journey – assessment; decision-making, planning and goal-setting; delivery, monitoring and evaluation of care; communicating and ensuring good communication between patients, carers and MDT members. It is essential that nurses have a good understanding of these conditions, current evidence and 'best practice', and awareness of areas where practice development, research and technological innovation are revolutionising the patient experience, quality of life and survival, carer and community contribution to management.

References

Andrews, K, Murphy, L, Munday, R, & Littlewood, C, 1996, Misdiagnosis of the vegetative state: retrospective study in a rehabilitation unit, *British Medical Journal*, vol. 313, no. 7048, pp. 13–16.

Ansell, BJ, & Keenan, JE, 1989, The Western Neuro Sensory Stimulation Profile: a tool for assessing slow-to-recover head-injured patients, *Archives of Physical Medicine and Rehabilitation*, vol. 70, no. 2, pp. 104–108.

Bauby, J-D, 1997, *The Diving Bell and the Butterfly: A Memoir of Life in Death*, Vintage, New York.

Bauer, G, Gerstenbrand, F, & Rumpl, E, 1979, Varieties of the locked-in syndrome, *Journal of Neurology*, vol. 221, no. 2, pp. 77–91.

Beaumont, JG, Marjoribanks, J, Flury, S, & Lintern, T, 1999, Assessing auditory comprehension in the context of severe physical disability: the PACST, *Brain Injury*, vol. 13, no. 2, pp. 99–112.

British Medical Association, 2007, *Treatment of Patients in Persistent Vegetative State*, BMA Medical Ethics Department.

Casanova, E, Lazzari, RE, Lotta, S, & Mazzucchi, A, 2003, Locked-in syndrome: improvement in the prognosis after an early intensive multidisciplinary rehabilitation, *Archives of Physical Medicine and Rehabilitation*, vol. 84, no. 6, pp. 862–867.

Chapman, JE, 1991, *Use of an eye-operated computer system in locked-in syndrome*, CSUN Sixth Annual International Conference: Technology and Persons with Disabilities, Fairfax, Virginia 22032, USA.

Childs, NL, Mercer, WN, & Childs, HW, 1993, Accuracy of diagnosis of persistent vegetative state, *Neurology*, vol. 43, no. 8, pp. 1465–1467.

Chua, KS, Ng, YS, Yap, SG, & Bok, CW, 2007, A brief review of traumatic brain injury rehabilitation, *Annals of the Academy of Medicine, Singapore*, vol. 36, no. 1, pp. 31–42.

Cullen, N, Chundamala, J, Bayley, M, & Jutai, J, 2007, The efficacy of acquired brain injury rehabilitation, *Brain Injury*, vol. 21, no. 2, pp. 113–132.

Davenport, RJ, Dennis, MS, & Warlow, CP, 1995, Improving the recording of the clinical assessment of stroke patients using a clerking pro forma, *Age and Ageing*, vol. 24, no. 1, pp. 43–48.

Dikeman, KJ, & Kazandijan, MS, 1996, *Communication and Swallowing Management of Tracheostomized and Ventilator-Dependent Adults*, Singular Publishing Group.

Frey, LA, White Jr, KP, & Hutchinson, TE, 1990, Eye-gaze word processing, *IEEE Transactions on Systems, Man and Cybernetics*, vol. 20, no. 4, pp. 944–950.

Gill-Thwaites, H, 1997, The Sensory Modality Assessment Rehabilitation Technique – a tool for assessment and treatment of patients with severe brain injury in a vegetative state, *Brain Injury*, vol. 11, no. 10, pp. 723–734.

Gill-Thwaites, H, 2006, Lotteries, loopholes and luck: misdiagnosis in the vegetative state patient, *Brain Injury*, vol. 20, no. 13–14, pp. 1321–1328.

Gill-Thwaites, H, & Munday, R, 1999, The Sensory Modality Assessment and Rehabilitation Technique (SMART): a comprehensive and integrated assessment and treatment protocol for the vegetative state and minimally responsive patient, *Neuropsychological Rehabilitation*, vol. 9, no. 3/4, pp. 305–320.

Gill-Thwaites, H, & Munday, R, 2004, The Sensory Modality Assessment and Rehabilitation Technique (SMART): a valid and reliable assessment for vegetative state and minimally conscious state patients, *Brain Injury*, vol. 18, no. 12, pp. 1255–1269.

Haig, AJ, Katz, RT, & Sahgal, V, 1987, Mortality and complications of the locked-in syndrome, *Archives of Physical Medicine and Rehabilitation*, vol. 68, no. 1, pp. 24–27.

Intercollegiate Stroke Working Party, 2008, *National Clinical Guideline for Stroke*, 3rd edn, Royal College of Physicians, London.

Katz, DI, 2001, *Minimally Conscious States*, http://www.kurzweilai.net/meme/frame.html?maine=/articles/art0161.html 12-5-2009

Laureys, S, Boly, M, & Maquet, P, 2006, Tracking the recovery of consciousness from coma, *Journal of Clinical Investigation*, vol. 116, no. 7, pp. 1823–1825.

Law, JH, Barnhart, K, Rowlett, W, de la Rocha O, & Lowenberg, S, 1993, Increased frequency of obstructive airway abnormalities with long-term tracheostomy, *Chest*, vol. 104, no. 1, pp. 136–138.

Leon-Carrion, J, van Eeeckhout P, Dominguez-Morales, MR, & Perez-Santamaria, FJ, 2002, The locked-in syndrome: a syndrome looking for a therapy, *Brain Injury*, vol. 16, no. 7, pp. 571–582.

Mackenzie, S, Gale, E, & Munday, R, 2005, Putney Auditory Single Word Yes/No Assessment (PASWORD). Development of a reliable test of yes/no at a single word level in patients unable to participate in assessments requiring a specific motor response: an exploratory study, *International Journal of Language and Communication Disorders*, vol. 41, pp. 225–234.

Magee, WL, 2007, Development of a music therapy assessment tool for patients in low awareness states, *NeuroRehabilitation*, vol. 22, no. 4, pp. 319–324.

Magee, WL, & Andrews, K, 2007, Multi-disciplinary perceptions of music therapy in complex neuro-rehabilitation, *International Journal of Therapy and Rehabilitation*, vol. 14, no. 2, pp. 70–74.

Millwood, J, Mackenzie, S, Munday, R, Pierce, E, & Fiske, J, 2005, A report from an investigation of abnormal oral reflexes, lip trauma and awareness levels in patients with profound brain damage, *Journal of Disability and Oral Health*, vol. 6, no. 2, pp. 72–78.

National Health and Medical Research Council, 2008, *Ethical guidelines for the care of people in post-coma unresponsiveness (vegetative state) or a minimally responsive state*, Australian Government.

Naude, K, & Hughes, M, 2005, Considerations for the use of assistive technology in patients with impaired states of consciousness, *Neuropsychological Rehabilitation*, vol. 15, no. 3–4, pp. 514–521.

Patterson, JR, & Grabois, M, 1986, Locked-in syndrome: a review of 139 cases, *Stroke*, vol. 17, no. 4, pp. 758–764.

Pierce, E, & McLaren, S, 2003, *Multidisciplinary Evaluation of Neuro-dependency (MEND)*, Royal Hospital for Neuro-disability, London.

Pierce, E, Cowan, P, & Stokes, M, 2001, Managing faecal retention and incontinence in neurodisability, *British Journal of Nursing*, vol. 10, no. 9, pp. 592–601.

Plum, F, & Posner, JB, 1966, *The Diagnosis of Stupor and Coma*, F.A. Davis Co, Philadelphia.

Sasaki, CT, Suzuki, M, Horiuchi, M, & Kirchner, JA, 1977, The effect of tracheostomy on the laryngeal closure reflex, *Laryngoscope*, vol. 87, no. 9 Pt 1, pp. 1428–1433.

Scherb, CA, Rapp, CG, Johnson, M, & Maas, M, 1998, The nursing outcomes classi-fication: validation by rehabilitation nurses, *Rehabilitation Nursing*, vol. 23, no. 4, pp. 174–178, 191.

Smith, E, & Delargy, M, 2005, Locked-in syndrome, *British Medical Journal*, vol. 330, no. 7488, pp. 406–409.

Taylor, CM, Aird, VH, Tate, RL, & Lammi, MH, 2007, Sequence of recovery during the course of emergence from the minimally conscious state, *Archives of Physical Medicine and Rehabilitation*, vol. 88, no. 4, pp. 521–525.

Thaxton, L, & Myers, MA, 2002, Sleep disturbances and their management in patients with brain injury, *Journal of Head Trauma Rehabilitation*, vol. 17, no. 4, pp. 335–348.

Varricchio, CG, 2006, Measurement issues in quality-of-life assessments, *Oncology Nursing Forum*, vol. 33, no. 1 Suppl, pp. 13–21.

Wade, DT, Hewer, RL, Skilbeck, CE, & David, RM, 1985, *Principles of Assessment in Stroke*, Chapman and Hall, London.

Whyte, J, DiPasquale, MC, & Vaccaro, M, 1999, Assessment of command-following in minimally conscious brain injured patients, *Archives of Physical Medicine and Rehabilitation*, vol. 80, no. 6, pp. 653–660.

Wilson, SL, & Gill-Thwaites, H, 2000, Early indication of emergence from vegetative state derived from assessments with the SMART – a preliminary report, *Brain Injury*, vol. 14, no. 4, pp. 319–331.

Chapter 11

Rehabilitation and recovery processes

Jane Williams and Julie Pryor

Key points

- Rehabilitation following stroke is a journey that the stroke survivor, their family and loved ones follow for a variable duration of time.
- Rehabilitation optimises the stroke survivor's participation in their life and surroundings.
- Nursing's contribution to patient rehabilitation is significant and specific.
- A rehabilitative approach to care should be commenced as soon as possible after the stroke event.
- Rehabilitation should focus on and be responsive to individual patients and their circumstances.

I was frightened as I was no longer in charge of my life. They [the rehabilitation team] helped me not to be frightened.

The stroke team cannot be faulted. They put our lives into a liveable place from the trauma and feeling of being shelved as useless.

(Courtesy of patients from a UK,
National Health Service hospital stroke service)

Introduction

What is rehabilitation?

Following stroke, most patients embark on a rehabilitation journey, an 'individual, active and dynamic process' (Barnes & Ward 2000, p. 6) aimed at ameliorating the person's experience of disability and reducing the burden of care. A person may not become aware of the need to embark on this intensely personal journey until they realise that the problems resulting from stroke are not going away (Easton 1999). Furthermore, each person's journey is unique in that the significance of the experience of stroke and its meaning for the individual is shaped by individual context and biography (Alaszewski et al. 2004; Faircloth et al. 2004).

For health care professionals, however, rehabilitation must begin at the patient's first point of contact with a health service and inform all decision-making thereafter. Rehabilitation requires that all health care professionals possess and act upon an awareness of how what does, and does not, happen today affects the patient's desired tomorrow (Plaisted 1978). As such, rehabilitation is more than a series of intermittent interventions done to patients by health professionals. It is a continuous process that is underpinned by 'the principle of patient empowerment' (Ozer 1999, p. 44). This requires active patient participation (Demain et al. 2006; van Vliet & Wulf 2006) and is enhanced by a self-management approach (Jones 2006) that fosters a 'can do' attitude. Theories of learning and change are as fundamental to rehabilitation as understanding of health and illness models. More specifically, rehabilitation focuses on:

- Maintenance and restoration of functioning
- Promotion of health, and
- Prevention and minimisation of disability

Defining rehabilitation

The term 'functioning' is 'an umbrella term for body functions, body structures'; 'activities' refers to 'execution of a task or action by an individual'; and 'participation' to 'a person's involvement in a life situation' (World Health Organisation (WHO) 2001, pp. 212–213). The term 'disability' is 'an umbrella term for impairments, activity limitation' and 'difficulties an individual may have in executing activities'; 'participation restrictions' are 'problems an individual may experience in involvement in life situations' (World Health Organisation (WHO) 2001, p. 213). These terms from the International Classification of Functioning, Disability and Health – ICF (2001) are used because of the wide interest in the ICF as a framework for rehabilitation (Bartlett et al. 2006; Grill et al. 2005; Scheuringer et al. 2005; Stucki et al. 2005b; Wade 2005; Worral 2005) and in particular stroke rehabilitation (Salter et al. 2005a, 2005b, 2005c; Tempest & McIntyre 2006). The model was endorsed by the World Health Assembly in 2001 and can be found at http://www.who.int/classification/icf. ICF highlights how a person's health conditions interact dynamically with contextual factors to create functioning or disability (Figure 11.1).

In relation to stroke, a person may have an impairment of sensation, an activity limitation in eating and a participation restriction by not being invited to family celebrations. Contextual factors might include personal factors such as outgoing personality and environmental factors such as attitudes of family members.

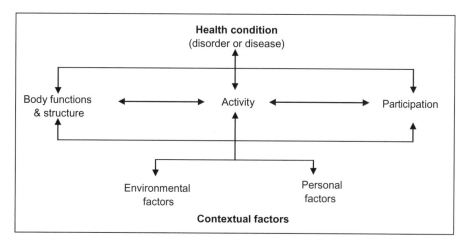

Figure 11.1 International Classification of Functioning, Disability and Health. Reproduced with permission from World Health Organisation (WHO), 2001, *International Classification of Functioning, Disability and Health (ICF),* World Health Organisation, Geneva.

The framework of the ICF can be used to provide conceptual underpinnings of the rehabilitation diagnosis, including its assessment procedures and interventions (Bartlett et al. 2006; Lettinga et al. 2006; Rentsch et al. 2003). This does not mean, however, that standardised rehabilitation interventions are used for everyone. Rehabilitation uses interventions that range from a macro to a micro level (Whyte & Hart 2003). This multiplicity of levels of interventions and the many interactions between them mean that rehabilitation is not an exact science, with a broad range of characteristics capable of influencing patient outcomes. For example, patient outcomes can be affected at the macro level by characteristics such as team functioning; at the micro level, by issues such as the timing of an upper limb training programme (Kwakkel 2006; Strasser et al. 2005).

Equally important is patient motivation (Maclean et al. 2000) and the extent of active patient engagement in rehabilitation. Rehabilitation interventions need to integrate and optimise the efforts of the person experiencing stroke and those guiding and supporting that person (family, friends as well as health and community workers). Importantly, rehabilitation services need to ensure they are client-centred. From a study of rehabilitation clients, Cott (2004, p. 1418) reports client-centred rehabilitation as characterised by:

- 'Individualization of programmes to the needs of each client in order to prepare them for life in the real world
- Mutual participation with health professionals in decision-making and goal-setting
- Outcomes that are meaningful to the client
- Sharing of information and education that is appropriate, timely and according to the client's wishes
- Emotional support

- Family and peer involvement throughout the rehabilitation process; and
- Coordination and continuity across the multiple service sectors'

It therefore follows that the behaviours of health care professionals and patients as well as interactions between them contribute to the effectiveness of rehabilitation. 'It is important that professionals communicate effectively so that their interventions are grounded in and support the survivor's goals and strategies' (Alaszewski et al. 2004, p. 1067).

Rehabilitation as an intervention

The nature of rehabilitation as an intervention is complex and multifactorial requiring multiple inputs from skilled and expert individuals. It has proven difficult to explain and explore the process and this has resulted in the development of many different definitions, service design and delivery models. Despite this, the evidence base for various rehabilitation approaches, individual therapies and service provision is growing all the time. In the UK the National Clinical Guidelines for Stroke (Intercollegiate Stroke Working Party 2008) provide recommendations based on the best available evidence. There are a wealth of international resources available, for example the Canadian Evidence Based Review of Stroke Rehabilitation database (EBRSR 2009), Cochrane Stroke Group (CSRG 2009), American Stroke Association (ASA 2009), National Stroke Foundation – Australia (NSF 2009) and Scottish Intercollegiate Guidelines Network (Scottish Intercollegiate Guidelines Network (SIGN) 2005). The evidence available for clinicians is overwhelming; consensus guidelines provide an invaluable tool and their use may result in improved outcomes (Duncan et al. 2005; Reker et al. 2002).

Initiation of rehabilitation

Rehabilitation needs to be a primary focus of care in the Emergency Department, in acute care, in rehabilitation wards and in the community. This is a challenge given the priority demanded for patients' more life-threatening problems. Nonetheless, the evidence in support of what Stucki, and colleagues (2005a, p. 353) refer to as 'the new paradigm of "early rehabilitation"' is compelling. In a study of 830 post-stroke (moderate and severe) patients in five inpatient rehabilitation facilities in the USA, Horn et al (2005, p. S101) found that 'earlier admission to rehabilitation, higher-level activities early in the rehabilitation process, tube feeding and newer medications are associated with better stroke outcomes'. The authors point out that their finding of participation in early gait activities and 'higher-order more challenging therapy activities' even for low-functioning patients challenges conventional thinking in rehabilitation (Horn et al. 2005, p. S111). It seems that improvements in lower-level functions can be achieved by focusing on higher-order activities. Furthermore, 'fewer days from stroke symptom onset to rehabilitation admission is associated with better functional outcomes at discharge and shorter LOS [length of stay]' (Maulden et al. 2005, p. S34). This assumption is currently being tested through AVERT (A Very Early Rehabilitation Trial; Bernhardt et al. 2006). Similarly, Salter et al (2009) found that 'patients admitted to stroke rehabilitation within 30 days of first-ever, unilateral stroke experienced greater functional gain and shorter length of stay than those whose admission to rehabilitation was delayed beyond 30 days'. Most importantly, the commencement of rehabilitation should not be delayed until transfer to a specialised rehabilitation service.

The nursing rehabilitation role

Rehabilitation is the responsibility of every nurse and as 'rehabilitators par excellence' (Henderson 1980, p. 146), nurses fulfil the roles of coach (Australasian Rehabilitation Nurses' Association 2003; Price 1997; Pryor 2005; Pryor & Smith 2002; Thompson 1990) and travelling companion for patients on their rehabilitation journey as well as coordinator of staff input into patient rehabilitation (Burton 1999). In the Emergency Department, by focusing on the maintenance of function and prevention of complications, nursing contributes to the person's rehabilitation (Box 11.1). In acute care, the main goals of rehabilitation interventions provided by nurses are the maintenance and restoration of functioning, prevention of complications and early mobilisation (Stucki et al. 2005a, p. 355).

By focusing on the maintenance of function nurses can prevent 'imposed dependence' (Gignac & Cott 1998, p. 741). This is of utmost importance in relation to older people and while not all stroke patients are elderly, it is important to note that hospitalisation is hazardous for older people (Mahoney et al. 1998; Sager et al. 1996) (Box 11.2). This makes care of the older stroke patient, who often has one or more co-morbid health conditions, very complex.

Box 11.1 Rehabilitative stroke nursing interventions for emergency and acute settings.

- Physiological monitoring
- Positioning
- Joint and limb protection
- Recognition, assessment and management of dysphagia
- Assessment and management of tissue viability
- Prevention of complications (e.g. aspiration pneumonia, DVT, constipation, hospital-acquired infections)
- Assessment and management of risk (e.g. falls)
- Management of urinary continence problems without (where possible) catheterisation
- Early education and information sharing (patient and family)
- Consideration of cultural differences
- Concordance with secondary prevention measures
- Medication management and self-medication programmes
- Commencing collection and collation of background information (housing, leisure, hobbies etc.)
- Ensuring the patient has adequate rest and sleep
- Psychological support to minimise trauma
- Onward referral to a specialist setting/team

> **Box 11.2** Hazards of hospitalisation.
>
> - Hospital-acquired infections
> - Weight loss and nutritional inadequacies
> - Loss of physical conditioning (strength and endurance)
> - Falls
> - Social isolation
> - Depression
> - Fatigue and sleep disturbance

An essential adjunct to rehabilitation interventions in non-specialised rehabilitation settings is the early identification of patients who would benefit from input from a specialised rehabilitation team. Early referral to that team may enable in-reach into the acute setting by the rehabilitation team.

In the specialty rehabilitation setting, nursing's contribution is central to optimal patient outcomes. Various studies of nursing practice in these settings reveal that nurses enable patients to reclaim self-care by adopting an informed 'hands-off' approach (Hill & Johnson 1999; O'Connor 2000; Pryor 2005; Pryor & Smith 2002), instead of 'doing for' or 'doing to' patients. Teaching is a significant factor in assisting patients to reclaim self-care (Burton 2000; Kirkevold 1997; Pryor 2005; Pryor & Smith 2002). An important adjunct to teaching is helping patients and families cope with, and adjust to, what has happened to them (Faircloth et al. 2004; Long et al. 2002; Pryor 2005).

Across all settings, nursing is responsible for patient and family education as well as the coordination of each patient's rehabilitation. This involves:

- Explaining the nature and purpose of rehabilitation to patients and families
- Explaining the roles of health care professionals, patients and families in rehabilitation
- Explaining the differences between acute care and rehabilitation
- Setting goals, that are relevant to the patient, with the patient
- Ensuring the timely communication of information between patient and/or family and health care professionals
- Ensuring the timely and appropriate communication of information between health care professionals
- Harmonising the efforts of patients and health care professionals

The importance of a coordinated approach to teamwork is highlighted by the Stroke Unit Trialists' Collaboration (2007). Being the only discipline to have a 24-hour presence and with the responsibility for monitoring patient well-being as well as the effectiveness of therapeutic interventions provided by the whole team, nursing assumes this responsibility. Sometimes an invisible contribution, coordination is most noticed when it is lacking.

Outcomes of rehabilitation

The outcomes of rehabilitation are of interest to 'patients [and their families], payers, and society as a whole' (DeJong et al. 2004, p. 678). At policy level, reduction in disability and improvement in participation in life by stroke survivors are the ultimate aims of rehabilitation (D'Alisa et al. 2005). At the point of rehabilitation service delivery, the desired outcome of rehabilitation is achievement of goals mutually agreed by the patient and the health care team. These goals are generally short-term goals that represent the steps required to achieve the patient's long term goal. Goals should be those that rehabilitation services can contribute to within available resources. It is commonly recommended that these goals are SMART; that is, Specific, Measurable, Achievable, Relevant and Time-limited.

The person's ultimate goal, however, is 'return to the existence they had lived before the stroke' (Hafsteinsdottir & Grypdonck 1997, p. 580). Unfortunately, this is not always possible, regardless of how much intervention is provided by the rehabilitation team. Nonetheless, successful rehabilitation is based on what matters to the person who has had a stroke (Alaszewski et al. 2004). An essential starting point is the re-establishment of a 'person's sense of control over his or her body and life' (Ozer 1999, p. 43).

Goal-directed rehabilitation

The use of goals is a hallmark of rehabilitation. Goal-setting identifies what is important to patients and a patient's goals provide the rationale for all actions undertaken by health care professionals. Engaging patients (and when patients are unable, their families) in the goal-setting process is an essential first step in the re-establishment of a person's sense of control. Engaging patients should also ensure that the patient's priorities become the team's priorities. Through engagement in the goal-setting process patients learn about their body structures and functions as well as the rehabilitation therapies and activities for addressing their impairments, activity limitation and participation restrictions. Some patients also gain a deeper appreciation of what is important to them. In addition, patients learn how to identify functional improvements and goal attainment. Molly (Case example 11.1) illustrates how targeted goal-setting can achieve what is required to enable patients to move from hospital to home.

Although 'evidence regarding the generalisability of goal planning to improve patient outcomes in rehabilitation is inconsistent at best' (Levack et al. 2006b, p. 752), goal-setting is widely supported as a pragmatic approach that fits with the problem-solving and educational processes of rehabilitation (Wade 1999).

Case example 11.1 Molly.

Molly had been an inpatient on a stroke rehabilitation ward for six weeks. She was experiencing continence problems, particularly at night, and her goal was to achieve night-time control to enable her to go home with the community stroke rehabilitation team.

Various methods where discussed and tried. Molly wasn't able to transfer independently yet and her husband had health problems which meant he would be unable to assist her. Success was achieved with a female urinal. Molly was able to leave hospital and continue rehabilitation at home. She is making good progress.

Effective goal-setting can assist patients to move from pre-contemplation to action (van den Broek 2005). As such, goals can be a powerful mechanism for enhancing patient ownership of, and engagement in, their rehabilitation, as well as for evaluating rehabilitation outcomes (Levack et al. 2006a). Most importantly, it is an ethical as well as practical imperative for rehabilitation to focus on what drives the patient (McClain 2005).

Given the importance of early rehabilitation, the initial purpose of goal-setting may be to facilitate patient readiness for rehabilitation. By listening, nurses can find out about a patient's life, noting what the patient values, with a view to understanding the patient's 'idealised self-image', a concept that McGrath and Adams (2005) suggest influences all of a person's actions. Carver and Scheier's control-process model of self-regulation suggests that 'at all times the behaviour [of a patient] is directed toward reducing the discrepancy between the person's goal and existing circumstances' (Siegert et al. 2004, p. 1175). In relation to this, Siegert and colleagues (2004) make explicit the importance of setting concrete goals that enable patients and health care workers to work towards a patient's super-ordinate goals and idealised self-image. Equally important, however, is an appreciation that it is the patient's perception of the rate of progress towards goal achievement in relation to their desired rate that results in a change in emotion or affect (McGrath & Adams 2005; Siegert & Taylor 2004). McGrath and Adams (2005) report positive changes in the affect of neurological patients following engagement in goal planning based on Carver and Scheier's model. Negative affect and goal disengagement, however, can arise from slower than expected progress towards goal attainment (Siegert & Taylor 2004).

Mauk's (Easton 1999; Mauk 2006) model of post-stroke recovery highlights the importance of setting goals that are appropriate for the patient's stage of recovery. Similar to Prochaska and colleagues' (1992) transtheoretical model of change, Mauk's model recognises the need for patients to realise that rehabilitation requires them to act. According to Mauk (2006, p. 259) patient engagement in post-stroke rehabilitation is contingent upon a patient realising that 'the effects of his or her stroke may not all go away'. Tension between lack of patient readiness for rehabilitation and the evidence supporting benefits of early rehabilitation makes a priority of research to determine the most effective ways to use goals to enhance patient rehabilitation.

Nonetheless, several factors seem to be emerging as central to effective goal-setting with patients. These are that:

- Patient engagement in the process is an imperative and any organisational policy or protocol for goal-setting must be flexible enough to ensure that patients can engage in the manner that best suits them, rather than the manner that best suits the organisation. This includes flexibility about whether the patient meets with one or more health care professionals to set goals.
- Discussion should start by establishing the patient's long term goals.
- The process must enable patients to maintain hope that their long-term goals can be achieved. Long-term goals should only be revised by patients, not health care professionals.

- The link between shorter-term goals and actions of health care professionals must be made explicit to the patient and their family.
- Short-term goals must be measurable.
- Short-term goals should identify who, in addition to the patient and perhaps their family, will be responsible for guiding and supporting the patient to achieve the goal and how they will do this.
- For patients who experience variations in their energy, strength, balance and/ or safety throughout the day or week, short-term goals should be linked to appropriate times of the day or days of the week.
- Progress toward goal achievement must be evaluated regularly so the next round of goals can be set. One to two weeks seems to be the norm, but this too requires further research.
- Patients and all health care professionals working with the patients must have ready access to their documented goals.
- Goals and evidence of goal attainment can be used as an educational tool to make explicit progress towards patients' long-term goals. The use of time-limited and measurable short-term goals enables the use of graphs to demonstrate goal achievement across time.

Recovery processes

Maximising recovery is the focus of care as soon as the stroke happens. Recovery processes are, in turn, optimised through the adoption of rehabilitation. Rehabilitation should commence as soon as possible and this, of course, includes utilising a rehabilitative approach in the acute phase. The exact nature of effective stroke rehabilitation is still not clear but should address physical, psychological, behavioural, cultural, spiritual and social issues for the individual and, equally importantly, their family. There is evidence that intensity of rehabilitation is vital in the early stages and should be provided by specialist teams (Diserens et al. 2006; Indredavik et al. 1999). Rehabilitation encompasses natural recovery through central nervous system reorganisation (plasticity) and functional recovery, both of which are influenced by rehabilitation (this is further explained in Chapter 2). Many factors affect the progress and recovery an individual may make, and ensuring that there are opportunities to practise regained skills through consistent management is vital. This is a pivotal role for nurses.

It has been estimated that one-third of stroke patients make significant improvements and a further third survive with continuing severe disability (Gladman & Sackley 1998). These groups require specific stroke treatment and interventions. Different therapeutic modalities are being researched to demonstrate which are most effective and for whom. Stroke rehabilitation has been referred to as a 'black box' of interventions (Kalra & Eade 1995). Dobkin and Carmichael (2005) conceptualise the interacting principles of 'restitution, substitution or compensation'. Restitution means that the pre-stroke ability has been restored, for example swallowing problems that have resolved. Substitution, as the word suggests, refers to using another means to achieving the same end, for example learning to write with the left hand when previously the person was right handed. Compensation is a technique used to work around the problem when neither restitution nor substitution is possible or appropriate. An example might be using a hip-hitching movement to facilitate walking.

The World Health Organisation's updated ICF model (referred to earlier in this chapter) provides a useful framework to consider a person's adjustment and adaptation to their stroke. The ICF is based on a *biopsychosocial model*, an integration of medical and social aspects. Through this synthesis, the ICF provides a coherent view of different perspectives of health: biological, individual and social. The effects of stroke on an individual and their family affect every level of the biopsychosocial model and the ICF can be very helpful in assisting the development of person- and family-centred programmes of rehabilitation.

Targeting rehabilitation at those most likely to benefit is challenging. Garraway and colleagues (1981) classified stroke patients into three groups. Firstly, there are those who are likely to make spontaneous recovery without substantial rehabilitation and return home promptly. Secondly, there are those with poor prognostic indicators (i.e. depressed level of consciousness), who generally do not achieve functional independence and require continuing care. However, this group may benefit from rehabilitation aimed at reducing their care needs or improving certain aspects of their quality of life (i.e. posture and seating). The final group consists of a middle band of stroke survivors, who are most likely to gain from intensive rehabilitation and make significant functional improvement. However, focusing solely on functional recovery risks overlooking emotional and psychosocial problems (Davidoff et al. 1992). As the ICF model indicates, these factors can play 'a much more important role in stroke outcome than most people realise' (Johnston et al. 1992).

Stroke is considered to be a family illness or a 'family dilemma' (Evans et al. 1992, 1994; Greveson & James 1991) as both the patient and their family embark on a journey for which they need information and support in physical, emotional and spiritual terms. The outcomes of stroke are many, varied and often unpredictable. How the patient and their family are helped through the acute phases of stroke care will influence their experience in transition to rehabilitation and may affect any future contact with stroke services.

Transfer to rehabilitation

Transfer from an acute to rehabilitation setting is an important event for patients. Transfer to rehabilitation indicates to patients that health care professionals believe further recovery is possible. Nonetheless, transfer from one service or health care team to another can be very stressful for patients and their families. The move from a familiar to unfamiliar environment, from known to unknown service providers requires patients and their families to become familiar with new routines and establish relationships with new staff.

To minimise patients' experiences of relocation stress syndrome (Gordon 2000), education about the nature and purpose of rehabilitation and an

---

Box 11.3   Six phases of the post-stroke journey (Mauk 2006).

- Agonising
- Fantasising
- Realising
- Blending
- Framing
- Owning

---

explanation of the roles of health care professionals, patients and families in rehabilitation should be provided to patients and their families. In particular, the differences between acute and rehabilitation settings should be highlighted. Without this knowledge, patients can take several days to understand what to expect from staff and what staff expect of them (Pryor 2005). In addition to verbal explanations, this information must be made available in written format for patients and families to consider in their own time. Inclusion of contact details for more information is essential.

Even when this education is provided, some patients are simply not ready to engage in rehabilitation. Some insight into why this may be the case is provided by Mauk's (2006) six-phase model of post-stroke recovery (Box 11.3).

Initially, patients engage in agonising (which is about survival) and fantasising (which is about protection of self from the shock of what has happened) before they realise that the effects of stroke 'may not all just go away'(p. 259). Mauk reports this as 'the pivotal point in recovery'(p. 259), because positive adaptation cannot occur until the patient has this realisation. Facing this reality enables patients to own their stroke and learn what is needful. Blending, framing and owning involve adaptation, reflection and moving on.

Nurses can enhance patient readiness to learn by listening to patients and families and helping them make sense of what has happened. Kirkevold (1997), in her study of nursing's contribution to stroke rehabilitation, referred to this as nursing's interpretive function, whereby nurses help patients and families make sense of what has happened to them, what is currently happening to them and what may happen in the future. In a similar study, Burton (2000) found nurses to be facilitators of personal recovery.

Much can be done to ensure continuity of care between acute and rehabilitation settings. A visit from staff in the rehabilitation unit before transfer out of the acute ward is an essential first step. This will ensure that information provided to prepare the patient and family for rehabilitation is accurate. It will also ensure the patient and family know at least one familiar face (but preferably more) upon arrival in rehabilitation. Pre-transfer education about rehabilitation allows the patient and family time to absorb the information provided, generate questions and have questions answered before transfer. A pre-transfer tour of the rehabilitation unit enables patients and family to see rehabilitation in action and may assist them to become ready for the active role that is expected of them.

Most importantly, patients need to understand that, unlike the intermittent nature of acute care interventions rehabilitation is a continuous process that

---

Case example 11.2 John.

Following transfer to the rehabilitation unit an introductory meeting was set within the first week. This enabled John and his family to ask more detailed questions about the stroke, likely progress and the rehabilitation process. His grown-up children live away and a method of communication was agreed to ensure they felt kept up to date. John was happy for his son to be next-of-kin and a password system was set up to ensure confidentiality was maintained and information was only provided to this named relative. This reassured both the family and John. A further meeting date was set for four weeks' time as it was anticipated John would require a lengthy period of rehabilitation. This enabled the family to organise the time to attend.

---

requires active patient participation with all clinical staff (Pryor 2005). It needs to be made explicit that rehabilitation is not done *to* patients, but *by* patients. Such explanations can assist patients to take ownership of their stroke and learn what is needed.

The need to prepare patients for rehabilitation should not be underestimated. Mismatches between nurses', patients' and family understandings of rehabilitation have been recognised for many years (Jones et al. 1997; Long et al. 2001; Thompson 1990), along with the acknowledgement that patients need to be educated about rehabilitation (Arts et al. 2000; Berger 1999, 2000; Elescha-Adams & McKintyre 1983; Greneger 2003; Nypaver et al. 1996; Pryor 2005; Pryor & Smith 2002; Sheppard 1994; Sondermeyer & Pryor 2006). John (Case example 11.2) shows the level of discussion with families that is required.

Rehabilitation provision

Service models

In the UK components of an integrated stroke service have been described most recently within the National Stroke Strategy (Department of Health 2007), having developed from previous documents, notably Standard Five of the National Service Framework for Older People (Department of Health 2001) and, more recently, supported in the National Audit Office report, *Reducing Brain Damage: Faster Access to Better Stroke Care* (National Audit Office 2005, pp. 20–21). The term 'integrated' refers to a smooth transition for the patient between phases of the journey following stroke and encompasses:

- Emergency response
- Hyperacute management
- Acute care
- Rehabilitation
- Transfer home or to residential services
- Longer-term management
- Stroke prevention

The debate regarding the organisation of stroke care is ongoing. In 1993, Langhorne and colleagues (1993) produced a meta-analysis which demonstrated that patients managed in a specialised stroke unit were less likely to die. In the following year, the Stroke Unit Trialists' Collaboration (SUTC) was set up (Dennis & Langhorne 1994) under the auspices of the Cochrane Collaboration. The collaborators wanted to answer the questions: what are stroke units and do they reduce disability in stroke survivors? The SUTC's review (Stroke Unit Trialists' Collaboration 1997) concluded 'stroke patients who received organised inpatient (stroke unit) care were more likely to be alive, independent and living at home one year after the stroke than those receiving conventional care. The apparent benefits were not restricted to any particular sub group of patients or models of stroke unit care. No systematic increase in length of stay in a hospital or institution was observed.'

The recommendations that stroke care should be provided by an organised, multidisciplinary team working within a discrete area continue to be considered best practice (Cifu & Stewart 1999; Stroke Unit Trialists' Collaboration 2007).

It is thought that the essential characteristics of a stroke unit are (Stroke Unit Trialists' Collaboration 1999):

- Coordinated, multidisciplinary rehabilitation
- Staff with a special interest in stroke
- Routine involvement of carers in the rehabilitation process
- Regular programmes of education and training

There are many different models of stroke care and The Stroke Association (1999) state that access to stroke services is 'a matter of chance'. The wide geographical variations in organisation of and access to stroke services have also been evident in each round of the UK National Sentinel Stroke Audit.

The planning of stroke services was previously thought to be 'impossible' (Osberg et al. 1990) due to a lack of information on the exact numbers of stroke patients and the costs of care. The situation improved in the UK with the advent of the Quality and Outcomes Framework (QuOF) data collected in primary care from general practitioners. Planning and organisation of stroke services should be provided across a range of settings: wards, units, care homes and individuals' own homes, and based on the geography of the area, demography and epidemiology of the local population. Comparison of models of stroke care and collaboration in research will enhance the identification of important and effective components of stroke care. In the UK, high grade evidence will be facilitated through the UK Stroke Research Network (see http://www.uksrn.ac.uk). While planning stroke services, the nature of the care provided in that service has to be outlined across the range of minor to very severe strokes with services able to meet the very different needs of these groups and their families.

In the UK the biennial National Sentinel Audits indicate progress in relation to rehabilitation service provision for stroke patients. Key findings of the 2008 audit are set out in Box 11.4.

Box 11.4 The national picture (Intercollegiate Stroke Working Party 2008).

- Only 22% of hospitals are able to provide stroke specialist early supported discharge
- Only 32% of hospitals have specialist community stroke rehabilitation teams
- Staffing ratios and skill mix across the range of professionals vary greatly in rehabilitation units
- A large number of stroke rehabilitation programmes exclude patients on the basis of their having no rehabilitation potential

---

Length of rehabilitation

The length of time that rehabilitation should be offered is unclear. The Stroke Association (1997) called for all stroke survivors to 'receive an annual review at which remaining disabilities are assessed and appropriate treatment is provided to ensure that recovery is sustained and any potential for further progress is fulfilled'. The long-term problems encountered by stroke survivors and their families will be influenced by the success of early rehabilitation and cross-organisational working will help to ensure that people receive an appropriate level of support.

The effectiveness and ongoing costs of rehabilitation for growing numbers of stroke survivors is not known. Osberg and colleagues (1990), in their study of characteristics of patients referred to as cost outliers who did not benefit from stroke rehabilitation, concluded that they 'consume a disproportionate share of all inpatient rehabilitation resources'. Gladman and Sackley (1998) counter this with references to the costs in terms of quality of life, asking, 'What are small changes in severe disability worth to the patient?'

Living after stroke without creating dependency on services is important. The Expert Patient Programme in the UK (The Expert Patient Programme 2009) and initiatives in other countries target resources towards self-management and gaining life skills to cope with this chronic condition. True success in rehabilitation surely must be when an individual feels they have the ability to direct and control their lives. The UK National Audit Office (2005) report states that 'most of the burden of stroke is in the cost of rehabilitation and life after stroke'. It is therefore imperative that hospital-based stroke services provide early rehabilitation by an inter-professional team with the necessary expertise and experience for optimal cost-effectiveness. The National Service Framework for Older People (Department of Health 2001) outlines a stroke pathway which includes early multidisciplinary assessment and a plan for rehabilitation agreed with the patient. The transition from hospital to home forms an important part of post-stroke care and evidence regarding the effectiveness of early supported discharge is emerging.

However, there is currently no consistency in how rehabilitation services are provided between organisations. Many different types of units and approaches are employed and the National Sentinel Stroke Audits also highlight the greatly differing staffing ratios and disciplines involved. These issues have been highlighted in the National Stroke Strategy (Department of Health 2007) and further work is required in consideration of effectiveness and efficiency of various service models, workforce issues and training and development requirements.

Adjustment to life after stroke

As previously discussed, formal rehabilitation aims to optimise recovery but for many stroke survivors and their families this is just the start of the long journey of adjustment to and coping with residual deficits. The literature relating to the longer-term aspects of rehabilitation and adjustment to life after stroke reflects the many negative or emotive aspects of the experience, for example:

> *The world of a stroke survivor is grounded in experiences of loss and effort which are inextricably connected.*
>
> (Secrest & Thomas 1999)

> *Stroke constitutes a formidable burden of disability and misery, having severe and long-lasting physical, emotional and social consequences for both patient and family.*
>
> (King's Fund 1988)

Stroke treatment and in particular rehabilitation tends to focus on improving function. In discussions with stroke survivors they are more likely to define recovery as a return to previously valued activities (Doolittle 1992). These discrepancies may cause tension between the multiprofessional team, patient and family. Bethoux and colleagues (1999) suggest that post-stroke quality of life deteriorates in some aspects over time and warn that some stroke survivors may 'idealise the pre-stroke condition'.

Many personal accounts of the experience of stroke have been published in book, newspaper, magazine and in television documentary format. These emotive and insightful stories provide additional information and may increase public awareness about stroke illness. The patient's experience of stroke is likely to be coloured by the amount of recovery made (Bartlett et al. 2006). The course of an illness has been referred to as a trajectory (Wiener & Dodd 1993) or the 'unfolding of an illness'. In stroke, the illness trajectory is uncertain and each patient's experience unique. Adapting to and acceptance of the stroke illness is crucial to recovery (Backe et al. 1996). The patient's ability to absorb information is very important and initial conversations with nurses 'constitute a vital contribution to achieving recovery' (Gibbon & Little 1995). Nilsson et al. (1997) describe the phenomenon as 'to meet with stroke' and continue 'this experience seems to challenge the whole of the individual's being'. Grasping the situation in which they find themselves takes over the patient's life and continues well after discharge from hospital. Encouraging patients and their families to see 'acquired disability as a time of transition rather than simply of loss' (Ellis-Hill et al. 2008) will support patients on their post-stroke journey.

Case example 11.3 Rehabilitation, from a user's perspective (Health talk online 2009).

Anyway, the bus came along and I went up the steps with my bag and there was an old lady [laughter] just inside. I mean, she must have been about 90 and she said, 'Come on dear, I'll help you'; [laughter] I thought, 'Oh my goodness, you know, there's this dear old lady, years and years older than me, helping me'. And, I did that a few times and I felt very proud of myself. I felt I was independent and then I set myself a goal for walking and we've got a shopping centre which is probably about 10 minutes, 15 minutes walk along, you know, when you can walk normally. But on the way, there's a bus shelter with seats inside and there are some stone walls along the way as well and then when you get further on into the shopping centre, there's another bus stop and there's another seat. So I thought, 'One day, I'll make it to those shops' and I did. One day I made it. I sat at the bus stop for about a quarter of an hour, to calm myself down and I made it a little further on and I sat on a wall and I got up and I made it to the next bus centre, the bus stop and the seat, I sat down. I went in a shop and bought things and I came back the same way and I did the same thing. I stopped and I sat, I walked and then when I thought it was really bad, I just stood where I was and I didn't move and then I continued walking and I, I'd done it. I'd made it. I'd made it to the shops on my own and I was getting to feel, and then of course, it was after that I started my driving and I, that was the real big thing, you know, I was independent.

Stroke survivors and their families are often extremely resilient and resourceful. Patient stories are a wonderful way of hearing how individual people have adjusted and learned to get on with life after stroke. There are many interesting and insightful stories from stroke survivors that can be accessed on http://www.healthtalkonline.org (Health talk online 2009): see, for example, Case example 11.3.

Conclusion

Rehabilitation is a pivotal aspect of a stroke patient's care and has to commence at an appropriate level *immediately* after the stroke occurs to maximise benefit. It is clear that one size does not fit all and the provision of a person- and family-centred programme of rehabilitation will ensure that the stroke survivor is assisted to recover and adjust in the way most meaningful for them. This requires flexibility of service models, periods of timely rehabilitation, expert workforce and most importantly, innovative cross-organisational commissioning to ensure that physical, social and psychological needs are met.

References

Alaszewski, A, Alaszewski, H, & Potter, J, 2004, The bereavement model, stroke and rehabilitation: a critical analysis of the use of a psychological model in professional practice, *Disability and Rehabilitation*, vol. 26, no. 18, pp. 1067–1078.

Arts, SE, Francke, AL, & Hutten, JB, 2000, Liaison nursing for stroke patients: results of a Dutch evaluation study, *Journal of Advanced Nursing*, vol. 32, no. 2, pp. 292–300.

ASA, 2009, *American Stroke Association*, ASA.

Australasian Rehabilitation Nurses' Association, 2003, *Rehabilitation Nursing: Competency standards for registered nurses*, Australasian Rehabilitation Nurses' Association, Putney, NSW.

Backe, M, Larsson, K, & Fridlund, B, 1996, Patients' conceptions of their life situation within the first week after a stroke event: a qualitative analysis, *Intensive and Critical Care Nursing*, vol. 12, no. 5, pp. 285–294.

Barnes, MP, & Ward, AB, 2000, *Textbook of Rehabilitation Medicine*, Oxford University Press, Oxford.

Bartlett, DJ, Macnab, J, Macarthur, C, Mandich, A, Magill-Evans, J et al., 2006, Advancing rehabilitation research: an interactionist perspective to guide question and design, *Disability and Rehabilitation*, vol. 28, no. 19, pp. 1169–1176.

Berger, M, 1999, Let's visit – on the road to rehabilitation, *Journal of Australasian Rehabilitation Nurses Association*, vol. 2, no. 2, pp. 7–9.

Berger, M., 2000, *The Self-Identified Needs of Carers for Clients Referred to an Inpatient Rehabilitation Programme*, Royal Rehabilitation Centre Sydney Monograph Series 3, Ryde, NSW.

Bernhardt, J, Dewey, H, Collier, J, Thrift, A, Lindley, R et al., 2006, A Very Early Rehabilitation Trial (AVERT), *International Journal of Stroke*, vol. 1, pp. 169–171.

Bethoux, F, Calmels, P, & Gautheron, V, 1999, Changes in the quality of life of hemiplegic stroke patients with time: a preliminary report, *American Journal of Physical Medicine and Rehabilitation*, vol. 78, no. 1, pp. 19–23.

Burton, CR, 1999, An exploration of the stroke co-ordinator role, *Journal of Clinical Nursing*, vol. 8, no. 5, pp. 535–541.

Burton, CR, 2000, A description of the nursing role in stroke rehabilitation, *Journal of Advanced Nursing*, vol. 32, no. 1, pp. 174–181.

Cifu, DX, & Stewart, DG, 1999, Factors affecting functional outcome after stroke: a critical review of rehabilitation interventions, *Archives of Physical Medicine and Rehabilitation*, vol. 80, no. 5 Suppl 1, pp. S35–S39.

Cochrane Stroke Review Group at http://www.dcn.ed.ac.uk/csrg/

Cott, C, 2004, Client-centred rehabilitation: client perspectives, *Disability and Rehabilitation*, vol. 26, no. 24, pp. 1411–1422.

D'Alisa, S, Baudo, S, Mauro, A, & Miscio, G, 2005, How does stroke restrict participation in long-term post-stroke survivors? *Acta Neurological Scandinavica*, vol. 112, no. 3, pp. 157–162.

Davidoff, G, Keren, O, Ring, H, & Solzi, P, 1992, Who goes home after a stroke: a case control study, *NeuroRehabilitation*, vol. 2, no. 2, pp. 53–63.

DeJong, G, Horn, SD, Gassaway, JA, Slavin, MD, & Dijkers, MP, 2004, Toward a taxonomy of rehabilitation interventions: using an inductive approach to examine the 'black box' of rehabilitation, *Archives of Physical Medicine and Rehabilitation*, vol. 85, no. 4, pp. 678–686.

Demain, S, Wiles, R, Roberts, L, & McPherson, K, 2006, Recovery plateau following stroke: fact or fiction? *Disability and Rehabilitation*, vol. 28, no. 13–14, pp. 815–821.

Dennis, M, & Langhorne, P, 1994, So stroke units save lives: where do we go from here? *BMJ*, vol. 309, no. 6964, pp. 1273–1277.

Department of Health, 2001, *The National Service Framework for Older People*, Department of Health, London.

Department of Health, 2007, *National Stroke Strategy*, Department of Health, London.

Diserens, K, Michel, P, & Bogousslavsky, J, 2006, Early mobilisation after stroke: review of the literature, *Cerebrovascular Diseases*, vol. 22, no. 2–3, pp. 183–190.

Dobkin, B, & Carmichael, T, 2005, Principles of recovery after stroke, in *Recovery after Stroke*, M Barnes, B Dobkin, & J Bogousslavsky, eds., Cambridge University Press, Cambridge, pp. 47–49.

Doolittle, ND, 1992, The experience of recovery following lacunar stroke, *Rehabilitation Nursing*, vol. 17, no. 3, pp. 122–125.

Duncan, PW, Zorowitz, R, Bates, B, Choi, JY, Glasberg, JJ et al., 2005, Management of Adult Stroke Rehabilitation Care: a clinical practice guideline, *Stroke*, vol. 36, no. 9, pp. e100–e143.

Easton, KL, 1999, The poststroke journey: from agonizing to owning, *Geriatric Nursing.*, vol. 20, no. 2, pp. 70–75.

EBRSR, 2009, *Canadian Evidence Based Review of Stroke Rehabilitation*, EBRSR. At http://www.ebrsr.com/ accessed 20/11/2009.

Elescha-Adams, M, & McKintyre, K, 1983, Facilitating the patient's entry into the rehabilitation setting, *Rehabilitation Nursing*, vol. 8, no. 5, pp. 22–46.

Ellis-Hill, C, Payne, S, & Ward, C, 2008, Using stroke to explore the life thread model: an alternative approach to understanding rehabilitation following an acquired disability, *Disability and Rehabilitation*, vol. 30, no. 2, pp. 150–159.

Evans, RL, Griffith, J, Haselkorn, JK, Hendricks, RD, Baldwin, D et al., 1992, Post-stroke family function: an evaluation of the family's role in rehabilitation, *Rehabilitation Nursing*, vol. 17, no. 3, pp. 127–131.

Evans, RL, Connis, RT, Bishop, DS, Hendricks, RD, & Haselkorn, JK, 1994, Stroke: a family dilemma, *Disability and Rehabilitation*, vol. 16, no. 3, pp. 110–118.

Faircloth, CA, Boylstein, C, Rittman, M, Young, ME, & Gubrium, J, 2004, Sudden illness and biographical flow in narratives of stroke recovery, *Sociology of Health and Illness*, vol. 26, no. 2, pp. 242–261.

Garraway, WM, Akhtar, AJ, Smith, DL, & Smith, ME, 1981, The triage of stroke rehabilitation, *Journal of Epidemiology and Community Health*, vol. 35, no. 1, pp. 39–44.

Gibbon, B, & Little, V, 1995, Improving stroke care through action research, *Journal of Clinical Nursing*, vol. 4, no. 2, pp. 93–100.

Gignac, MA, & Cott, C, 1998, A conceptual model of independence and dependence for adults with chronic physical illness and disability, *Social Science and Medicine*, vol. 47, no. 6, pp. 739–753.

Gladman, JR, & Sackley, CM, 1998, The scope for rehabilitation in severely disabled stroke patients, *Disability and Rehabilitation*, vol. 20, no. 10, pp. 391–394.

Gordon, M, 2000, *Manual of Nursing Diagnosis*, Mosby, St Louis.

Greneger, R, 2003, Relocation stress syndrome in rehabilitation transfers: a review of the literature, *Journal of the Australasian Rehabilitation Nurses Association*, vol. 6, pp. 8–13.

Greveson, G, & James, O, 1991, Improving long-term outcome after stroke – the views of patients and carers, *Health Trends*, vol. 23, no. 4, pp. 161–162.

Grill, E, Ewert, T, Chatterji, S, Kostanjsek, N, & Stucki, G, 2005, ICF Core Sets development for the acute hospital and early post-acute rehabilitation facilities, *Disability and Rehabilitation*, vol. 27, no. 7/8, pp. 361–366.

Hafsteinsdottir, TB, & Grypdonck, M, 1997, Being a stroke patient: a review of the literature, *Journal of Advanced Nursing*, vol. 26, no. 3, pp. 580–588.

Health talk online, at http://www.healthtalkonline.org; accessed 12 May 2009.

Henderson, VA, 1980, Preserving the essence of nursing in a technological age, *Journal of Advanced Nursing*, vol. 5, no. 3, pp. 245–260.

Hill, MC, & Johnson, J, 1999, An exploratory study of nurses' perceptions of their role in neurological rehabilitation, *Rehabilitation Nursing*, vol. 24, no. 4, pp. 152–157.

Horn, SD, DeJong, G, Smout, RJ, Gassaway, J, James, R et al., 2005, Stroke rehabilitation patients, practice, and outcomes: is earlier and more aggressive therapy better? *Archives of Physical Medicine and Rehabilitation*, vol. 86, no. 12 Suppl 2, pp. S101–S114.

Indredavik, B, Bakke, F, Slordahl, SA, Rokseth, R, & Haheim, LL, 1999, Treatment in a combined acute and rehabilitation stroke unit: which aspects are most important? *Stroke*, vol. 30, no. 5, pp. 917–923.

Intercollegiate Stroke Working Party, 2008, *National Sentinel Audit for Stroke 2008. National and Local Results for the Process of Stroke Care Audit 2008*, Royal College of Physicians, London.

Johnston, MV, Kirshblum, S, & Shiflett, SC, 1992, Prediction of outcomes following rehabilitation of stroke patients, *NeuroRehabilitation*, vol. 2, no. 4, pp. 72–97.

Jones, F, 2006, Strategies to enhance chronic disease self-management: how can we apply this to stroke? *Disability and Rehabilitation*, vol. 28, no. 13–14, pp. 841–847.

Jones, M, O'Neill, P, Waterman, H, & Webb, C, 1997, Building a relationship: communications and relationships between staff and stroke patients on a rehabilitation ward, *Journal of Advanced Nursing*, vol. 26, no. 1, pp. 101–110.

Kalra, L, & Eade, J, 1995, Role of stroke rehabilitation units in managing severe disability after stroke, *Stroke*, vol. 26, no. 11, pp. 2031–2034.

King's Fund, 1988, *Consensus Conference – Stroke*, Kings Fund, London.

Kirkevold, M, 1997, The role of nursing in the rehabilitation of acute stroke patients: toward a unified theoretical perspective, *Advances in Nursing Science*, vol. 19, no. 4, pp. 55–64.

Kwakkel, G, 2006, Impact of intensity of practice after stroke: issues for consideration, *Disability and Rehabilitation*, vol. 28, no. 13/14, pp. 823–830.

Langhorne, P, Williams, BO, Gilchrist, W, & Howie, K, 1993, Do stroke units save lives? *Lancet*, vol. 342, no. 8868, pp. 395–398.

Lettinga, AT, van Twillert S, Poels, BJ, & Postema, K, 2006, Distinguishing theories of dysfunction, treatment and care. Reflections on 'describing rehabilitation interventions', *Clinical Rehabilitation*, vol. 20, no. 5, pp. 369–374.

Levack, WM, Dean, SG, Siegert, RJ, & McPherson, KM, 2006a, Purposes and mechanisms of goal planning in rehabilitation: the need for a critical distinction, *Disability and Rehabilitation*, vol. 28, no. 12, pp. 741–749.

Levack, WM, Taylor, K, Siegert, RJ, Dean, SG, McPherson, KM et al., 2006b, Is goal planning in rehabilitation effective? A systematic review, *Clinical Rehabilitation*, vol. 20, no. 9, pp. 739–755.

Long, AF, Kneafsey, R, Ryan, J, Berry, J, & Howard, R, 2001, *Teamworking in rehabilitation: exploring the role of the nurse*, English National Board for Nursing, Health Visiting and Midwifery, London. Researching Professional Education, Research Reports Series Number 19.

Long, AF, Kneafsey, R, Ryan, J, & Berry, J, 2002, The role of the nurse within the multi-professional rehabilitation team, *Journal of Advanced Nursing*, vol. 37, no. 1, pp. 70–78.

Maclean, N, Pound, P, Wolfe, C, & Rudd, A, 2000, Qualitative analysis of stroke patients' motivation for rehabilitation, *BMJ*, vol. 321, no. 7268, pp. 1051–1054.

Mahoney, JE, Sager, MA, & Jalaluddin, M, 1998, New walking dependence associated with hospitalization for acute medical illness: incidence and significance, *Journals of Gerontology A Biological Science Medical Science*, vol. 53, no. 4, pp. M307–M312.

Mauk, KL, 2006, Nursing interventions within the Mauk Model of Poststroke Recovery, *Rehabilitation Nursing*, vol. 31, no. 6, pp. 257–263.

Maulden, SA, Gassaway, J, Horn, SD, Smout, RJ, & DeJong, G, 2005, Timing of initiation of rehabilitation after stroke, *Archives of Physical Medicine and Rehabilitation*, vol. 86, no. 12 Suppl 2, p. S34-S40.

McClain, C, 2005, Collaborative rehabilitation goal setting, *Topics in Stroke Rehabilitation*, vol. 12, no. 4, pp. 56–60.

McGrath, JA, Adams, L, 2005, Patient centered goal planning: a systemic therapy, *Topics in Stroke Rehabilitation*, vol. 6, no. 2, pp. 43–50.

National Audit Office, 2005, *Reducing Brain Damage – Faster Access to Better Stroke Care*, The Stationery Office, London.

Nilsson, I, Jansson, L, & Norberg, A, 1997, To meet with a stroke: patients' experiences and aspects seen through a screen of crises, *Journal of Advanced Nursing*, vol. 25, no. 5, pp. 953–963.

NSF, 2009, *National Stroke Foundation*, NSF.

Nypaver, JM, Titus, M, & Brugler, CJ, 1996, Patient transfer to rehabilitation: just another move? *Rehabilitation Nursing*, vol. 21, no. 2, pp. 94–97.

O'Connor, SE, 2000, Nursing interventions in stroke rehabilitation: a study of nurses' views of their pattern of care in stroke units, *Rehabilitation Nursing*, vol. 25, no. 6, pp. 224–230.

Osberg, JS, Haley, SM, McGinnis, GE, & DeJong, G, 1990, Characteristics of cost outliers who did not benefit from stroke rehabilitation, *American Journal of Physical Medicine and Rehabilitation*, vol. 69, no. 3, pp. 117–125.

Ozer, MN, 1999, Patient participation in the management of stroke rehabilitation, *Topics in Stroke Rehabilitation*, vol. 6, no. 1, pp. 43–59.

Plaisted, LM, 1978, Rehabilitation nurse, in *Disability and Rehabilitation Handbook*, RM Goldenson, ed., McGraw-Hill, New York.

Price, E, 1997, *An exploration of the nature of therapeutic nursing in a general rehabilitation team (inpatient)*, Albany, Unpublished Masters thesis, Massey University.

Prochaska, JO, DiClemente, CC, & Norcross, JC, 1992, In search of how people change. Applications to addictive behaviors, *American Psychologist*, vol. 47, no. 9, pp. 1102–1114.

Pryor, J, 2005, *A grounded theory of nursing's contribution to inpatient rehabilitation*, Deakin University.

Pryor, J, & Smith, C, 2002, A framework for the role of Registered Nurses in the specialty practice of rehabilitation nursing in Australia, *Journal of Advanced Nursing*, vol. 39, no. 3, pp. 249–257.

Reker, DM, Duncan, PW, Horner, RD, Hoenig, H, Samsa, GP et al., 2002, Postacute stroke guideline compliance is associated with greater patient satisfaction, *Archives of Physical Medicine and Rehabilitation*, vol. 83, no. 6, pp. 750–756.

Rentsch, HP, Bucher P, Dommen Nyffeler I, Wolf C, Hefti H et al., 2003, The implementation of the 'International Classification of Functioning, Disability and Health' (ICF) in daily practice of neurorehabilitation: an interdisciplinary project at the Kantonsspital of Lucerne, Switzerland, *Disability and Rehabilitation*, vol. 25, no. 8, pp. 411–421.

Sager, MA, Franke, T, Inouye, SK, Landefeld, CS, Morgan, TM et al., 1996, Functional outcomes of acute medical illness and hospitalization in older persons, *Archives of Internal Medicine*, vol. 156, no. 6, pp. 645–652.

Salter, K, Jutai, JW, Teasell, R, Foley, NC, & Bitensky, J, 2005a, Issues for selection of outcome measures in stroke rehabilitation: ICF body functions, *Disability and Rehabilitation*, vol. 27, no. 4, pp. 191–207.

Salter, K, Jutai, JW, Teasell, R, Foley, NC, Bitensky, J et al., 2005b, Issues for selection of outcome measures in stroke rehabilitation: ICF activity, *Disability and Rehabilitation*, vol. 27, no. 6, pp. 315–340.

Salter, K, Jutai, JW, Teasell, R, Foley, NC, Bitensky, J et al., 2005c, Issues for selection of outcome measures in stroke rehabilitation: ICF participation, *Disability and Rehabilitation*, vol. 27, no. 9, pp. 507–528.

Salter, K, Jutai, J, Hartley, M, Foley, N, Bhogal, S et al., 2009, Impact of early vs delayed admission to rehabilitation on functional outcomes in persons with stroke, *Journal of Rehabilitation Medicine*, vol. 38, pp. 113–117.

Scheuringer, M, Grill, E, Boldt, C, Mittrach, R, Muller, P et al., 2005, Systematic review of measures and their concepts used in published studies focusing on rehabilitation in the acute hospital and in early post-acute rehabilitation facilities, *Disability and Rehabilitation*, vol. 27, no. 7/8, pp. 419–429.

Scottish Intercollegiate Guidelines Network (SIGN), 2005, *Management of Patients with Stroke: Rehabilitation, Prevention and Management of Complications, and Discharge Planning*, SIGN, Edinburgh.

Secrest, JA, & Thomas, SP, 1999, Continuity and discontinuity: the quality of life following stroke, *Rehabilitation Nursing*, vol. 24, no. 6, pp. 240–246.

Sheppard, B, 1994, Patients' views of rehabilitation, *Nursing Standard*, vol. 9, no. 10, pp. 27–30.

Siegert, RJ, & Taylor, WJ, 2004, Theoretical aspects of goal-setting and motivation in rehabilitation, *Disability and Rehabilitation*, vol. 26, no. 1, pp. 1–8.

Siegert, RJ, McPherson, KM, & Taylor, WJ, 2004, Toward a cognitive-affective model of goal-setting in rehabilitation: is self-regulation theory a key step? *Disability and Rehabilitation*, vol. 26, no. 20, pp. 1175–1183.

Sondermeyer, J, & Pryor, J, 2006, 'You're going to Rehab': a study into the experiences of patients moving from acute care settings to an inpatient rehabilitation unit, *Journal of the Australasian Rehabilitation Nurses Association*, vol. 9, no. 2, pp. 23–27.

Strasser, DC, Falconer, JA, Herrin, JS, Bowen, SE, Stevens, AB et al., 2005, Team functioning and patient outcomes in stroke rehabilitation, *Archives of Physical Medicine and Rehabilitation*, vol. 86, no. 3, pp. 403–409.

Stroke Unit Trialists' Collaboration, 1997, Collaborative systematic review of the randomised controlled trials of organised inpatient (stroke unit) care after stroke, *British Medical Journal*, vol. 314, no. 7088, pp. 1151–1159.

Stroke Unit Trialists' Collaboration, 1999, *Organised inpatient(stroke unit) care for stroke. (Cochrane review)*, Update Software, The Cochrane Library, Oxford. Issue 1.

Stroke Unit Trialists' Collaboration, 2007, *Organised inpatient (stroke unit) care for stroke (Cochrane Review)*, Issue 4: Art No. CD000197, Oxford.

Stucki, G, Stier-Jarmer, M, Grill, E, & Melvin, J,. 2005a, Rationale and principles of early rehabilitation care after an acute injury or illness, *Disability and Rehabilitation*, vol. 27, no. 7/8, pp. 353–359.

Stucki, G, Ustun, B, & Melvin, J, 2005b, Applying the ICF for the acute hospital and early post-acute rehabilitation facilities, *Disability and Rehabilitation*, vol. 27, no. 7/8, pp. 349–352.

Tempest, S, & McIntyre, A, 2006, Using the ICF to clarify team roles and demonstrate clinical reasoning in stroke rehabilitation, *Disability and Rehabilitation*, vol. 28, no. 10, pp. 663–667.

The Expert Patient Programme, at http://www.expertpatients.co.uk; accessed 12 May 2009.

The Stroke Association, 1997, *Stroke: National Tragedy, National Policy*, The Stroke Association, London.

The Stroke Association, 1999, *Stroke Care – A Matter of Chance*, The Stroke Association, London.

Thompson, TCL, 1990, *A qualitative investigation of rehabilitation nursing care in an inpatient unit using Leininger's theory*, Unpublished doctoral dissertation, Wayne State University, Michigan.

van den Broek, M, 2005, Why does neurorehabilitation fail? *Journal of Head Trauma Rehabilitation*, vol. 20, no. 5, pp. 464–473.

van Vliet, PM, Wulf, G, 2006, Extrinsic feedback for motor learning after stroke: what is the evidence? *Disability and Rehabilitation*, vol. 28, no. 13–14, pp. 831–840.

Wade, D, 1999, Rehabilitation therapy after stroke, *Lancet*, vol. 354, no. 9174, pp. 176–177.

Wade, DT, 2005, Describing rehabilitation interventions, *Clinical Rehabilitation*, vol. 19, no. 8, pp. 811–818.

Whyte, J, & Hart, T, 2003, It's more than a black box; it's a Russian Doll: defining rehabilitation treatments, *American Journal of Physical Medicine and Rehabilitation*, vol. 20, no. 369, p. 374.

Wiener, CL, & Dodd, MJ, 1993, Coping amid uncertainty: an illness trajectory perspective, *Scholarly Inquiry for Nursing Practice*, vol. 7, no. 1, pp. 17–31.

World Health Organisation (WHO), 2001, *International Classification of Functioning, Disability and Health (ICF)*, WHO, Geneva.

Worral, L, 2005, Unifying rehabilitation through theory development, *Disability and Rehabilitation*, vol. 27, no. 24, pp. 1515–1516.

Chapter 12

Stroke and palliative care: a difficult combination?

Christopher R. Burton and Sheila Payne

Key points

- Palliative care seeks to improve the quality of life of an individual and their family.
- It is important to recognise and manage physical, psychological and spiritual aspects of care.
- Many people die immediately or within a few months of a stroke.
- The collaboration of stroke and palliative care specialists will advance assessment and management post-stroke.

Case example 12.1 71 years old, fit and well until found unconscious in bed.

On admission treated with antibiotics and 'do not resuscitate' order placed. On day two CT scan showed large haemorrhage. Decision made not to commence artificial feeding and to withdraw antibiotics. Mr G was prescribed diamorphine to help with breathing during his last hours of life. Nurses on the unit contacted his friends, who were then able to be present at his death some four days later. Mr G's named nurse believed that he had a 'good death' that was well managed, largely because the nature and course of his death had been predictable.

Case example 12.2 84 years old, in a wheelchair due to previous stroke.

Admitted to the unit unconscious. CT scan showed massive haemorrhage. Husband expressed a wish that she not have life-prolonging treatment.
   On day 10, after consultation with her family, artificial feeding started and antibiotics given. On day 15, decided to cease treatment with antibiotics and to provide supportive nursing. Moved to another ward on day 25; husband requested artificial feeding be stopped. It continued, and she died forty-one days after her admission.

Introduction

Despite recent advances in both the treatment and management of stroke, a significant proportion of patients continue to die from the disease. For example, the case fatality rate, comprising those patients that die within 28 days, is variously reported to be between 20 and 30% (National Audit Office 2005). Although published before evidence of the clinical effectiveness of stroke unit care and thrombolysis was widely disseminated, variations in case fatality rates with stroke subtype have been reported: lacunar infarct (2%), partial anterior circulation infarct (4%), posterior circulation infarct (7%), and total anterior circulation infarct (39%) (Bamford et al. 1990).

Whilst absent from the first edition, more recent editions of the *National Clinical Guidelines for Stroke* have recognised the importance of palliative care, and have included relevant recommendations for practice (Intercollegiate Stroke Working Party 2008). However, the guidelines indicate the lack of evidence available to underpin practice recommendations. This chapter considers the role that palliative care can play in improving the care and experiences of both patients and families following a stroke. An overview of a recent research study (Payne et al. 2008) that identified the palliative care needs of acute stroke patients is provided. Developments in theoretical aspects of palliative care, and their implementation into UK health service policy, are introduced as the basis for new practice models which seek to integrate palliative and end of life care into mainstream stroke practice. The chapter concludes with a discussion of some of the challenges that may affect the degree to which this integration can be achieved.

Palliative care

From a practical perspective, the principles of palliative care will be familiar to many, and include:

- The provision of relief from pain and other distressing symptoms
- Affirms life and regards dying as a normal process
- Intends neither to hasten nor postpone death
- Integrates the psychological and spiritual aspects of patient care
- Offers a support system to help patients live as actively as possible until death
- Offers a support system to help the family cope during the patient's illness and in their own bereavement
- Uses a team approach to address the needs of patients and their families; including bereavement counselling, if indicated
- Will enhance quality of life, and may also positively influence the course of illness
- Is applicable early in the course of illness, in conjunction with other therapies that are intended to prolong life including investigations needed to better understand and manage distressing clinical complications

These principles are encapsulated within the World Health Organisation definition of palliative care (Sepulveda et al. 2002, p. 94):

Palliative care is an approach that improves the quality of life of patients and their families facing the problems associated with life-threatening illness, through the prevention and relief of suffering by means of early identification and impeccable assessment and treatment of pain and other problems, physical, psychosocial and spiritual.

This holistic definition is interesting in two key ways. Firstly, no mention is made of the word 'terminal'. Palliative care may then have a role in disease course where there is a risk of death, but no certainty that the patient will die. Secondly, explicit reference is made to the need for early intervention. Our initial experiences of conducting research into palliative care in stroke services indicated that clinicians in stroke services may have a tendency to equate palliative care with terminal care. This view is perhaps underpinned by a traditional interpretation of the role of palliative care: as a disease trajectory develops over time, so the intensity of curative interventions decreases and the intensity of palliative care interventions increases, and at some point along this trajectory the patient will be defined as terminally ill. In practice, however, accurate prognostication is difficult, and reliance on this model may mean that palliative care interventions are commenced too late for the patient and family to derive much benefit. Other models of palliative care reflect a more fluid relationship with curative interventions, where both curative and palliative care interventions are combined to different degrees over longer periods of time, as the patient's condition fluctuates (Payne et al. 2008).

The service delivery strategies in which the principles of palliative care are implemented into health services have been characterised by the National Council for Hospice and Specialist Palliative Care Services (2002, p. 2), who differentiate between:

- General palliative care which 'is provided by the usual professional carers of the patient and family with low to moderate complexity of palliative care need', and
- Specialist palliative care services which 'are provided for patients and their families with moderate to high complexity of palliative care need. They are defined in terms of their core service components, their functions and the composition of the multi-professional teams that are required to deliver them'

Supportive care means helping patients and their families cope with the disease and its treatment. There is increasing recognition that the principles of palliative care are an important component of a wide range of health care services, whether patients are terminally ill or not, and in diseases other than cancer, in order to support multidisciplinary teams in symptom management and ethical practice (Dunlop 2001).

Contemporary definitions of specialist end of life care are usually associated with cancer services, with generalist care delivered by the full range of service providers. An agreed definition of generalist end of life care is lacking (Shipman et al. 2008). In contrast, definitions of specialist practice discuss additional education and training, and focused clinical practice. A lack of capacity within specialist palliative care (Gomes & Higginson 2006), and a lack of evidence that specialist palliative care is effective or appropriate in non-cancer contexts, underpin the aims of the NHS End of Life Care Strategy (Department of Health 2008): to enhance the quality of generalist palliative care. Currently, specialist palliative care and hospice services are overwhelmingly targeted at cancer patients and they are unlikely to have sufficient resources or skills to extend to non-cancer services.

The NHS End of Life Care Programme has provided considerable impetus to the expansion of access to palliative care across patient groups. The End of Life Care Strategy recommends three tools that have largely been developed in the context of cancer care. The Macmillan Gold Standards Framework (Thomas 2004) supports the strategic evaluation of palliative care in community-based cancer care. The Liverpool Care Pathway (Ellershaw et al. 2001) provides generic practice recommendations for terminal palliative care. The Preferred Priorities of Care tool functions as a form of advance care plan to elicit patient choice in care location. However, the applicability of these initiatives to stroke services has not been systematically evaluated.

Relevance of palliative care to stroke

Whilst significant advances in the management and treatment of acute stroke have been made in recent years, the fact remains that post-stroke mortality remains high. The strategic thrust of stroke strategy focuses on improving access to evidence-based acute services. For example, the National Audit Office Report subtitled *Faster Access to Better Stroke Care* focuses on improvements in delivering rapid access to hyperacute stroke imaging and thrombolysis (National Audit Office 2005). Coupled with drives to increase the numbers of patients accessing thrombolytic therapy in the hyperacute phase of stroke, there is the expectation that acute stroke services will see increasing numbers of patients. Of those seen, up to one-third may die within one month of disease onset, if mortality rates continue as previously.

The *National Clinical Guidelines for Stroke* (Intercollegiate Stroke Working Party 2008) recommend that patients should have access to specialist palliative care expertise when needed, and all staff providing this care should have undergone appropriate training. The guidelines are ambiguous about how palliative care should be integrated within stroke services, and no distinction between those patients who die in the acute stage and those who die in the later stage of the disease pathway is made. In non-acute stroke, patients near the end of life have time to prepare for death, and professionals have an opportunity to assess, organise and implement appropriate interventions.

Both the delivery of the NHS End of Life Care Strategy, and the enactment of the Mental Capacity Act (Mental Capacity Act 2005) mean that stroke service staff are likely to encounter patients with 'Statements of Preferences' or

'Advance Decisions', or to participate in 'Advance Care Planning' (Henry & Seymour 2007). In addition, the cognitive and communication consequences of stroke suggest that the assessment of capacity, and the ongoing validity of Advance Decisions will be complex. Discussion of these issues with patients and families by staff who are comfortable and confident in addressing end of life topics will be essential.

What are the palliative care needs of stroke patients?

Palliative care may be of benefit in the management of some symptoms in stroke, such as pain and discomfort, incontinence, depression and anxiety, as well as supporting communication with patients and carers about prognosis, complicated decisions about feeding, hydration and family involvement (Le et al. 2008). However, there are few evidence-based recommendations to guide practice in this area. Furthermore, prospective information on the palliative care needs of any group of stroke patients is largely lacking, with a few exceptions (Le et al. 2008; Rogers & Addington-Hall 2005). A recent critical review of the international literature on palliative care for stroke patients was undertaken (Stevens et al. 2007), identifying seven studies, four of which were completed within the United Kingdom. No robust intervention studies were found. A synthesis of the studies provided the following information:

- Many patients who died after stroke did not receive optimal symptom control (Addington-Hall et al. 1995; Anderson et al. 1995)
- Patients were not perceived to receive 'sufficient' help to overcome psychological morbidity (Addington-Hall et al. 1995, 1998)
- Informal caregivers report difficulty accessing information about the patient's medical condition (Addington-Hall et al. 1995)
- The caring experience was distressful, not generally felt to be rewarding, with high reporting of insufficient help and assistance (Addington-Hall et al. 1998; Anderson et al. 1995)
- Palliative care strategies may have a role in the care of stroke patients, and should be systematically provided on the basis of need (Jack et al. 2004; Rogers & Addington-Hall 2005)

The review highlights that palliative care is a seriously neglected area of stroke research, which pales in comparison to research in acute care and rehabilitation. Effective and appropriate models of care delivery that suggest which palliative care interventions would be appropriate, and how these should be assimilated within the total package of care and interventions provided to patients, are unavailable. There is some evidence that hospital staff feel palliative care may be inappropriate for acute patients (Gott et al. 2001), but whether this reflects a good understanding of the principles and practice of palliative care, or a lack of awareness of the potential of specialist palliative care is unclear.

To address the gaps in the literature, the UK Stroke Association funded a study to explore the palliative care needs of acute stroke patients (Payne et al.

2008). The study was exploratory, and used a standardised assessment to identify the range and severity of palliative care needs in a prospective sample of 196 patients with a wide range of stroke severities. The assessment tool was developed in 2004, by the Sheffield Palliative Care Studies Group, to screen patients with advanced illness, regardless of diagnosis, for referral into specialist palliative care. It is composed of five domains as follows:

- Physical symptoms
- Psychological issues
- Religious and spiritual issues
- Independence and activity issues
- Family and social issues

The development of the assessment tool was underpinned by an extensive literature review (Ahmed et al. 2004) and interviews with cancer and heart failure patients (Bestall et al. 2004), and was refined through testing in patients referred to palliative care services. Interviews in a smaller subsample of patients and family members were also conducted to explore their perspectives in more depth, and identify preferences for the organisation and delivery of palliative care (Ahmed et al. 2008). Casenotes were audited where possible to identify referrals to palliative care services, and to explore the management of palliative care related issues. Our study concluded with focus groups of stroke service staff to explore the study findings, and identify organisational, professional and practical issues in the delivery of palliative care to stroke patients.

We identified a wide range of physical palliative care needs, with significant proportions of patients experiencing them (Payne et al. 2008). Nearly 50% of patients had some form of pain or headache. Our review of casenotes indicated that nearly all patients had their pain assessed at some point during the acute phase of their stroke. However, the interviews performed suggested that the management of pain (spasms and tingling) in non-specialist stroke settings, for example when patients were located on general wards outside the stroke units, may be problematic, possibly reflecting a lack of stroke specialist knowledge or expertise. Four out of five stroke patients experienced fatigue-related symptoms or restlessness. This is important given the shift towards more intensive and early mobilisation after stroke (Indredavik et al. 1999), and early supported discharge (Department of Health 2007).

Approximately one-half of all patients in our study experienced some form of low mood, anxiety, confusion or poor concentration (Payne et al. 2008). In comparison 20–30% of patients with advanced cancer have formal diagnosis of mental health problems, the most common being depression (Hotopf et al. 2002). In addition, it is worth noting that nearly one in five patients expressed some degree of agreement with the item 'feeling that life's not worth living'. The evidence of the high prevalence of post-stroke depression is strong (Intercollegiate Stroke Working Party 2008). These data would suggest the importance of providing opportunities for patients to debrief their experiences, and to provide access to appropriate psychological care where appropriate.

Some needs (such as fatigue) are part of both the palliative care and rehabilitation literatures. For example, Stone et al. (2003) report the incidence of fatigue to be 56% in a sample (n = 576) of patients with cancer and receiving chemotherapy. Our data suggest that the prevalence of fatigue in stroke is much higher. Cancer professionals appear to view fatigue as a combined effect of both the disease and associated interventions, and that it is largely untreated. Treatment recommendations made by a sample (n = 368) of professionals in cancer care included rest and relaxation (90%), improved dietary intake (83%), transfusion (67%), exercise (59%), physiotherapy (34%) and corticosteroids (27%). However, the context of the stroke and cancer literatures is different, and approaches to meeting these needs will also be different. The evidence base for both pharmacological and non-pharmacological interventions for fatigue is poor (Stone 2002). Unfortunately, little intervention research in post-stroke fatigue is available (McGeough et al. 2009), although studies of aetiology suggest fatigue is similarly multifactorial (Jaracz et al. 2007), and both the factors and the interventions to address them will differ.

The importance of stroke as a family event was clearly highlighted in our study. Over 50% of patients were worried about the effect of their illness on other family members. A systematic review has indicated the prevalence of patients' fears about feeling a burden to others, including family members (McPherson et al. 2007). It appeared that family networks were coping with the impact of stroke. Nearly 80% of families felt that family support was sufficient, or that the family network could provide the support that they felt they needed (Low et al. 1999). It should be noted, however, that these patients were hospitalised, and any impact of the significant challenges faced by patients and families during transfer of care, and renegotiating life with stroke in community settings (Burton 2000; Hafsteinsdottir & Grypdonck 1997) may not have begun to be manifest.

Where patients were recognised or acknowledged as dying, family members were keen to ensure that the death was peaceful and dignified. The importance of the management of distressing symptoms for the benefit of both patients and family members alike was discussed in interviews. Inevitably, dealing with families in crisis appeared to be complex for staff, and there was potential for there to be negative family experiences, which may not necessarily have reflected the quality of communication about impending death. Uncertainty in prognosis is inevitable in stroke care, and this can be difficult for patients, families and professionals alike. Communication between patients, family members and professionals was consistently highlighted as central to a positive experience of stroke. Honesty and clarity of information was required, even where prognoses were bleak. Patients and family members appeared to attach as much importance to the style of communication as to the substance of the transfer of information. Where decisions had been made to shift the focus from active intervention to more supportive care, families and patients still wanted to be included in the dialogue with professionals. Fears of further strokes were evident, and patients needed opportunities to discuss these fears. The impact of stroke, and the necessary readjustment and mobilisation of resources in families suggests that services need to consider in greater depth the family network, rather than cursory acknowledgement of a 'carer'. There was recognition amongst patients and family members that staff work pressures may limit opportunities for communication, but strategies for management of that time were highlighted, including the use of pre-prepared questions, and identification of a nominated individual to 'manage' communication with staff. It is essential that time for communication is realistically incorporated into stroke workforce planning models.

Palliative care dilemmas

A striking feature of our interviews with stroke service staff, quotations from which are included in this section, was the confidence that staff had in being able to provide many aspects of stroke care. This perhaps should have been unsurprising given the similarities between some aspects of stroke and palliative care. For example, stroke practice has a long history of engagement with family members, and the importance of the 'carers' perspective' is consistently highlighted in policy documents. Nevertheless, some concerns were identified, which are perhaps best characterised in the following quotations from interviews with staff about providing palliative care:

I think the problem is with a stroke that you treat someone for two or three weeks and then decide, no, it's not working and you withdraw your treatment. I think that's what most people find uncomfortable ... they're not going to die from the stroke then, they're going to die because you're not feeding them, you're not hydrating them. And I think that that's the uncomfortable part of our job.
(Palliative care dilemmas – withdrawal of treatment)

Because stroke is so individual to each individual person. For the first two or three weeks we give people everything and as health care professionals we're not very good at saying 'this isn't working' and then you get the family dynamics where, if you try to be positive and you know, you do try to prepare them but the patients do open their eyes or whatever, and it's sort of not back tracking on what you're saying, but it's about that 'this patient isn't going to progress any further'. Quality of life is so individual ...
(Palliative care dilemmas – difficulty in identifying and communicating poor prognoses)

I mean when you get ... towards end of life, we're often stuck right in the middle of people who are perhaps 'well, TLC-ish' you know. I think that's what we're saying, that that decision is very, very slow in the making almost to the point where the patient has almost passed away when that decision is made.
(Palliative care dilemmas – making treatment decisions)

These quotations reinforce the complexity of providing palliative care within the context of stroke services. The *National Clinical Guidelines for Stroke* (Intercollegiate Working Party for Stroke 2008) recognise the importance of education and training for staff providing palliative care, and this may provide an opportunity for skill acquisition or development. However, this has to be supported by an appropriate organisational context which enables the implementation of education and training outcomes.

Organisational challenges

The context in which stroke services are currently provided is significant. This is, quite rightly, underpinned by a rehabilitation and patient activation philosophy – with the result that the resources, skills and experience to provide appropriate palliative care interventions to acute stroke patients may not be readily available. It may be impractical to expect staff to possess equivalent skills in functional goal-setting approaches to care with some patients, and also to actively discuss prognosis, palliation and associated ethical issues with patients and families. Given demand on UK cancer services, it is unlikely that reliance upon specialist services to additionally support stroke care will be a realistic option.

A tested model for the integration of generalist palliative care into stroke services is lacking, although one potential strategy, oriented at acute care, from the NHS End of Life Care Strategy is available: the Liverpool Care Pathway – LCP (Ellershaw et al. 2001). The LCP is multiprofessional, and focuses on the integration of a goal-oriented approach to care planning. The applicability of the LCP to the needs of stroke patients has not been systematically evaluated, although there are early suggestions that its incorporation can improve prescribing practice and communication about prognosis (Jack et al. 2004). Experience suggests that whilst many acute stroke units have access to the LCP through NHS Trust end of life care strategies, many challenges remain. These challenges include: variable implementation and translation of organisational end of life policy to stroke unit care; practical difficulties in identifying when to commence the LCP; and an absence of any supportive or end of life care before the patient is in the last days and hours of life.

Conclusion

Strengthening the contribution of palliative care within stroke settings provides opportunities for inter-disciplinary learning, research and development, which engage both the stroke and palliative care clinical and academic communities. Examples of the integration of rehabilitation and palliative care have already been established with cancer services (National Institute for Health and Clinical Excellence (NICE) 2004). The NHS End of Life Care Strategy does provide some strategic direction for an integrated approach to service delivery. Uncertainty about prognostication in stroke practice, and the anticipated increasing admission rates of people with severe stroke to acute stroke services, suggests that integration should focus on the routine combination of both active intervention and general supportive care, even when the stroke patient is not dying.

The findings from our study reported in this chapter would indicate that clinical issues such as fatigue, pain, the fear of dying and the loss of independence need to be addressed, and that the relative merits of alternative practice frameworks to facilitate this integration flexibly (i.e. regardless of whether an explicit decision to actively withdraw intervention has been made) need to be established. Unfortunately, existing practice frameworks such as the Liverpool Care Pathway which focus primarily on terminal care will provide only partial solutions to this integration.

Acknowledgements

The authors would like to thank Professor Julia Addington-Hall for supplying the case examples at the start of the chapter.

References

Addington-Hall, J, Lay, M, Altman, D, & McCarthy, M, 1995, Symptom control, communication with health professionals, and hospital care of stroke patients in the last year of life as reported by surviving family, friends, and officials, *Stroke*, vol. 26, no. 12, pp. 2242–2248.

Addington-Hall, J, Lay, M, Altman, D, & McCarthy, M, 1998, Community care for stroke patients in the last year of life: results of a national retrospective survey of surviving family, friends and officials, *Health and Social Care in the Community*, vol. 6, no. 2, pp. 112–119.

Ahmed, N, Bestall, JC, Ahmedzai, SH, Payne, SA, Clark, D et al., 2004, Systematic review of the problems and issues of accessing specialist palliative care by patients, carers and health and social care professionals, *Palliative Medicine*, vol. 18, no. 6, pp. 525–542.

Ahmed, N, Bestall, JC, Payne, SA, Noble, B, & Ahmedzai, SH, 2008, The use of cognitive interviewing methodology in the design and testing of a screening tool for supportive and palliative care needs, *Supportive Care Cancer*, vol. 17, no. 6, pp. 665–673.

Anderson, CS, Linto, J, & Stewart-Wynne, EG, 1995, A population-based assessment of the impact and burden of caregiving for long-term stroke survivors, *Stroke*, vol. 26, no. 5, pp. 843–849.

Bamford, J, Sandercock, P, Dennis, M, Burn, J, & Warlow, C, 1990, A prospective study of acute cerebrovascular disease in the community: the Oxfordshire Community Stroke Project – 1981–86. 2. Incidence, case fatality rates and overall outcome at one year of cerebral infarction, primary intracerebral and subarachnoid haemorrhage, *Journal of Neurology, Neurosurgery and Psychiatry*, vol. 53, no. 1, pp. 16–22.

Bestall, JC, Ahmed, N, Ahmedzai, SH, Payne, SA, Noble, B et al., 2004, Access and referral to specialist palliative care: patients' and professionals' experiences, *International Journal of Palliative Nursing*, vol. 10, no. 8, pp. 381–389.

Burton, CR, 2000, A description of the nursing role in stroke rehabilitation, *Journal of Advanced Nursing*, vol. 32, no. 1, pp. 174–181.

Department of Health, 2007, *National Stroke Strategy*, Department of Health, London.

Department of Health, 2008, *End of Life Care Strategy. Promoting High Quality Care for All Adults at the End of Life*, Department of Health, London.

Dunlop, R, 2001, Specialist palliative care and non-malignant diseases, in *Palliative Care for Non-Cancer Patients*, JM Addington-Hall, & IJ Higginson, eds., Oxford University Press, Oxford.

Ellershaw, J, Smith, C, Overill, S, Walker, SE, & Aldridge, J, 2001, Care of the dying: setting standards for symptom control in the last 48 hours of life, *Journal of Pain and Symptom Management*, vol. 21, no. 1, pp. 12–17.

Gomes, B, & Higginson, IJ, 2006, Factors influencing death at home in terminally ill patients with cancer: systematic review, *British Medical Journal*, vol. 332, no. 7540, pp. 515–521.

Gott, MC, Ahmedzai, SH, & Wood, C, 2001, How many inpatients at an acute hospital have palliative care needs? Comparing the perspectives of medical and nursing staff, *Palliative Medicine*, vol. 15, no. 6, pp. 451–460.

Hafsteinsdottir, TB, & Grypdonck, M, 1997, Being a stroke patient: a review of the literature, *Journal of Advanced Nursing*, vol. 26, no. 3, pp. 580–588.

Henry, C, & Seymour, J, 2007, *Advance Care Planning: A Guide for Health and Social Care Professionals*, NHS End of Life Care Programme, Leicester.

Hotopf, M, Chidgey, J, Addington-Hall, J, & Ly, KL, 2002, Depression in advanced disease: a systematic review. Part 1. Prevalence and case finding, *Palliative Medicine*, vol. 16, no. 2, pp. 81–97.

Indredavik, B, Bakke, F, Slordahl, SA, Rokseth, R, & Haheim, LL, 1999, Treatment in a combined acute and rehabilitation stroke unit: which aspects are most important? *Stroke*, vol. 30, no. 5, pp. 917–923.

Intercollegiate Stroke Working Party, 2008, *National Clinical Guidelines for Stroke*, Royal College of Physicians, London.

Jack, C, Jones, L, Jack, BA, Gambles, M, Murphy, D et al., 2004, Towards a good death: the impact of the care of the dying pathway in an acute stroke unit, *Age and Ageing*, vol. 33, no. 6, pp. 625–626.

Jaracz, K, Mielcarek, L, & Kozubski, W, 2007, Clinical and psychological correlates of poststroke fatigue. Preliminary results, *Neurologia i Neurochirurgia Polska*, vol. 41, no. 1, pp. 36–43.

Le, BH, Pisasale, M, & Watt, J, 2008, Palliative care in stroke, *Palliative Medicine*, vol. 22, no. 1, pp. 95–96.

Low, JT, Payne, S, & Roderick, P, 1999, The impact of stroke on informal carers: a literature review, *Social Science and Medicine*, vol. 49, no. 6, pp. 711–725.

McGeough, E, Pollock, A, Smith, LN, Dennis, M, Sharpe, M, Lewis, S, Mead, GE. Interventions for post-stroke fatigue. Cochrane Database of Systematic Reviews 2009, Issue 3. Art. No.: CD007030. DOI: 10.1002/14651858.CD007030.pub2

McPherson, CJ, Wilson, KG, & Murray, MA, 2007, Feeling like a burden to others: a systematic review focusing on the end of life, *Palliative Medicine*, vol. 21, no. 2, pp. 115–128.

Mental Capacity Act, 2005, (C.9), HMSO, London.

National Audit Office, 2005, *Reducing Brain Damage – Faster Access to Better Stroke Care*, The Stationery Office, London.

National Council for Hospice and Specialist Palliative Care Services, 2002, *Definitions of Supportive and Palliative Care*, National Council for Hospice and Specialist Palliative Care Services, London.

National Institute for Health and Clinical Excellence (NICE), 2004, *Improving Supportive and Palliative Care for Adults with Cancer*, National Institute for Health and Clinical Excellence, London.

Payne, S, Seymour, J, & Ingleton, C, 2008, *Palliative Care Nursing*, 2nd edn, McGraw Hill, Maidenhead.

Rogers, A, & Addington-Hall, JM, 2005, Care of the dying stroke patient in the acute setting, *Journal of Research in Nursing*, vol. 10, no. 2, pp. 153–167.

Sepulveda, C, Marlin, A, Yoshida, T, & Ullrich, A, 2002, Palliative care: the World Health Organization's global perspective, *Journal of Pain and Symptom Management*, vol. 24, no. 2, pp. 91–96.

Shipman, C, Gysels, M, White, P, Worth, A, Murray, SA et al., 2008, Improving generalist end of life care: national consultation with practitioners, commissioners, academics, and service user groups, *British Medical Journal*, vol. 337, p. a1720.

Stevens, T, Payne, SA, Burton, C, Addington-Hall, J, & Jones, A, 2007, Palliative care in stroke: a critical review of the literature, *Palliative Medicine*, vol. 21, no. 4, pp. 323–331.

Stone, P, 2002, The measurement, causes and effective management of cancer-related fatigue, *International Journal of Palliative Nursing*, vol. 8, no. 3, pp. 120–128.

Stone, P, Ream, E, Richardson, A, Thomas, H, Andrews, P et al., 2003, Cancer-related fatigue – a difference of opinion? Results of a multicentre survey of healthcare professionals, patients and caregivers, *European Journal of Cancer Care*, vol. 12, no. 1, pp. 20–27.

Thomas, K, 2004, *The Gold Standards Framework. A Programme for Community Palliative Care*, Macmillan Cancer Relief, London.

Chapter 13

Reducing the risk of stroke

Peter Humphrey, Jo Gibson and Stephanie Jones

> **Key points**
>
> - Primary and secondary prevention are key measures to reduce stroke incidence, and thus reduce death and disability from stroke.
> - Secondary prevention measures are important in all patients with TIA or stroke.
> - Specialist services to assess, diagnose and treat patients urgently after TIA or stroke are crucial in order to gain the maximum benefit from secondary prevention.
> - Most acute UK hospitals now have a neurovascular service.
> - Only a third of neurovascular clinics currently see, assess and manage patients within seven days.
> - Only a third of stroke patients are discharged from hospital on the recommended combination of aspirin and dipyridamole.

I've been telling him to do something for years: he smokes too much and drinks too much [...] maybe tomorrow [...] maybe now he'll listen, do it today.

(Margaret, wife of John, who was admitted with a left middle cerebral artery stroke)

Introduction

There has been a decline in the incidence of stroke over the past 20 years, probably due to improvements in the management of vascular risk factors, and the use of antiplatelet agents, anticoagulants and surgery where appropriate (Rothwell et al. 2004). Stroke patients are also at high risk of other cardiovascular events such as myocardial infarction and limb ischaemia, and many interventions to reduce stroke risk will also reduce their risk of these related events. The development of such interventions has made the reduction of stroke risk an important element of acute and long-term nursing interventions for stroke patients.

Secondary prevention is important after a person has experienced a completed stroke, regardless of its severity, and also after transient ischaemic attack (TIA). However, the short-lived nature of symptoms in TIA may result in delayed or missed opportunities for secondary prevention, especially as many patients present late or not at all.

As flagged in Chapter 3, it is important to understand the pathophysiology of stroke if rational treatment and appropriate secondary prevention is to be initiated. For example, carotid stenosis and atrial fibrillation are likely to be the cause of embolic cortical ischaemic stroke rather than deep white matter subcortical ischaemic stroke (Hankey et al. 1991; Kappelle et al. 1988; Kumar & Caplan 2007). It is therefore crucial to accurately diagnose the aetiology of stroke or TIA and its anatomical site, before secondary prevention can be addressed. As explained in Chapter 3, most strokes are classified as ischaemic in aetiology, arising from atherothrombosis affecting the cerebral circulation, or from embolisation from other sources of thrombus (for example in atrial fibrillation). These account for around 85% of all strokes in the UK, with the remainder due to haemorrhagic causes.

Primary prevention

Stroke is a common condition, which is costly in terms of its financial impact on health care resources and in its impact on the lives of people who experience a stroke and their families. The implementation of evidence-based measures to reduce the incidence of stroke can be highly effective in reducing these financial and human costs. Yet until recently, acute treatment and rehabilitation after stroke has dominated research, health policy and clinical practice in cerebrovascular diseases. Whilst acute care and rehabilitation are undoubtedly important, a more straightforward strategy to reduce the burden of death and disability imposed by stroke is to implement measures to prevent and hence reduce the incidence of stroke (Wolf 1998). Two main approaches are:

- *primary prevention* – the use of measures to reduce the development of cerebrovascular disease in the general population by reducing exposure to causal and risk factors
- *secondary prevention* – identifying and targeting interventions at those who are known to be at higher risk, and the use of early diagnosis and treatment (Tones & Green 2004)

Many modifiable risk factors have been identified for ischaemic stroke, similar to those for other atherothrombotic conditions such as coronary heart disease and peripheral vascular disease. The implementation of effective measures to address these risk factors in the general population, that is, in those who have never had a stroke or TIA, will reduce the risk of development of significant cerebrovascular disease and thus reduce stroke incidence.

Risk factors

The major modifiable risk factors are hypertension, smoking, diabetes mellitus, physical activity, exercise, raised blood lipid levels, obesity and dietary factors such as dietary sodium intake, consumption of fish and fruit and vegetables.

Hypertension

Raised diastolic blood pressure (BP) is known to be associated with increased stroke risk, with a 46% increase in relative risk for every 7.5 mmHg increase in diastolic pressure. Conversely, the use of antihypertensives to reduce blood pressure leads to a corresponding fall in stroke incidence (42% relative risk reduction for an average blood pressure reduction of 5.8 mmHg). This relationship is apparent even at diastolic pressures considered as normal (under 90 mmHg) (Collins et al. 1990). In those with isolated systolic hypertension, most common in older people (systolic BP above 160 but diastolic below 90 mmHg), antihypertensive medication has been shown to reduce stroke risk by 36% over 4.5 years (SHEP Cooperative Research Group 1991). Similarly, in the 60–79-year age group, every 10 mmHg reduction in systolic BP will reduce stroke risk by approximately one-third (Lawes et al. 2004).

It is also known that restricting the consumption of dietary salt is beneficial in the treatment of existing hypertension, resulting in typical reductions in systolic pressure of around 5 mmHg in patients on low sodium versus high sodium diets (Jurgens & Graudal 2004). Some patients experience benefits of greater magnitude, to the extent that they can stop or reduce their antihypertensive medication (Hooper et al. 2004). However, for people with normal blood pressure, reduction in salt intake is of little benefit, resulting in a clinically insignificant mean reduction in systolic blood pressure of only 1.27 mmHg (Jurgens & Graudal 2004); nor does a low sodium diet affect these people's five-year risk of newly developing hypertension (Hooper et al. 2004). There is also no reliable long-term evidence that reduction of salt intake in those without symptomatic vascular disease reduces cardiovascular morbidity and mortality (Scientific Advisory Committee on Nutrition 2003), although it may be beneficial for secondary prevention after stroke or other cardiovascular events.

Tobacco use

There is a strong relationship between cigarette smoking and stroke incidence, with tobacco use increasing relative risk by some 50%. The increase in risk is dose-dependent, with people who are heavier users of tobacco being at highest risk (Shinton & Beevers 1989), independent of other risk factors. However, the individual's risk of stroke and other vascular diseases falls rapidly on cessation of smoking, reaching the same level as those who have never smoked within five years of quitting (Wolf et al. 1988). Smoking cessation is most likely to be successful if a combination of professional support (Rice & Stead 2004) and pharmacological therapy, either nicotine replacement therapy (Silagy et al. 2004) or bupropion (Hughes et al. 2003), is used. More recently introduced, varenicline (http://www.nps.org.au/__data/assets/pdf_file/0012/ 17031/varenicline.pdf) is showing promise but long-term evaluation has yet to be undertaken. Such interventions increase quit rates typically 1.5- to 2-fold compared with control groups.

Physical activity

Exercise has a beneficial effect on stroke risk factors such as hypertension, obesity, dyslipidaemia and glucose tolerance. Both moderate and heavy exercise/activity have been shown to significantly reduce the relative risk of both ischaemic and haemorrhagic strokes (Lee et al. 2003).

Dyslipidaemia

Elevated total cholesterol and elevated low-density lipoprotein (LDL) cholesterol are both associated with increased stroke risk. Randomised trials of statin therapy have shown typical relative risk reductions for stroke of 25% (Straus et al. 2002) to 30% (Warshafsky et al. 1999). The benefits of statin therapy are thought to be partly due to its ability to stabilise atheromatous plaque, reducing its thrombogenicity, as well as its effect on dyslipidaemia *per se*. Other lipid-lowering therapies, such as fibrates, resins or dietary modification, have not been demonstrated to reduce stroke risk (Bucher et al. 1998).

Diabetes mellitus

Although the presence of diabetes mellitus itself (type 1 or type 2) is an independent risk factor for stroke, there is no evidence that stroke risk is increased by poor glycaemic control itself (Diabetes Control and Complications Trial Research Group (DCCTRG) 1993; UK Prospective Diabetes Study Group 1998; University Group Diabetes Program 1970). It is thought that the increased stroke rate in people with diabetes is caused by excess incidence of hypertension and hyperlipidaemia compared with people without diabetes (Straus et al. 2002).

Dietary measures

Obesity has been demonstrated, by prospective cohort study, to be an independent risk factor for stroke. Men with a body mass index (BMI) of 30 or greater have twice the stroke risk of those with a BMI of 20–29, and each unit increase in BMI is associated with a 6% increase in relative risk of stroke (Kurth et al. 2002). Other dietary measures which may reduce stroke risk include reducing dietary sodium intake in hypertension, consumption of fish and fish oils (Skerrett & Hennekens 2003), and consumption of fruit and vegetables (Johnsen et al. 2003). There is also a possible link between raised plasma homocysteine and increased stroke risk (Perry et al. 1995). It is known that plasma homocysteine can be reduced by intake of dietary or supplemental folic acid (Boushey et al. 1995) but there is no evidence that this measure reduces stroke risk.

Medical therapy: antiplatelet and antithrombotic agents

The use of antiplatelet agents such as aspirin is only recommended for reduction of stroke risk in people who are known to have vascular disease. In people who have coronary artery disease or peripheral arterial disease, as well as in those who have had a stroke or TIA, antiplatelet therapy with aspirin reduces stroke risk (Antiplatelet Trialists' Collaboration 1994). A newer agent, clopidogrel, is useful for patients who are unable, through true intolerance, to take aspirin (CAPRIE Steering Committee 1996). Clopidogrel and aspirin have never been compared head-to-head, but clopidogrel may confer slightly greater long-term reduction in risk. Current clinical guidelines do not recommend its use in preference to aspirin except in people who are intolerant of low-dose aspirin and either have experienced an occlusive vascular event or have symptomatic peripheral arterial disease (National Institute for Health and Clinical Excellence (NICE) 2005). A combination of aspirin and clopidogrel does not confer any significant benefit in reducing vascular events; it does, however, increase the risk of haemorrhage compared with clopidogrel alone (Diener et al. 2004).

People with atrial fibrillation have a high risk of stroke from embolisation of cardiac thrombus. Anticoagulation with warfarin significantly reduces their risk (odds ratio versus placebo: 0.3). Aspirin is also moderately effective with an odds ratio versus placebo of 0.68, but is not as effective as warfarin in head-to-head studies (odds ratio 0.64). Anticoagulant therapy is associated with an increased risk of haemorrhage, but this does not outweigh the benefits of reduced stroke risk (Aguilar & Hart 2005).

Secondary prevention: identifying those at risk of stroke

Whilst primary prevention addresses stroke risk in the whole population, secondary prevention focuses on measures to reduce the risk of a major cerebral ischaemic event in people who are already known to have significant cerebrovascular disease. The target population for secondary prevention measures is those people who have had a TIA or stroke, and also those who are known to have significant cerebrovascular disease in the absence of symptoms. The annual incidence of TIA in the UK is estimated at 0.035% (Coull et al. 2004) to 0.04% (Dennis et al. 1989). This is equivalent to about 21 000 people per year in the UK. Many more people have a stroke from which they quickly and fully recover. A large (n = 10 112) telephone survey in the US revealed that TIA prevalence was 2.3% (Johnston et al. 2003). Many (54%) had hemispheric symptoms; and 9% had amaurosis fugax (transient loss of vision in one eye) alone. In addition, a further 3.2% of respondents reported having experienced symptoms consistent with a TIA but had not sought medical attention. Of those who had sought advice on experiencing a TIA, 36% waited more than 24 hours before doing so (Johnston et al. 2003). These results suggest that only one in every four people who has a TIA seeks medical advice within 24 hours, and that almost 60% of TIAs are never reported to a health professional, perhaps because of the transient nature of the symptoms and a lack of understanding of their potential seriousness. Others do seek medical advice but the TIA may be still undiagnosed (Koudstaal et al. 1989). These figures represent a serious public health challenge, and barrier to effective stroke prevention.

It is imperative that people who experience symptoms of a TIA seek urgent medical advice. TIA is an important indicator of future stroke risk, even more so than a previous completed stroke. Three-month stroke risk is estimated to be eight times higher in those who have had a TIA than after a first completed stroke (Kennedy et al. 2002), with the early (three-month) risk of stroke after TIA being variously reported as 10–20.1% (Coull et al. 2004; Eliasziw et al. 2004; Johnston et al. 2000). Half of such strokes are estimated to occur within two days of the first TIA (Johnston et al. 2000). Prevention of these very early strokes is challenging, since many patients delay seeking medical advice after a TIA for 24 hours or more. However, the results of the EXPRESS study (Rothwell et al., 2007) suggest that the early initiation of existing services after TIA and minor stroke can reduce subsequent stroke risk by around 80%. The recent development and validation of prognostic scores to predict people's risk of very early stroke after TIA may also be an important tool in emergency management (Johnston et al. 2007). It is also known that there is a 25.1% risk of any further adverse event, including recurrent TIA, stroke, hospitalisation for cardiac arrhythmia, and death, in the three months following a TIA (Johnston et al. 2000). Although stroke risk is highest in the first few months after a TIA, there is also an increased long-term risk of stroke (3.4% per year after the first year) and of myocardial infarction (3.1%) (Hankey et al. 1991). The annual death rate after TIA is about 7%, of which two-thirds are due to stroke or cardiac disease (Hankey et al. 1991). The total five-year risk of further stroke after any first cerebral ischaemic event (TIA or stroke) is estimated at 30–43% (Mant et al. 2004). Even in 'low-risk' patients who have survived the initial high-risk period after a TIA, the ten-year risk of major vascular events (stroke, myocardial infarction or vascular death) is 42.8% (Clark et al. 2003). Short- and long-term secondary risk reduction measures are therefore essential to reduce this burden of excess mortality and morbidity.

In addition to those who have already been identified as having had a TIA or stroke, many more people in the general population have severe asymptomatic cerebrovascular disease and thus may also benefit from secondary risk reduction measures. However, as these people have, by definition, no symptoms, they may never be identified as being at risk of stroke. There is no systematic programme of screening in the UK for asymptomatic carotid disease, although it has been argued that this is a necessary measure to reduce the incidence of stroke (Toole 2004). As a result of lack of symptoms, or lack of recognition and self-reporting of symptoms, many people who are at high risk of stroke and who would benefit from secondary risk reduction measures are thus never identified and treated by health services.

The availability of rapid access neurovascular services for patients with suspected TIA or stroke was mandated in the UK by the National Service Framework for Older People (Department of Health 2001), and more recently by the National Stroke Strategy (Department of Health 2007). The current guidelines specify that eligible patients should be assessed in a neurovascular clinic and have necessary stroke risk reduction measures implemented within seven days of their TIA or first stroke for lower-risk patients, and within 24 hours for those at highest risk (Department of Health 2007). This is essential for specialist investigations such as carotid duplex ultrasound scanning to be accessed, but also, more fundamentally, because the diagnosis of TIA is by no means straightforward (Koudstaal et al. 1989; Kraaijeveld et al. 1984). Not all patients with carotid territory TIA or stroke present with classic symptoms, and the symptoms of TIA are, by definition, transient and often unwitnessed. Indeed, 40% of patients in one series who were referred to a regional neurovascular clinic with a non-specialist physician's diagnosis of TIA had not, in fact, had a TIA (Martin et al. 1997). If the diagnosis of TIA is not correctly made, then some patients may receive inappropriate treatment after a non-cerebrovascular event, giving rise to the unnecessary use of health care resources and possibly exposing the patient to avoidable risk, such as adverse drug reactions. Other patients who have had a genuine TIA or stroke may not have their condition recognised, investigated and treated appropriately. Currently, over 91% of UK acute general hospitals have a stroke unit, with 95% having a neurovascular clinic service for rapid assessment and management of TIA and stroke in those patients who do not require immediate hospital admission. Of these, only 35% are able to see and investigate outpatients within 7 days, let alone within the recommended 24-hour time span for higher-risk patients (Intercollegiate Stroke Working Party 2008). Therefore, nearly two-thirds of acute hospitals in the UK are currently unable to provide the urgent investigation and treatment needed after TIA or stroke other than via inpatient admission and investigation.

It follows that, if a patient is to obtain the urgent assessment, investigation and advice they need after a TIA or stroke, they (or a relative or friend) must:

- Firstly recognise the significance of their symptoms
- Seek early medical advice

The health professional they consult must then, in turn: appreciate the importance of:

- The presenting symptoms
- The necessity for urgent investigation and treatment, and
- Be aware of local emergency pathways and neurovascular service provision

Even if these criteria are fulfilled, the patient still has, in the UK, at best around a one-in-three chance of being able to gain access to the rapid assessment and treatment that they need. It is little wonder, therefore, that many people in the UK go on to have further disabling or fatal stroke after a TIA or first stroke, without ever having had the opportunity to address their stroke risk factors.

Transient ischaemic attack

The most commonly used definition of a transient ischaemic attack (TIA) is nearly 30 years old (National Institutes of Health 1975). This definition limits

TIA to '*a sudden, focal neurologic deficit that lasts for less than 24 hours, is of presumed vascular origin, and which is confined to an area of the brain or eye perfused by a specific artery*'. A deficit which has not completely resolved within 24 hours, even if it is partially resolved by this time, is defined as a stroke. However, the 24-hour limit was chosen for convenience rather than because of any relationship to the natural history and underlying pathology of the condition. Some 50% of TIAs resolve in under 30 minutes, yet only 13.8% of all patients presenting with any cerebrovascular event experience complete resolution of their symptoms within the 1–24-hour time interval (Levy 1988). Short-lived TIAs, whose symptoms last less than one hour, are rarely associated with any demonstrable ischaemic lesion on computed tomography (CT) scanning. However, those patients who have had a 'TIA' of several hours' duration, but which has since completely resolved, often do have cerebral ischaemic lesions which are indistinguishable from those found after disabling stroke. It has therefore been suggested that the diagnosis of TIA should be redefined. Under the proposed new definition, any symptoms which last for more than one hour, or which are associated with ischaemic lesions on CT scanning, or both, should be reclassified as a stroke (Albers et al. 2002).

This distinction is not a trivial one. Treatments for acute stroke, notably thrombolysis, should be administered as soon as possible for greatest benefit, and within 3 hours or, at most, 4.5 hours (Hacke et al. 2008) of the onset of symptoms. Using the classic definition of TIA, some patients whose symptoms have not yet resolved at 3 hours after onset may still recover within the ensuing 21 hours, and would therefore be deemed not to have had a stroke. People with symptoms of ischaemic stroke should receive thrombolysis as soon as possible, and clinicians should not wait 24 hours to establish the differential diagnosis of TIA or stroke. This means that some patients who have a TIA will receive thrombolysis. Revising the definition means that the diagnosis is clarified earlier, enabling treatment decisions to be made. The proposed new definition is thus both a closer reflection of the underlying pathology, and a pragmatic step towards improving access to treatment for acute stroke. In practice, however, many patients do not seek medical advice for several hours or even days after the onset of symptoms, particularly if their symptoms are mild or have resolved within minutes.

The extent to which TIA is a useful marker for cerebrovascular disease is also the subject of debate. Although early (one month) stroke risk is high after TIA, most people who have carotid stenosis and subsequently develop a stroke have never had, or become aware of, any prior symptoms. Others may have had minor symptoms which have been ignored or misinterpreted (by the patient themselves or by health professionals), have had atypical symptoms, or may perhaps have had a 'silent' TIA, occurring during sleep or causing transient focal cerebral ischaemia but without symptoms (Toole 2004). In addition, up to 10% of people aged over 65 years can be found to have previously silent cerebral infarctions on brain imaging (Brott et al. 1994). There is good evidence that treating asymptomatic (or 'presymptomatic'; Toole 2004) high-grade carotid stenosis with carotid endarterectomy will reduce the incidence of stroke (Halliday et al. 2004), although it must be borne in mind that this is at the cost of causing perioperative strokes in some patients. There is no screening programme for the condition and thus no systematic way of identifying those at risk. Asymptomatic stenosis is, at present, most often detected incidentally, perhaps during investigation for another condition or by initial detection of a carotid bruit (itself not a reliable sign).

Current guidelines in secondary stroke prevention

Secondary risk reduction is an important part of reducing the burden of stroke mortality and morbidity, and has therefore merited much attention in recent guidelines for clinical practice. However, stroke risk factors are often inadequately controlled after TIA or stroke (Joseph et al. 1999; Sappok et al. 2001), even in the hands of a specialist neurovascular clinic (Mouradian et al. 2002).

It is now recommended that all patients who have had an acute stroke or TIA should have an individualised plan for stroke risk reduction implemented within seven days of the event (Intercollegiate Stroke Working Party 2008; National Institute for Health and Clinical Excellence (NICE) 2008). Factors which need to be considered include lifestyle changes (smoking, exercise, diet and weight control, reducing salt and alcohol intake); blood pressure management; antithrombotic treatment; antilipid agents; assessment and treatment of carotid stenosis; and consideration of stopping hormone replacement therapy. Individuals' needs will vary, but, unless contraindicated, all patients should commence an antiplatelet agent or anticoagulant, and statin therapy if total serum cholesterol is more than 3.5 mmol/l. Some investigators also recommend that all patients, even those who are normotensive, should commence combination therapy with the antihypertensive drugs perindopril 4 mg and indapamide 2–2.5 mg (PROGRESS Collaborative Group 2001). Treating only overt hypertension or hyperlipidaemia in these individuals is not enough to reduce their stroke risk (Muir 2004). Certainly, their blood pressure should be monitored and antihypertensives started if it is persistently higher than 140/85 mmHg (or higher than 130/80 mmHg in people with diabetes mellitus). Antihypertensive medication should be tailored to achieve the lowest possible blood pressure without causing symptomatic hypotension.

Assessment and medical treatment of transient ischaemic attacks

An example of management of TIA in the UK is illustrated in Box 13.1. Over the past five years it has become clear that the speed of implementation of secondary preventative measures is a crucial factor in the prevention of further strokes. A stroke or TIA must be seen as a medical emergency and a sea change is required in stroke management if the full benefits of treatments are to materialise. Those at greatest risk of an early further stroke are those with large artery atherosclerosis, usually carotid stenosis, whereas those with small vessel disease, usually subcortical or lacunar, have the lowest risk of early recurrence (Lovett et al. 2004). The EXPRESS Study (Rothwell et al. 2007) has

---

Box 13.1 Vignette illustrating management of TIA in the UK.

Mr Vernon is a 78-year-old retired man who lives with his wife. He is a non-smoker, is not known to have diabetes or hypertension and is in good health. One day whilst he was driving home from shopping, his wife noticed that his driving was 'erratic' and 'jerky'. Mr Vernon himself had not noticed a problem, but after returning home he noticed that 10 minutes later he could not move his right leg. This lasted for about 20 minutes. He did not feel there was a need to seek advice but his wife phoned the general practitioner who arranged to see him and referred him to hospital. His blood pressure on presentation was 170/90 mmHg.

Questions

(a) What is Mr Vernon's ABCD2 score? (See below for explanation of ABCD2)
(b) What further investigations would you arrange?

Mr Vernon's blood tests were normal, with a total cholesterol of 4.6 mmol/l. ECG was also normal. He had a duplex scan of the carotid arteries and was found to have 1–14% right internal carotid artery stenosis and 15–49% left internal carotid artery stenosis.

Questions

(c) What further treatment and medication will Mr Vernon need?
(d) What other advice and long-term follow-up will be needed?

Answers

(a) The ABCD2 score is 5 (age = 1; BP = 1; clinical symptoms = 2; duration = 1; diabetes=0). This indicates a need for immediate assessment and implementation of secondary prevention measures within 48 hours at most.
(b) Mr Vernon will need full neurological assessment, blood tests, including glucose and cholesterol, further assessment of blood pressure, ECG, and carotid Duplex scan.
(c) Mr Vernon will need to commence long-term antihypertensive medication, a statin, aspirin 300 mg stat, followed by 75 mg/day. He will also need to take dipyridamole 200 mg twice daily for two years. Carotid endarterectomy is not indicated as the degree of ICA stenosis is moderate (15–49%).
(d) Mr Vernon must be advised to seek further immediate medical help if another similar episode occurs. He needs to refrain from driving his car for 4 weeks. Follow-up should be arranged according to local service arrangements to ensure he is taking the prescribed medication correctly and that his risk factors such as hypertension are controlled. He will also be entered into the GP's Stroke Register to facilitate long-term follow-up.

---

shown that to realise significant benefits from secondary prevention requires TIA or stroke patients to be seen immediately and preventative measures instituted there and then; anything less is often insufficient to prevent stroke.

The ABCD2 score helps to identify those at greatest risk of early stroke (Johnston et al. 2003; Rothwell et al. 2006); see Table 13.1. A score of 4 or more signifies a high risk of stroke in the next seven days. These patients need immediate assessment, with implementation of secondary preventative measures as soon as possible, within two days at most. Lower-risk patients (score 3 or less) need assessment within seven days and secondary prevention measures putting in place as soon as possible.

Most TIAs are embolic, arising from distal embolisation into the cerebral circulation from a tight (more than 70%; European Carotid Surgery Trialists' Collaborative Group (ECSTCG) 1991) stenosis of the internal carotid artery. However, a small number of attacks are haemodynamic (due to lack of blood flow) rather than embolic. These can often be identified by the clinical

Table 13.1 The ABCD2 score (Johnston et al. 2003; Rothwell et al. 2006).

		Score
Age	≥60 years	1
Blood pressure	Systolic ≥140 and/or diastolic ≥90	1
Clinical	Unilateral motor weakness	2
	Speech disturbance without weakness	1
	Other, e.g. amaurosis fugax	0
Duration of TIA	≥60 min	2
	10–59 min	1
	<10 min	0
Diabetes	Yes	1
	No	0
Total (maximum)		7

characteristics and only occur in the presence of severe arterial disease, usually in more than one vessel, for example if one or even both internal carotid arteries is occluded. Treatment with surgery or stenting to improve the blood flow to the brain or eye may ameliorate haemodynamic symptoms, although there is no sound evidence for this. Other measures such as antiplatelet therapy are not helpful in reducing the frequency of these symptoms. Haemodynamic TIAs may be associated with symptoms of pre-syncope as they may be triggered by a fall in blood pressure, or may exhibit other atypical symptoms.

Ageism

Stroke is primarily an illness of later life. There is good evidence that older people are not being investigated and treated as actively as younger people with ischaemic events (de Lusignan et al. 2006; Fairhead & Rothwell 2006). If the incidence of stroke is to be reduced then this needs to be addressed. The incidence of symptomatic carotid stenosis increases steeply with age but, despite good evidence of major benefit from carotid endarterectomy in elderly patients and a willingness to have surgery, there is a substantial under-investigation in routine clinical practice in patients aged more than 80 years with TIA or ischaemic stroke (Fairhead & Rothwell 2006). Although carotid endarterectomy is a robust long-term treatment, it is often forgotten that the major benefit of this operation is conferred in the reduction of stroke risk in the next 12–24 months. Provided the individual's life expectancy exceeds this, then carotid endarterectomy should be offered to people of almost all ages provided the individual is fit for surgery.

There is similar evidence of ageism for the use of anticoagulation in the elderly with atrial fibrillation and stroke (Brass et al. 1998) and for the use of statins. Anticoagulation in atrial fibrillation is safe and effective in those aged over 75 years (Mant et al. 2007); however, risk of falls and drug concordance must be considered.

Antiplatelet treatment

Three antiplatelet drugs are widely used for the prevention of ischaemic stroke: aspirin, dipyridamole and clopidogrel. Overall, antiplatelet therapy reduces the relative risk of vascular events by about 20% (Antithrombotic Trialists' Collaboration 2002).

- Low-dose aspirin (75–150 mg) is the standard treatment of choice; the initial starting dose should be a single 300 mg tablet followed by 75 mg a day long term.
- Dipyridamole alone reduces the risk of vascular events by 10%. It may cause headache in a third of patients at onset, but this may be relieved by simple analgesia such as paracetamol and often settles over a few weeks.
- The European Stroke Prevention Study 2 and ESPRIT Trial have confirmed that the combination of aspirin 75 mg a day and dipyridamole 200 mg twice daily is more effective than aspirin alone (Diener et al. 1996; Sudlow 2007; The ESPRIT Study Group 2006). NICE has recommended that this combination is given for two years after a TIA or ischaemic stroke; thereafter preventative therapy should revert to aspirin alone. However, this is based on cost-effectiveness rather than effectiveness *per se*.
- Clopidogrel (75 mg daily) may be used in those who are aspirin intolerant (CAPRIE Steering Committee 1996).

Aspirin and clopidogrel are both associated with a small excess risk of haemorrhage but this is far outweighed by the benefit of reduction in risk of cardiovascular and cerebrovascular events. Gastrointestinal bleeding is more likely with aspirin than clopidogrel, whereas clopidogrel may cause side-effects of rash or diarrhoea. Aspirin and esomeprazole may be superior to clopidogrel in preventing recurrent ulcer bleeding (Chan et al. 2005).

The combination of aspirin and clopidogrel has been compared with clopidogrel alone in the MATCH study: The reduction in the number of ischaemic events was exactly balanced by an increase in haemorrhagic complications (Diener et al. 2004). There may be some patients at high risk of ischaemic stroke who would benefit from this combination but this remains unclear (Howard et al. 2007), and at present there is no clinical indication for this combination in stroke patients unlike in patients with unstable angina or recent myocardial infarction. However, the CARESS trial of patients with symptomatic carotid stenosis showed fewer embolic signals on transcranial Doppler while on aspirin and clopidogrel compared with aspirin alone (Markus et al. 2005). The Express Study is, at the time of writing, trialling the use of a combination of aspirin and clopidogrel for one month only after the initial ischaemic event and then switching to aspirin and dipyridamole as per the NICE regime.

It a patient has persistent TIAs despite treatment with aspirin and dipyridamole, aspirin resistance is considered to be a possible factor in recurrent TIA and needs further research. Switching to clopidogrel alone may be considered although its benefit in this situation is unproven. In addition, the diagnosis of embolic TIAs should be reassessed, as the attacks might in fact be haemodynamic TIAs or have an unrelated cause.

Anticoagulation

Anticoagulation should be considered for all patients with atrial fibrillation (AF) and a previous TIA or stroke. Anticoagulation with warfarin reduces annual stroke risk from 12% to 4% – a relative risk reduction of 66% (EAFT (European Atrial Fibrillation Trial) Study Group 1993). In comparison, aspirin confers only a 17% relative risk reduction. The target international normalised ratio (INR) should be 2–3.5. There is good evidence that elderly people with AF are often not offered anticoagulation even if it is clearly the best option (Hart & Halperin 2001). The small risk of haemorrhagic complications on warfarin, though greater than those on aspirin, is far outweighed by the benefits in this situation, especially as people with untreated AF often have large ischaemic strokes with severe disability. Contraindications to anticoagulation (e.g. history of intracranial haemorrhage, recent gastrointestinal bleed or verified peptic ulcer, severe hypertension, dementia, frequent falls or a bleeding disorder) must be borne in mind.

Dual antiplatelet therapy with aspirin and clopidogrel is inferior to warfarin for preventing vascular events in atrial fibrillation (The ACTIVE Investigator 2006) and also confers greater risk of bleeding complications than warfarin.

The use of anticoagulation in patients with ischaemic stroke but no cardiac source of emboli remains unproven. There is no added benefit from anticoagulation over standard antiplatelet treatment for TIA and stroke patients in general (Powers 2001). This also applies to patients with a symptomatic intracranial arterial stenosis, or in the presence of the antiphospholipid antibody or lupus anticoagulant (APASS Investigators 2004; Chimowitz et al. 2005).

There is much debate about when to start anticoagulation with ischaemic stroke or TIA patients with atrial fibrillation. It seems safe to start anticoagulation immediately in those with TIAs or a mild ischaemic stroke but to delay initiating therapy for 10–14 days in those with moderate or severe clinical deficit (National Institute for Health and Clinical Excellence (NICE) 2008).

Short-term anticoagulation with rapidly acting intravenous agents such as heparin may be used for patients who are having frequent TIAs. Such patients are usually found to have a major cardiac source of emboli or a severe internal carotid stenosis. While there are no clinical trials to support this practice, clinical experience and expert consensus suggests this may be the only method of controlling symptoms until a more definitive treatment such as urgent carotid endarterectomy is sought.

Combining anticoagulation with antiplatelet therapy is rarely justified as this doubles the bleeding rate with minimal extra benefit (Gorelick 2007). New anticoagulant drugs such as Dabigatrine are being investigated, which may have similar efficacy to warfarin without the need for monitoring.

Treating high blood pressure

High blood pressure is known to be the most important risk factor for stroke with a doubling of the long-term risk of stroke for every 10–12 mmHg rise in systolic BP or 7–8 mmHg rise in diastolic BP (Lawes et al. 2004). It follows that treating hypertension is the most important factor for preventing stroke. In the PROGRESS study, treatment with a combination of perindopril and indapamide led to an overall reduction in blood pressure by 12 mmHg (systolic) and 5 mmHg (diastolic) and a reduction in relative risk of stroke of 43% (PROGRESS Collaborative Group 2001). A similar benefit was seen in normotensive patients. Treatment should begin immediately after a TIA but delayed for two weeks after a stroke. Trials of early blood pressure lowering in stroke are in progress.

In the past, there have been concerns that cerebral blood flow might be reduced by administration of antihypertensives in the long term after a stroke. However, it has been shown that the prognosis is much better if blood pressure is treated in this situation, even in patients who are normotensive (Heart Outcomes Prevention Evaluation (HOPE) Study Investigators 2000; PROGRESS Collaborative Group 2001; Schrader et al. 2005).

Audits of stroke care have shown that the poor control of blood pressure is the most important factor in stroke mortality; furthermore it is an avoidable and treatable risk factor (Rashid et al. 2003; Rudd et al. 2004). In general, blood pressure after stroke should be lowered to its lowest tolerated level, even below apparently normotensive levels, that is, 130/70 mmHg. A few patients, especially those with severe bilateral carotid occlusions and/or stenoses, may not be able to tolerate excessive drops in blood pressure and should receive treatment to lower their blood pressure as much as possible without giving rise to hypotensive symptoms. It is unclear whether the benefits from blood pressure treatment are generic or specific to the agents used in the above trials.

Lowering cholesterol levels

There is now robust data from large randomised placebo-controlled and comparative trials regarding the benefits of statins in patients with vascular disease (Cholesterol Treatment Trialists' Collaborators (CTTC) 2005; Heart Protection Study Collaborative Group (HPSCG) 2004; Sever et al. 2003). The relative risk reduction of vascular events was approximately 20–30%. This applied not only to those with elevated total cholesterol of over 5.2 mmol/l but also to those with random 'normal' total cholesterol as low as 3.5 mmol/l. Statins act as inhibitors of the enzyme HMG-CoA reductase which controls the rate-limiting step of the synthesis of cholesterol in the liver. They also exert an additional protective effect by stabilising atheromatous plaque in the arteries, thus reducing the risk of plaque rupture and thrombosis. More intensive statin therapy using high-dose statin, for example atorvastatin 80 mg, seems to give even greater benefits (Amarenco et al. 2006; Topol 2004).

Simvastatin 40 mg daily (now available in generic form and at a fraction of the cost of all other high-dose statins) is recommended for all TIA or stroke patients who have total cholesterol of over 3.5 mmol/l, unless contraindicated (Drugs and Therapeutics Bulletin 2007; Hankey 2006). It is cost-effective (Heart Protection Study Collaborative Group (HPSCG) 2006). The risk of statins is small, with less than 1 per 10 000 patient years developing a myopathy. The risk of neuropathy with statins is probably also overestimated (Heart Protection Study Collaborative Group (HPSCG) 2004).

Ezetimibe inhibits the absorption of cholesterol across the wall of the small intestine and can be considered in those who maintain elevated cholesterol after maximum doses of statins have been used (Drugs and Therapeutics Bulletin 2004).

The data regarding fibrates are limited in stroke. Fenofibrate may be useful especially in patients with high triglycerides, which may affect those with diabetes mellitus and the metabolic syndrome.

Smoking

Smoking is an independent risk factor for stroke (Donnan et al. 1993; Shinton & Beevers 1989). Stopping smoking reduces this risk (Peto et al. 1994). The experience of having a stroke or TIA may increase the patient's motivation to stop smoking. Ideally, other family members should be encouraged to also quit smoking if the stroke patient is to achieve long-term success. Nurses can appropriately deliver smoking cessation advice and support, with referral to cessation clinics or to community practitioners if needed. Pharmacological aids such as nicotine replacement, bupropion and varenicline will improve the chance of success and can normally be used safely after TIA or stroke. Counselling and other support are also available; for example, in Australia through Quitline and the Quitnow website. The manufacturers of varenicline (Chantix/Champix) offer a support package with website and blog. Specialist cessation services providing behavioural support (in groups or individually) for smokers who want help with stopping and specialist cessation counsellors are provided within many health services and/or occupational health services. GPs and health professionals should make use of opportunities to discuss quitting with smokers. Adjunct commercial programmes and self-help strategies also abound. A planned and staged approach may suit some smokers but spontaneous, opportunistic decisions are equally likely to be successful (West et al. 2000).

Diabetes mellitus

Diabetes mellitus is a proven risk factor for stroke; optimal control of blood glucose reduces the risk of vascular complications (Wilcox et al. 2007). Aggressive treatment of blood pressure and cholesterol is also paramount in these patients (Costa et al. 2006; Heart Outcomes Prevention Evaluation (HOPE)

Study Investigators 2000; Reckless 2006) and may be as or more important than strict glycaemic control.

General dietary measures

All patients with vascular disease should be advised about general dietary measures such as reducing salt and saturated fat intake, although such dietary changes, in general, have only a limited effect (Cappuccio 2007). Excessive alcohol predisposes to stroke, especially cerebral haemorrhage, and individuals should be advised to keep their intake below the UK recommended weekly units – 21 for men and 14 for women (Reynolds et al. 2003).

Advice about weight reduction and regular exercise may also be appropriate although there is little objective data to support this scientifically (Hankey 2006).

Numerous studies support an association between homocysteine levels and vascular disease. Attempts to reduce homocysteine with folic acid and vitamin B have so far met with disappointing results although more trials are in progress (Goldstein & Rothwell 2007). Supplements of vitamin A, C and E after a vascular event have been conclusively shown to be of no benefit (Heart Protection Study Collaborative Group (HPSCG) 2002).

Box 13.2 illustrates a common scenario of lifestyle patterns and risk factors.

Carotid endarterectomy (CEA)

Development of CEA

Hippocrates was the first person to document that TIAs may herald stroke, around 2400 years ago. For centuries, however, it was thought that strokes were caused only by haemorrhagic or occlusive disease of the intracerebral arteries, rather than the carotid arteries. A better understanding of the aetiology of stroke was achieved by the early twentieth century, when it was realised that carotid artery atheroma could lead to stroke via a process of distal embolisation into the intracerebral arteries (Hunt 1914). By the 1950s, the operation of carotid endarterectomy (CEA) began to develop. The first surgical CEA was performed by DeBakey in 1953 (DeBakey 1975). A year later Eastcott et al (1954) published an account of the first UK operation for carotid occlusive disease performing an end-to-end anastomosis of the common and distal internal carotid arteries.

Following this early work, CEA rapidly became the standard operation for carotid occlusive disease. It was widely used from the 1960s to the mid 1980s in both Europe and, more commonly, in the US, as a means of reducing the risk of stroke in patients with either asymptomatic or symptomatic carotid stenosis. It is estimated that about one million people worldwide had the operation between 1974 and 1985 (Barnett 1990, 1991) with about 1500 procedures being performed annually in Great Britain and Ireland by 1984

Box 13.2 Vignette 2.

Mr Chambers is a 50-year-old man who runs a local restaurant and works long hours. He smokes around 15 cigarettes per day and is not overweight. He feels he is in good health, takes no regular medication and rarely consults a doctor.

Mr Chambers had a transient episode of left-sided weakness, lasting only moments, which he ignored and later described as a 'little wobble'. Two days later, however, whilst at work, he had a further and more severe episode of left-sided weakness, and fell to the floor. He also had slurred speech. A colleague phoned for an ambulance and he was admitted to the Emergency Department for further assessment. On arrival at hospital his symptoms had resolved.

Mr Chambers had urgent carotid imaging which showed a stenosis of the right internal carotid artery of 80–89%, and 15–49% of the left internal carotid artery. His cholesterol was raised at 5.7 mmol/l, and his blood pressure was 160/70.

Questions

(a) What is Mr Chambers' diagnosis and ABCD2 score?
(b) What would you do to expedite further investigations?
(c) What is Mr Chambers' risk of stroke over the next three years with best medical treatment, or with urgent carotid endarterectomy in addition to best medical treatment?
(d) In addition to prescribed medication and surgical treatment, what further action can Mr Chambers take to reduce his risk of stroke?

Answers

(a) Mr Chambers' ABCD2 score is 5 (age = 0; BP 1; clinical symptom 2; duration 2 (recurrent event); diabetes 0. The diagnosis on arrival at hospital is recurrent TIA, as this is the second event within two days.
(b) Mr Chambers needs to be admitted to hospital, preferably to the stroke unit, in order to facilitate urgent investigations and treatment.
(c) Mr Chambers' three-year risk of stroke on best medical treatment may be estimated at 16.8%. With carotid endarterectomy this is reduced to 2.8%, but with an additional 7.5% surgical stroke/death rate (figures from ECST). Local audit data for stroke/death after carotid endarterectomy may vary from this.
(d) Mr Chambers must stop smoking, and may need advice and support to achieve this. Although he is not overweight, his long working hours and the nature of his job may mean that he needs to undertake some dietary changes. He may also need to modify his busy lifestyle in order to reduce stress and to take exercise.

(Murie & Morris 1986). However, by the mid 1980s, concern was mounting about the safety of CEA, due to the small but important risk of perioperative stroke. It was not known whether this risk outweighed the effectiveness of the operation in reducing future stroke risk, an especially important concern since the operation was intended mainly to reduce stroke risk rather than to relieve ongoing symptoms. At this time, several published case series reported huge variations in mortality and morbidity (i.e. stroke) rates, with a ten-fold difference in morbidity between the lowest and highest (Table 13.2).

High mortality and morbidity rates were a particular concern because of the lack of knowledge about the natural history of the condition with best medical treatment. It is also likely that the published series would have underestimated the true mortality and morbidity rates, due to publication bias. There was also disagreement about the most appropriate indications for CEA, with only one-third of the patients in one series having had an operation which was fully agreed to have been appropriate, when reviewed retrospectively by an expert panel (Winslow et al. 1988).

Table 13.2 Case series of outcomes of carotid endarterectomy.

Study	Mortality (%)	Mortality and morbidity (%)
Easton and Sherman (1977)	Not stated	21.1
Muuronen (1984)	3.6	14.5
Brott and Thalinger (1984)	2.8	9.5
Slavish et al. (1984)	2.7	8.0
Zeiger et al. (1987)	1.4	2.1

As a result of these concerns and the emergence of more rigorous standards of audit and research required to support treatment decisions, there was a backlash against CEA during the 1980s and a decline in its use. Having increased from 15 000 procedures in 1971 to 107 000 in 1985, there was a dramatic decline to 83 000 CEAs in 1986 in the United States (Pokras & Dyken 1988). The need for robust evidence of the effectiveness of CEA in reducing stroke incidence in both symptomatic and asymptomatic people was identified, and several randomised trials were set up in the mid to late 1980s.

CEA trials

The first randomised trial of CEA was the Joint Study of Extracranial Arterial Occlusion (Fields et al. 1970). Although this demonstrated a reduction in long-term risk of stroke after surgery, this reduction was outweighed by the study's high perioperative mortality and morbidity rates. Subsequently, the effectiveness of CEA in patients with recent symptoms of carotid artery disease has been evaluated in two major trials: the European Carotid Surgery Trial Collaborative – ECST (1991, 1998) and the North American Symptomatic Carotid Endarterectomy Trial (1991). ECST had a sample of 3024 patients; NASCET, 2885. Both trials randomised patients with recent (less than six months) symptoms of TIA or recovered stroke to two treatment arms: either current best medical treatment (BMT) alone, or BMT plus CEA. These trials were very similar in their aims and design, but with two important differences. First, the method of measurement of carotid stenosis was not the same, making direct comparison of the trials potentially confusing, as the values for carotid stenosis derived are not equivalent. Secondly, ECST stratified patients according to whether they had mild (0–29%), moderate (30–69%) and severe (70–99%) internal carotid artery stenosis, while NASCET had only two categories: moderate (0–69%) and severe (70–99%).

Despite methodological differences between the trials, they reported closely comparable results. Both trials found that for patients with recent carotid territory symptoms (amaurosis fugax or TIA) and an ipsilateral internal carotid stenosis of 70–99%, surgery was more effective than best medical treatment alone in reducing the long-term stroke/surgical death rate. In ECST the perioperative stroke or death rate for surgery was 7.5%, with an additional 2.8%

risk of postoperative ipsilateral stroke in the following three years, compared to a three-year risk of 16.8% in the control group (European Carotid Surgery Trialists' Collaborative Group (ECSTCG) 1991). In NASCET, the perioperative stroke or death rate for severe stenosis was 5.8%, with an additional 3.2% risk of stroke in the next two years, compared with 26% in the control group. Many of the strokes which occurred in both treatment arms were ones from which patients recovered quickly and fully, but the incidence of fatal or disabling strokes was also reduced in the surgical group, from 13.1% to 2.5% (North American Symptomatic Carotid Endarterectomy Trial Collaborators (NASCETC) 1991). For patients in ECST with stenosis of less than 30%, surgery was found to be less effective than best medical treatment, while for the patients in both studies with 30–69% stenosis, the outcomes of either treatment were evenly balanced.

Further analysis of the final results of both trials has suggested some additional refinements. Factors which confer a higher likelihood of benefit from CEA include: male sex, age more than 75 years, higher degree of stenosis (90–99%), hemispheric symptoms (sensorimotor TIA) rather than ocular symptoms, contralateral occlusion, carotid plaque irregularity, and other co-morbidities (Naylor et al. 2003). While some of these factors (e.g. older age) also confer a higher surgical risk of stroke or death, this is outweighed by the higher baseline risk of stroke with medical treatment alone in these patients. CEA for symptomatic carotid stenosis has also been evaluated in a Cochrane database review (Cina et al. 2000).

Both ECST and NASCET were well-conducted large-scale, multicentre clinical trials, with full randomisation to CEA or control, although, due to the nature of surgical intervention, blinding of the clinical team and patient was not possible. However, an attempt was made to overcome any potential bias in reporting and evaluating outcome events (stroke or death) by using a blinded clinical audit committee to classify them. Patients were followed up for three years or more, and complications arising from the process of preoperative investigation, particularly angiography, were included when assessing perioperative mortality and morbidity. Acknowledged to be methodologically robust, these trials were not without critics. Criticisms of both trials concerned, firstly, variations in the treatment for the medical arm of the trial. For example, the dose of aspirin given as an antiplatelet agent was left to the discretion of the clinician. The management of other risk factors for stroke, such as hypertension, was also unspecified and likely to vary substantially. Secondly, although the trials rightly focused on the crucial and robust end-points of stroke/death versus stroke-free survival, there was no assessment of quality of life, anxiety and depression in either arm of the trials. These were important factors to consider for these patients, who were faced with the paradox of undergoing potentially harmful surgery with no guarantee of long-term benefit (Rose 1981).

Application of CEA trial findings

An important concern for the application of the results in present-day practice is that best medical treatment has changed since ECST and NASCET reported their early results. It has been mooted that, although it would be ethically impossible to re-run the trials now, the results might be very different in the light of advances in best medical treatment. In the surgical arm of the trial, too, there have been changes. Few patients today undergo the previously standard investigation of carotid angiography, which itself confers a small risk of stroke. Most institutions now use duplex scanning, supplemented with magnetic resonance angiogram, both of which are non-invasive and hence virtually risk-free investigations. The use of imaging techniques to detect carotid stenoses has been evaluated in a Health Technology Assessment review (Wardlaw et al. 2006). None of the imaging methods are completely reliable and most units use two imaging investigations before deciding if any stenosis is greater than 70% (ECST) or 50% (NASCET) and should thus be considered for surgery. Magnetic resonance angiography (MRA) with contrast enhancement seems the most accurate, non-invasive, imaging method although there is little to choose between ultrasound, computerised tomography angiography (CTA) and MRA. Local facilities and expertise are likely to be important factors and all centres assessing carotid stenosis should regularly audit their results. Inter-observer and intra-observer variability for the measurement of carotid stenosis is probably more important than differences in imaging technique (Young et al. 1996). The UK National Stroke Strategy Imaging Guide has emphasised the importance of swift access to imaging and of ensuring high-quality, audited services (Department of Health 2008), whichever modality is used.

There have also been treatment innovations, such as the use of locoregional anaesthesia (LA) rather than general anaesthesia (GA). A major Europe-wide randomised trial of general versus local anaesthetic for CEA has demonstrated no difference in rates of major complications (stroke or death) for local versus general anaesthesia for CEA (GALA Trial Collaborative Group 2008). Local anaesthesia normally means a reduced length of hospital stay (36–48 hours rather than 3–4 days for GA) and therefore confers greater cost-benefit and is usually more acceptable to patients. However, some patients do not wish to have the procedure under LA or cannot tolerate it.

All patients who have had a non-disabling carotid territory event should also have assessment and treatment of carotid stenosis by duplex scanning, followed by carotid endarterectomy if surgery is indicated. If surgery is necessary, it should take place as early as possible, since stroke risk is highest immediately after a carotid territory event. The UK National Stroke Strategy (Department of Health 2007) has stated that carotid endarterectomy should be performed within 48 hours in patients with ABCD2 scores of 4 or more, and within seven days in other patients, in order to have the maximum effect on reducing the number of patients who go on to have a completed stroke after a carotid territory event. The NICE guidelines (National Collaborating Centre for Chronic Conditions (NCCCC) 2008) take a more conservative approach and recommend carotid endarterectomy is performed within two weeks of the event.

People who have not had previous symptoms of TIA or stroke but who have a carotid stenosis are also at risk of subsequent stroke. The Asymptomatic Carotid Surgery Trial – ACST (N = 3120) studied the balance of risks for CEA in thee patients (Halliday et al. 2004). For patients with 70% ICA stenosis or greater, CEA conferred lower long-term (five-year) risk of stroke than conservative treatment. The net five-year risks of stroke or death were 6.4% in the CEA group (including a 3.1% perioperative stroke/death rate), versus 11.8% in the conservative group. This benefit was confined, however, only to patients under the age of 75 years. For older patients, the five-year risk of death from other causes outweighed any potential impact from CEA. The authors cautioned that the results should only be applied to institutions where the perioperative risks were similar to those in the study centres. A higher rate of perioperative stroke/death would negate any benefits from the long-term reduction of stroke risk.

The potential benefit of CEA for asymptomatic carotid disease is limited by the difficulty of identifying patients who have a severe carotid stenosis but who have not had any carotid territory symptoms. In the absence of symptoms, the condition can only be detected either incidentally, or by screening. The introduction of such a screening programme is, however, not currently widely advocated.

Audit of CEA

Continuing audit of individuals', centres' and collective results in CEA is necessary. In the UK, the audit data compiled for the National Vascular Database (Vascular Society 2004) show that outcomes for CEA are comparable to the ECST results. The combined immediate stroke and mortality rate is 2.7%, although not all surgeons and centres contribute their data, and in some cases, data entry is incomplete. In a systematic review of 51 studies of the outcome of CEA, the risk of stroke and death has been found to range from 2.3% to 7.7%, although the mean risk was 5.6%, consistent with ECST and NASCET (Rothwell et al. 1996). In the light of this variability, those performing CEA should advise patients of their own track record, based on rigorous clinical audit, rather than quoting data from the clinical trials. There are still commonly long delays before surgery takes place.

Carotid angioplasty and stenting

Carotid stenting is a less invasive procedure than carotid endarterectomy and rarely causes cranial nerve injury, which occurs in around 8% of patients having CEA (Sajid et al. 2007). However, it is unclear whether carotid stenting is a safe and durable alternative to endarterectomy. It is important to remember that the carotid stenosis leads to stroke as a result of distal embolisation, rather than from reduced blood flow. The aim in interventions for carotid stenosis is therefore to safely remove the source of emboli, rather than improving blood flow to the brain.

The CAVATAS (Carotid and Vertebral Artery Transluminal Angioplasty Study) compared surgery to angioplasty and found a similar complication rate (CAVATAS Investigators 2001). However, the risk of interventional stroke in both groups was 10% – an unacceptably high level. Other randomised trials have also failed to show a benefit from stenting (Furlan 2006), although some individual centres have demonstrated low complication rates for carotid stenting especially if emboli protection devices are used to prevent embolic debris passing into the brain.

Meta-analysis of all carotid stenting trials shows it to be an unproven treatment: it may be appropriate for some patients who have a high risk of surgical complications. More trials are required to address the complications of the procedure and its long-term durability. This procedure should currently not be performed outside a clinical trial. Angioplasty for vertebral stenosis also remains unproven (Coward et al. 2007).

Public awareness and access to services

Many factors contribute to delays in seeking treatment for stroke and TIA, but the principal factor is believed to be a lack of public knowledge regarding symptoms and the need for a rapid response (Becker et al. 2001; Evenson et al. 2001; Yoon & Byles 2002). Achieving rapid patient presentation relies mainly on the public's ability to identify the symptoms of stroke and TIA and to contact the emergency medical services without delay (Ferro et al. 1994; Harraf et al. 2002). Patients need to appreciate the urgency with which they should seek help and the seriousness of their symptoms. The UK Stroke Association has highlighted this issue with its FAST (Face, Arm, Speech, Time to call) campaign, as has the US Brain Attack Coalition and the National Stroke Foundation in Australia.

Those with lower levels of education (Muller-Nordhorn et al. 2006; Yoon et al. 2001) have consistently shown poor levels of stroke knowledge. Other factors that have been shown to affect knowledge are age and ethnicity. Older age groups have poor knowledge of the risk factors (Pancioli et al. 1998) and symptoms of stroke and TIA (Kothari et al. 1997). A lack of knowledge among those who have already suffered a stroke is especially worrying. Why these groups have poorer levels of health knowledge is not fully understood, and warrants further attention, particularly as these groups are at higher risk of stroke than the general population.

Many people do not take early TIA or stroke symptoms seriously and wait for their symptoms to abate rather than seeking immediate medical advice (Williams et al. 1997). Most do not realise that they are experiencing stroke symptoms (Parahoo et al. 2003). Around 50% of the public state that they would contact the emergency medical services when stroke is suspected (Parahoo et al. 2003). However, as few as 18% of the public actually call the emergency services in this situation (Carroll et al. 2004).

The most effective way to increase knowledge about stroke has been in stroke and TIA risk factor screening, educational programmes and first aid training (DeLemos et al. 2003; Handschu et al. 2006; Stern et al. 1999). While it is appreciated that increasing knowledge does not automatically lead to a change in behaviour, an increase in knowledge may facilitate behaviour change (Rosenstock 2005).

Raising public awareness and educational interventions should be targeted in particular towards those at risk of stroke or TIA, that is, older members of the general population, ethnic minority groups and those with lower levels of education. These groups generally have lower levels of knowledge, and yet stroke disproportionately impacts upon these groups (Bonita et al. 1997; Sacco et al. 1989).

Delays in accessing treatment may also arise within the health care system itself. There may be delays in primary care, for example if the health professional who assesses the patient does not diagnose a TIA, or refer the patient appropriately. Furthermore, there may be problems at the point of referral from primary to secondary care, or within secondary care itself, if the patient is referred swiftly but investigation and treatment is delayed. Although referral for investigation of carotid stenosis should be treated as an urgent matter, it may still take weeks – if not months – for the patient to eventually have surgery after the initial presentation of symptoms (National Audit Office (NAO) 2005). The longer the delay, the more chance there is for a major stroke to occur in the interim. As a result of these factors, the practical difficulties of identifying patients with TIA, and investigating and treating them swiftly, are not proving easy to resolve. Secondary prevention can undoubtedly be effective, but it is useless if patients cannot or do not access it. Since the risk of subsequent stroke is highest in the first few days and weeks after the onset of TIA or stroke symptoms, the potential benefit of CEA reduces the longer the patient survives event-free. So if CEA is delayed, the risks of the procedure may outweigh the benefits.

Even in those patients who do access the appropriate services after TIA or stroke, patients' understanding of the importance of symptoms, acute treatment and the effectiveness of secondary prevention falls far short of what is required to ensure optimal uptake of specialist stroke care. Primary and secondary care need to work together with specific written and verbal individualised instructions given to every patient (Maasland et al. 2007).

Secondary prevention of stroke in less common aetiologies and patient groups

Intracerebral haemorrhage

The prevention of further bleeds after an intracerebral haemorrhage needs to initially consider the aetiology. The common causes are hypertension, often due to rupture of microaneurysms, cerebral amyloid in blood vessels (increasingly recognised in the elderly population), alcohol excess, arteriovenous malformations, drug abuse, for example amphetamines, proprietary drugs such as warfarin and thrombolytic agents, vasculitis, bleeding into tumours, haematological disorders, Moyamoya disease or cerebral vein thrombosis (The European Stroke Initiative Writing Committee 2006). The treatment clearly needs to be directed at the primary cause. Treatment of blood pressure remains the mainstay, with advice about alcohol intake as appropriate.

Subarachnoid haemorrhage

Subarachnoid haemorrhage (SAH) is usually due to aneurysm rupture, most of which occur round the circle of Willis. Rarer causes of subarachnoid haemorrhage include idiopathic, perimesencephalic haemorrhage and arteriovenous malformations. Aneurysms which have ruptured have a high mortality and re-bleeding rate; management has changed dramatically in the past five years and coiling rather than surgery is now the treatment of choice. The complication rates for coiling are much less than for surgery; furthermore the risk of late epilepsy is much less than after surgery (Molyneux et al. 2002). However, the need for retreatment of coiled patients is higher (Campi et al. 2007). Calcium antagonists (usually nimodipine) should be started early to reduce the risk of delayed ischaemia after SAH (Rinkel et al. 2005).

Stroke in those aged less than 45 years

Less than 5% of all strokes occur in those under 45 years. Young stroke is rarely due to atheromatous disease (Bogousslavsky & Caplan 2001). All such cases should be assessed by those with expertise in this age group, not only to identify the rare aetiologies but also to prevent the over-diagnosis of stroke or TIA which will otherwise have a devastating effect on the individual's future health perception and outcome (Martin et al. 1997).

The most common causes of TIA or stroke at young age are cardioembolic disease or cervical artery dissection: each accounts for about 25% of all young strokes. A further 25% are due to the numerous other rare causes of stroke (Nedeltchev et al. 2005), but the final quarter are idiopathic.

Young women and pregnancy

Oral contraceptives should be avoided in any women with a history of stroke. Young women who have had a stroke and then become pregnant, however, seem to have a low risk of recurrence during this or any subsequent pregnancy. The risk is higher in those with stroke of definite cause and in the puerperium but even here the absolute risk is small (Lamy et al. 2000). A history of stroke should not therefore be a bar to subsequent pregnancies.

Cerebral venous thrombosis

This has similar symptoms to ischaemic stroke, except that epilepsy (both focal and generalised) tends to occur in up to 50% of patients with cerebral venous thrombosis and may precede other stroke symptoms (epilepsy in arterial stroke occurs in less than 5%). The causes are different to arterial stroke and include haematological or prothrombotic conditions, infection or inflammatory disease, tumours, the puerperium, the Pill and head injury. Anticoagulation, usually short term, is the treatment of choice to prevent progression (Stam 2005) and seems to be beneficial even in those with haemorrhagic infarcts.

Conclusion

There are many effective measures which people can take to reduce their risk of stroke, whether via primary or secondary prevention. However, the processes of enabling people firstly to identify themselves as being at risk of cerebrovascular disease, and then to access the help they need in order to reduce their stroke risk, are far from straightforward. The significance of TIA in identifying those at highest risk of further cerebrovascular events is not fully understood, but services need to be organised to deal promptly with those TIAs which suggest a high risk of stroke.

There is strong evidence that timely investigation and implementation of the interventions described above will substantially reduce the individual's risk of first or subsequent stroke. It is, however, important to remember that patients who have had a TIA, or who have apparently fully recovered from a stroke, have other health care needs apart from secondary prevention. TIA or stroke itself generates anxiety and affects the individual's health perception and status. A TIA is a potentially distressing syndrome in its own right, not just because of its implication that the patient is at high risk of having a further stroke.

References

Aguilar, M, & Hart, R, 2005, Antiplatelet therapy for preventing stroke in patients with non-valvular atrial fibrillation and no previous history of stroke or transient ischemic attacks, *Cochrane Database of Systematic Reviews* no. 4, CD001925.

Albers, GW, Caplan, LR, Easton, JD, Fayad, PB, Mohr, JP et al., 2002, Transient ischemic attack–proposal for a new definition, *New England Journal of Medicine*, vol. 347, no. 21, pp. 1713–1716.

Amarenco, P, Bogousslavsky, J, Callahan, A, III, Goldstein, LB, Hennerici, M et al., 2006, High-dose atorvastatin after stroke or transient ischemic attack, *New England Journal of Medicine*, vol. 355, no. 6, pp. 549–559.

Antiplatelet Trialists' Collaboration, 1994, Collaborative overview of randomised trials of antiplatelet therapy – I: Prevention of death, myocardial infarction, and stroke by prolonged antiplatelet therapy in various categories of patients, *British Medical Journal*, vol. 308, no. 6921, pp. 81–106.

Antithrombotic Trialists' Collaboration, 2002, Collaborative meta-analysis of randomised trials of antiplatelet therapy for prevention of death, myocardial infarction and stroke in high risk patients, *British Medical Journal*, vol. 324, no. 7329, pp. 71–86.

APASS Investigators, 2004, Antiphospholipid antibodies and subsequent thrombo-occlusive events in patients with ischemic stroke, *Journal of the American Medical Association*, vol. 291, pp. 576–584.

Barnett, HJ, 1990, Symptomatic carotid endarterectomy trials, *Stroke*, vol. 21, no. 11 Suppl, pp. 1112–1115.

Barnett, HJM, 1991, Evaluating methods for prevention in stroke, *Annals of the Royal College of Physicians and Surgeons of Canada*, vol. 24, pp. 33–42.

Becker, K, Fruin, M, Gooding, T, Tirschwell, D, Love, P et al., 2001, Community-based education improves stroke knowledge, *Cerebrovascular Diseases*, vol. 11, no. 1, pp. 34–43.

Bogousslavsky, J, & Caplan, LR, 2001, *Uncommon Causes of Stroke*, Cambridge University Press, Cambridge.

Bonita, R, Broad, JB, & Beaglehole, R, 1997, Ethnic differences in stroke incidence and case fatality in Auckland, New Zealand, *Stroke*, vol. 28, no. 4, pp. 758–761.

Boushey, CJ, Beresford, SA, Omenn, GS, & Motulsky, AG, 1995, A quantitative assessment of plasma homocysteine as a risk factor for vascular disease. Probable benefits of increasing folic acid intakes, *Journal of the American Medical Association*, vol. 274, no. 13, pp. 1049–1057.

Brass, LM, Krumholz, HM, Scinto, JD, Mathur, D, & Radford, M, 1998, Warfarin use following ischemic stroke among Medicare patients with atrial fibrillation, *Archives of Internal Medicine*, vol. 158, no. 19, pp. 2093–2100.

Brott, T, & Thalinger, K, 1984, The practice of carotid endarterectomy in a large metropolitan area, *Stroke*, vol. 15, no. 6, pp. 950–955.

Brott, T, Tomsick, T, Feinberg, W, Johnson, C, Biller, J et al., 1994, Baseline silent cerebral infarction in the Asymptomatic Carotid Atherosclerosis Study, *Stroke*, vol. 25, no. 6, pp. 1122–1129.

Bucher, HC, Griffith, LE, & Guyatt, GH, 1998, Effect of HMGcoA reductase inhibitors on stroke. A meta-analysis of randomized, controlled trials, *Annals of Internal Medicine*, vol. 128, no. 2, pp. 89–95.

Campi, A, Ramzi, N, Molyneux, AJ, Summers, PE, Kerr, RS et al., 2007, Retreatment of ruptured cerebral aneurysms in patients randomized by coiling or clipping in the International Subarachnoid Aneurysm Trial (ISAT), *Stroke*, vol. 38, no. 5, pp. 1538–1544.

Cappuccio, FP, 2007, Salt and cardiovascular disease, *British Medical Journal*, vol. 334, no. 7599, pp. 859–860.

CAPRIE Steering Committee, 1996, A randomised, blinded, trial of clopidogrel versus aspirin in patients at risk of ischaemic events (CAPRIE). CAPRIE Steering Committee, *Lancet*, vol. 348, no. 9038, pp. 1329–1339.

Carroll, C, Hobart, J, Fox, C, Teare, L, & Gibson, J, 2004, Stroke in Devon: knowledge was good, but action was poor, *Journal of Neurology, Neurosurgery and Psychiatry*, vol. 75, no. 4, pp. 567–571.

CAVATAS Investigators, 2001, Endovascular versus surgical treatment in patients with carotid stenosis in the Carotid and Vertebral Artery Transluminal Angioplasty Study (CAVATAS): a randomised trial, *Lancet*, vol. 357, no. 9270, pp. 1729–1737.

Chan, FK, Ching, JY, Hung, LC, Wong, VW, Leung, VK et al., 2005, Clopidogrel versus aspirin and esomeprazole to prevent recurrent ulcer bleeding, *New England Journal of Medicine*, vol. 352, no. 3, pp. 238–244.

Chimowitz, MI, Lynn, MJ, Howlett-Smith, H, Stern, BJ, Hertzberg, VS et al., 2005, Comparison of warfarin and aspirin for symptomatic intracranial arterial stenosis, *New England Journal of Medicine*, vol. 352, no. 13, pp. 1305–1316.

Cholesterol Treatment Trialists' Collaborators (CTTC), 2005, Efficacy and safety of cholesterol-lowering treatment: prospective meta-analysis of data from 90 056 participants in 14 randomised trials of statins, *Lancet*, vol. 366, no. 9493, pp. 1267–1278.

Cina, CS, Clase, CM, & Haynes, RB, 2000, Carotid endarterectomy for symptomatic carotid stenosis, *Cochrane Database of Systematic Reviews* no. 2, CD001081.

Clark, TG, Murphy, MF, & Rothwell, PM, 2003, Long term risks of stroke, myocardial infarction, and vascular death in 'low risk' patients with a non-recent transient ischaemic attack, *Journal of Neurology Neurosurgery and Psychiatry*, vol. 74, no. 5, pp. 577–580.

Collins, R, Peto, R, MacMahon, S, Hebert, P, Fiebach, NH et al., 1990, Blood pressure, stroke, and coronary heart disease. Part 2, Short-term reductions in blood pressure: overview of randomised drug trials in their epidemiological context, *Lancet*, vol. 335, no. 8693, pp. 827–838.

Costa, J, Borges, M, David, C, & Vaz, CA, 2006, Efficacy of lipid lowering drug treatment for diabetic and non-diabetic patients: meta-analysis of randomised controlled trials, *British Medical Journal*, vol. 332, no. 7550, pp. 1115–1124.

Coull, AJ, Lovett, JK, & Rothwell, PM, 2004, Population based study of early risk of stroke after transient ischaemic attack or minor stroke: implications for public education and organisation of services, *British Medical Journal*, vol. 328, no. 7435, pp. 326–328.

Coward, LJ, McCabe, DJ, Ederle, J, Featherstone, RL, Clifton, A et al., 2007, Long-term outcome after angioplasty and stenting for symptomatic vertebral artery stenosis compared with medical treatment in the Carotid And Vertebral Artery Transluminal Angioplasty Study (CAVATAS): a randomized trial, *Stroke*, vol. 38, no. 5, pp. 1526–1530.

de Lusignan, S, Belsey, J, Hague, N, Dhoul, N, & van Vlymen J, 2006, Audit-based education to reduce suboptimal management of cholesterol in primary care: a before and after study, *Journal of Public Health*, vol. 28, no. 4, pp. 361–369.

DeBakey, ME, 1975, Successful carotid endarterectomy for cerebrovascular insufficiency. Nineteen-year follow-up, *Journal of the American Medical Association*, vol. 233, no. 10, pp. 1083–1085.

DeLemos, CD, Atkinson, RP, Croopnick, SL, Wentworth, DA, & Akins, PT, 2003, How effective are 'community' stroke screening programs at improving stroke knowledge and prevention practices? Results of a 3-month follow-up study, *Stroke*, vol. 34, no. 12, p. e247–e249.

Dennis, MS, Bamford, JM, Sandercock, PA, & Warlow, CP, 1989, Incidence of transient ischemic attacks in Oxfordshire, England, *Stroke*, vol. 20, no. 3, pp. 333–339.

Department of Health, 2001, *The National Service Framework for Older People*, Department of Health, London.

Department of Health, 2007, *National Stroke Strategy*, Department of Health, London.

Department of Health, 2008, *Implementing the National Stroke Strategy – An Imaging Guide*, Department of Health, London.

Diabetes Control and Complications Trial Research Group (DCCTRG), 1993, The effect of intensive treatment of diabetes on the development and progression of long term complications in insulin dependent diabetes mellitus, *New England Journal of Medicine*, vol. 329, pp. 977–986.

Diener, HC, Cunha, L, Forbes, C, Sivenius, J, Smets, P et al., 1996, European Stroke Prevention Study. 2. Dipyridamole and acetylsalicylic acid in the secondary prevention of stroke, *Journal of Neurological Sciences*, vol. 143, no. 1–2, pp. 1–13.

Diener, HC, Bogousslavsky, J, Brass, LM, Cimminiello, C, Csiba, L et al., 2004, Aspirin and clopidogrel compared with clopidogrel alone after recent ischaemic stroke or transient ischaemic attack in high-risk patients (MATCH): randomised, double-blind, placebo-controlled trial, *Lancet*, vol. 364, no. 9431, pp. 331–337.

Donnan, GA, You, R, Thrift, A, & McNeil, JJ, 1993, Smoking as a risk factor for stroke, *Cerebrovascular Diseases*, vol. 3, pp. 129–138.

Drugs and Therapeutics Bulletin, 2004, Ezetimibe – a new cholesterol-lowering drug, *Drugs and Therapeutics Bulletin 2004*, vol. 42, Sept., pp. 65–67.

Drugs and Therapeutics Bulletin, 2007, Which statin, what dose? *Drugs and Therapeutics Bulletin 2007*, vol. 45, May, pp. 33–37.

EAFT (European Atrial Fibrillation Trial) Study Group, 1993, Secondary prevention in non-rheumatic atrial fibrillation after transient ischaemic attack or minor stroke, *Lancet*, vol. 342, pp. 1255–1262.

Eastcott, HH, Pickering, GW, & Rob CG, 1954, Reconstruction of internal carotid artery in a patient with intermittent attacks of hemiplegia, *Lancet*, vol. 267, no. 6846, pp. 994–996.

Easton, JD, & Sherman, DG, 1977, Stroke and mortality rate in carotid endarterectomy: 228 consecutive operations, *Stroke*, vol. 8, no. 5, pp. 565–568.

Eliasziw, M, Kennedy, J, Hill, MD, Buchan, AM, & Barnett, HJ, 2004, Early risk of stroke after a transient ischemic attack in patients with internal carotid artery disease, *Canadian Medical Association Journal*, vol. 170, no. 7, pp. 1105–1109.

European Carotid Surgery Trialists' Collaborative Group (ECSTCG), 1991, MRC European Carotid Surgery Trial: interim results for symptomatic patients with severe (70–99%) or with mild (0–29%) carotid stenosis. European Carotid Surgery Trialists' Collaborative Group, *Lancet*, vol. 337, no. 8752, pp. 1235–1243.

European Carotid Surgery Trialists' Collaborative Group (ECSTCG), 1998, Randomised trial of endarterectomy for recently symptomatic carotid stenosis: final results of the MRC European Carotid Surgery Trial (ECST), *Lancet*, vol. 351, no. 9113, pp. 1379–1387.

Evenson, KR, Rosamond, WD, & Morris, DL, 2001, Prehospital and in-hospital delays in acute stroke care, *Neuroepidemiology*, vol. 20, no. 2, pp. 65–76.

Fairhead, JF, & Rothwell, PM, 2006, Underinvestigation and undertreatment of carotid disease in elderly patients with transient ischaemic attack and stroke: comparative population based study, *British Medical Journal*, vol. 333, no. 7567, pp. 525–527.

Ferro, JM, Melo, TP, Oliveira, V, Crespo, M, Canhao, P et al., 1994, An analysis of the admission delay of acute stroke, *Cerebrovascular Diseases*, vol. 4, pp. 72–75.

Fields, WS, Maslenikov, V, Meyer, JS, Hass, WK, Remington, RD et al., 1970, Joint study of extracranial arterial occlusion. V. Progress report of prognosis following surgery or nonsurgical treatment for transient cerebral ischemic attacks and cervical carotid artery lesions, *Journal of the American Medical Association*, vol. 211, no. 12, pp. 1993–2003.

Furlan, AJ, 2006, Carotid-artery stenting – case open or closed? *New England Journal of Medicine*, vol. 355, no. 16, pp. 1726–1729.

GALA Trial Collaborative Group, 2008, General anaesthesia versus local anaesthesia for carotid surgery (GALA): a multicentre, randomised controlled trial, *Lancet*, vol. 372, no. 9656, pp. 2132–2142.

Goldstein, LB, & Rothwell, PM, 2007, Primary prevention and health services delivery, *Stroke*, vol. 38, no. 2, pp. 222–224.

Gorelick, PB, 2007, Combining aspirin with oral anticoagulant therapy: is this a safe and effective practice in patients with atrial fibrillation? *Stroke*, vol. 38, no. 5, pp. 1652–1654.

Hacke, W, Kaste, M, Bluhmki, E, Brozman, M, Davalos, A et al., 2008, Thrombolysis with alteplase 3 to 4.5 hours after acute ischemic stroke, *New England Journal of Medicine*, vol. 359, pp. 1317–1329.

Halliday, A, Mansfield, A, Marro, J, Peto, C, Peto, R et al., 2004, Prevention of disabling and fatal strokes by successful carotid endarterectomy in patients without recent neurological symptoms: randomised controlled trial, *Lancet*, vol. 363, no. 9420, pp. 1491–1502.

Handschu, R, Reitmayer, M, Raschick, M, Erbguth, F, Neundorfer, B et al., 2006, First aid in acute stroke : introducing a concept of first action to laypersons, *Journal of Neurology*, vol. 253, no. 10, pp. 1342–1346.

Hankey, GJ, 2006, *Stroke Treatment and Prevention*, Cambridge University Press, Cambridge.

Hankey, GJ, Slattery, JM, & Warlow, CP, 1991, The prognosis of hospital-referred transient ischaemic attacks, *Journal of Neurology, Neurosurgery and Psychiatry*, vol. 54, no. 9, pp. 793–802.

Harraf, F, Sharma, AK, Brown, MM, Lees, KR, Vass, RI et al., 2002, A multicentre observational study of presentation and early assessment of acute stroke, *British Medical Journal*, vol. 325, no. 7354, p. 17.

Hart, RG, & Halperin, JL, 2001, Atrial fibrillation and stroke: concepts and controversies, *Stroke*, vol. 32, no. 3, pp. 803–808.

Heart Outcomes Prevention Evaluation (HOPE) Study Investigators, 2000, Effects of ramipril on cardiovascular and microvascular outcomes in people with diabetes mellitus: results of the HOPE study and MICRO-HOPE substudy, *Lancet*, vol. 355, p. 253.

Heart Protection Study Collaborative Group (HPSCG), 2002, MRC/BHF Heart Protection Study of cholesterol lowering with simvastatin in 20 536 high-risk individuals: a randomised placebo-controlled trial, *Lancet*, vol. 360, no. 9326, pp. 7–22.

Heart Protection Study Collaborative Group (HPSCG), 2004, Effects of cholesterol-lowering with simvastatin on stroke and other major vascular events in 20 536 people with cerebrovascular disease or other high risk conditions, *Lancet*, vol. 363, pp. 757–767.

Heart Protection Study Collaborative Group (HPSCG), 2006, Lifetime cost effectiveness of simvastatin in a range of risk groups and age groups derived from a randomised trial of 20,536 people, *British Medical Journal*, vol. 333, p. 1145.

Hooper, L, Bartlett, C, Davey, SG, & Ebrahim, S, 2004, Advice to reduce dietary salt for prevention of cardiovascular disease, *Cochrane Database of Systematic Reviews*, no. 1, CD003656.

Howard, G, McClure, LA, Krakauer, JW, & Coffey, CS, 2007, Stroke and the statistics of the aspirin/clopidogrel secondary prevention trials, *Current Opinion in Neurology*, vol. 20, no. 1, pp. 71–77.

Hughes, JR, Stead, LF, & Lancaster, T, 2003, Antidepressants for smoking cessation, *Cochrane Database of Systematic Reviews* no. 2, CD000031.

Hunt, JR, 1914, The role of the carotid arteries in the causation of vascular lesions of the brain, with remarks on certain special features of the symptomatology, *American Journal of the Medical Sciences*, vol. 147, pp. 704–713.

Intercollegiate Stroke Working Party, 2008, *National Sentinel Stroke Audit. Phase 1 Organisational audit 2008*. Report for England, Wales and Northern Ireland, Royal College of Physicians, London.

Johnsen, SP, Overvad, K, Stripp, C, Tjonneland, A, Husted, SE et al., 2003, Intake of fruit and vegetables and the risk of ischemic stroke in a cohort of Danish men and women, *American Journal of Clinical Nutrition*, vol. 78, no. 1, pp. 57–64.

Johnston, SC, Gress, DR, Browner, WS, & Sidney, S, 2000, Short-term prognosis after emergency department diagnosis of TIA, *Journal of the American Medical Association*, vol. 284, no. 22, pp. 2901–2906.

Johnston, SC, Fayad, PB, Gorelick, PB, Hanley, DF, Shwayder, P et al., 2003, Prevalence and knowledge of transient ischemic attack among US adults, *Neurology*, vol. 60, no. 9, pp. 1429–1434.

Johnston, SC, Rothwell, PM, Nguyen-Huynh, MN, Giles, MF, Elkins, JS et al., 2007, Validation and refinement of scores to predict very early stroke risk after transient ischaemic attack, *Lancet*, vol. 369, no. 9558, pp. 283–292.

Joseph, LN, Babikian, VL, Allen, NC, & Winter, MR, 1999, Risk factor modification in stroke prevention: the experience of a stroke clinic, *Stroke*, vol. 30, no. 1, pp. 16–20.

Jurgens, G, Graudal, NA, 2004, Effects of low sodium diet versus high sodium diet on blood pressure, renin, aldosterone, catecholamines, cholesterols, and triglyceride, *Cochrane Database of Systematic Reviews* no. 1, CD004022.

Kappelle, LJ, Koudstaal, PJ, van Gijn, J, Ramos, LM, & Keunen, JE, 1988, Carotid angiography in patients with lacunar infarction. A prospective study, *Stroke*, vol. 19, no. 9, pp. 1093–1096.

Kennedy, J, Hill, MD, Eliasziw, M, Buchan, AM, & Barnett, HJ, 2002, Short-term prognosis following acute cerebral ischaemia, *Stroke*, vol. 33, p. 382.

Kothari, R, Sauerbeck, L, Jauch, E, Broderick, J, Brott, T et al., 1997, Patients' awareness of stroke signs, symptoms, and risk factors, *Stroke*, vol. 28, no. 10, pp. 1871–1875.

Koudstaal, PJ, Gerritsma, JG, & van Gijn J, 1989, Clinical disagreement on the diagnosis of transient ischemic attack: is the patient or the doctor to blame? *Stroke*, vol. 20, no. 2, pp. 300–301.

Kraaijeveld, CL, van Gijn J, Schouten, HJ, & Staal, A, 1984, Interobserver agreement for the diagnosis of transient ischemic attacks, *Stroke*, vol. 15, no. 4, pp. 723–725.

Kumar, S, & Caplan, LR, 2007, Why identification of stroke syndromes is still important, *Current Opinion in Neurology*, vol. 20, no. 1, pp. 78–82.

Kurth, T, Gaziano, JM, Berger, K, Kase, CS, Rexrode, KM et al., 2002, Body mass index and the risk of stroke in men, *Archives of Internal Medicine*, vol. 162, no. 22, pp. 2557–2562.

Lamy, C, Hamon, JB, Coste, J, & Mas, JL, 2000, Ischemic stroke in young women: risk of recurrence during subsequent pregnancies. French Study Group on Stroke in Pregnancy, *Neurology*, vol. 55, no. 2, pp. 269–274.

Lawes, CM, Bennett, DA, Feigin, VL, & Rodgers, A, 2004, Blood pressure and stroke: an overview of published reviews, *Stroke*, vol. 35, no. 3, pp. 776–785.

Lee, CD, Folsom, AR & Blair, SN, 2003, Physical activity and stroke risk. A meta analysis, *Stroke*, vol. 34, pp. 2475–2481.

Levy, DE, 1988, How transient are transient ischemic attacks? *Neurology*, vol. 38, no. 5, pp. 674–677.

Lovett, JK, Coull, AJ, & Rothwell, PM, 2004, Early risk of recurrence by subtype of ischemic stroke in population-based incidence studies, *Neurology*, vol. 62, no. 4, pp. 569–573.

Maasland, L, Koudstaal, PJ, Habbema, JD, & Dippel, DW, 2007, Knowledge and understanding of disease process, risk factors and treatment modalities in patients with a recent TIA or minor ischemic stroke, *Cerebrovascular Diseases*, vol. 23, no. 5–6, pp. 435–440.

Mant, J, Wade, D, & Winner, S, 2004, Health care needs assessment: stroke, in *Health Care Needs Assessment: The Epidemiologically Based Needs Assessment Reviews*, 2nd edn, A Stevens et al., eds., Radcliffe Medical Press, Oxford.

Mant, J, Hobbs, FD, Fletcher, K, Roalfe, A, Fitzmaurice, D et al., 2007, Warfarin versus aspirin for stroke prevention in an elderly community population with atrial fibrillation (the Birmingham Atrial Fibrillation Treatment of the Aged Study, BAFTA): a randomised controlled trial, *Lancet*, vol. 370, no. 9586, pp. 493–503.

Markus, HS, Droste, DW, Kaps, M, Larrue, V, Lees, KR et al., 2005, Dual antiplatelet therapy with clopidogrel and aspirin in symptomatic carotid stenosis evaluated using doppler embolic signal detection: the Clopidogrel and Aspirin for Reduction of Emboli in Symptomatic Carotid Stenosis (CARESS) trial, *Circulation*, vol. 111, no. 17, pp. 2233–2240.

Martin, PJ, Young, G, Enevoldson, TP, & Humphrey, PR, 1997, Overdiagnosis of TIA and minor stroke: experience at a regional neurovascular clinic, *Quarterly Journal of Medicine*, vol. 90, no. 12, pp. 759–763.

Molyneux, A, Kerr, R, Stratton, I, Sanderock, P, Clarke, M et al., 2002, International Subarachnoid Aneurysm Trial (ISAT) of neurosurgical clipping versus endovascular coiling in 2143 patients with ruptured intracranial aneurysms: a randomised trial, *Lancet*, vol. 360, no. 9342, pp. 1267–1274.

Mouradian, MS, Majumdar, SR, Senthilselvan, A, Khan, K, & Shuaib, A, 2002, How well are hypertension, hyperlipidemia, diabetes, and smoking managed after a stroke or transient ischemic attack? *Stroke*, vol. 33, no. 6, pp. 1656–1659.

Muir, KW, 2004, Secondary prevention for stroke and transient ischaemic attacks, *British Medical Journal*, vol. 328, no. 7435, pp. 297–298.

Muller-Nordhorn, J, Nolte, CH, Rossnagel, K, Jungehulsing, GJ, Reich, A et al., 2006, Knowledge about risk factors for stroke: a population-based survey with 28,090 participants, *Stroke*, vol. 37, no. 4, pp. 946–950.

Murie, JA, & Morris, PJ, 1986, Carotid endarterectomy in Great Britain and Ireland, *British Journal of Surgery*, vol. 73, no. 11, pp. 867–870.

Muuronen, A, 1984, Outcome of surgical treatment of 110 patients with transient ischemic attack, *Stroke*, vol. 15, no. 6, pp. 959–964.

National Audit Office (NAO), 2005, *Reducing Brain Damage – Faster Access to Better Stroke Care*, The Stationery Office, London.

National Collaborating Centre for Chronic Conditions (NCCCC), 2008, *Stroke: National Clinical Guideline for Diagnosis and Initial Management of Acute Stroke And Transient Ischaemic Attack (TIA)*, Royal College of Physicians (RCP), London.

National Institute for Health and Clinical Excellence (NICE), 2005, *Technological Appraisal 90 Clopidogrel and Dipyridamole for the Prevention Of Artherosclerotic Events*, NICE, London.

National Institute for Health and Clinical Excellence (NICE), 2008, *Stroke: The Diagnosis and Acute Management of Stroke and Transient Ischaemic Attacks*, NICE, London.

National Institutes of Health, 1975, A classification and outline of cerebrovascular diseases, *Stroke*, vol. 6, pp. 564–616.

Naylor, AR, Rothwell, PM, & Bell, PR, 2003, Overview of the principal results and secondary analyses from the European and North American randomised trials of endarterectomy for symptomatic carotid stenosis, *European Journal of Vascular and Endovascular Surgery*, vol. 26, no. 2, pp. 115–129.

Nedeltchev, K, der Maur, TA, Georgiadis, D, Arnold, M, Caso, V et al., 2005, Ischaemic stroke in young adults: predictors of outcome and recurrence, *Journal of Neurology, Neurosurgery and Psychiatry*, vol. 76, no. 2, pp. 191–195.

North American Symptomatic Carotid Endarterectomy Trial Collaborators (NASCETC), 1991, Beneficial effect of carotid endarterectomy in symptomatic patients with high-grade stenosis, *New England Journal of Medicine*, vol. 325, pp. 445–453.

Pancioli, AM, Broderick, J, Kothari, R, Brott, T, Tuchfarber, A et al., 1998, Public perception of stroke warning signs and knowledge of potential risk factors, *Journal of the American Medical Association*, vol. 279, no. 16, pp. 1288–1292.

Parahoo, K, Thompson, K, Cooper, M, Stringer, M, Ennis, E et al., 2003, Stroke: awareness of the signs, symptoms and risk factors – a population-based survey, *Cerebrovascular Diseases*, vol. 16, no. 2, pp. 134–140.

Perry, IJ, Refsum, H, Morris, RW, Ebrahim, SB, Ueland, PM et al., 1995, Prospective study of serum total homocysteine concentration and risk of stroke in middle-aged British men, *Lancet*, vol. 346, no. 8987, pp. 1395–1398.

Peto, R, Lopez, AD, Boreham, J, Thun, M, & Heath Jr, C, 1994, *Mortality from Smoking in Developed in Developed Countries 1950–2000: Indirect Estimates from National Vital Statistics*, Oxford University Press, Oxford.

Pokras, R, & Dyken, ML, 1988, Dramatic changes in the performance of endarterectomy for diseases of the extracranial arteries of the head, *Stroke*, vol. 19, no. 10, pp. 1289–1290.

Powers, WJ, 2001, Oral anticoagulant therapy for the prevention of stroke, *New England Journal of Medicine*, vol. 345, no. 20, pp. 1493–1495.

PROGRESS Collaborative Group, 2001, Randomised trial of a perindopril-based blood pressure lowering regimen among 6105 individuals with previous stroke or transient ischaemic attack, *Lancet*, vol. 358, pp. 1033–1041.

Rashid, P, Leonardi-Bee, J, & Bath, P, 2003, Blood pressure reduction and secondary prevention of stroke and other vascular events: a systematic review, *Stroke*, vol. 34, no. 11, pp. 2741–2748.

Reckless, JP, 2006, Diabetes and lipid lowering: where are we? *British Medical Journal*, vol. 332, no. 7550, pp. 1103–1104.

Reynolds, K, Lewis, B, Nolen, JD, Kinney, GL, Sathya, B et al., 2003, Alcohol consumption and risk of stroke: a meta-analysis, *Journal of the American Medical Association*, vol. 289, no. 5, pp. 579–588.

Rice, VH, & Stead, LF, 2004, Nursing interventions for smoking cessation, *Cochrane Database of Systematic Reviews* no. 1, CD001188.

Rinkel, GJ, Feigin, VL, Algra, A, van den Bergh, WM, Vermeulen, M et al., 2005, Calcium antagonists for aneurysmal subarachnoid haemorrhage, *Cochrane Database of Systematic Reviews* no. 1, CD000277.

Rose, G, 1981, Strategy of prevention: lessons from cardiovascular disease, *British Medical Journal*, vol. 282, no. 6279, pp. 1847–1851.

Rosenstock, IM, 2005, Why people use health services, *Milbank Quarterly*, vol. 83, pp. 1–32.

Rothwell, PM, Slattery, J, & Warlow, CP, 1996, A systematic review of the risks of stroke and death due to endarterectomy for symptomatic carotid stenosis, *Stroke*, vol. 27, no. 2, pp. 260–265.

Rothwell, PM, Eliasziw, M, Gutnikov, SA, Warlow, CP, & Barnett, HJ, 2004, Endarterectomy for symptomatic carotid stenosis in relation to clinical subgroups and timing of surgery, *Lancet*, vol. 363, no. 9413, pp. 915–924.

Rothwell, PM, Giles, MF, Flossmann, E, & Nielsen, E, 2006, A simple score (ABCD) to identify individuals at high early risk of stroke after transient ischemic attack, *Journal of Emergency Medicine*, vol. 30, no. 2, pp. 251–252.

Rothwell, PM, Giles, MF, Chandratheva, A, Marquardt, L, Geraghty, O et al., 2007, Effect of urgent treatment of transient ischaemic attack and minor stroke on early recurrent stroke (EXPRESS study): a prospective population-based sequential comparison, *Lancet*, vol. 370, no. 9596, pp. 1432–1442.

Rudd, AG, Lowe, D, Hoffman, A, Irwin, P, & Pearson, M, 2004, Secondary prevention for stroke in the United Kingdom: results from the National Sentinel Audit of Stroke, *Age and Ageing*, vol. 33, no. 3, pp. 280–286.

Sacco, RL, Foulkes, MA, Mohr, JP, Wolf, PA, Hier, DB et al., 1989, Determinants of early recurrence of cerebral infarction. The Stroke Data Bank, *Stroke*, vol. 20, no. 8, pp. 983–989.

Sajid, MS, Vijaynagar, B, Singh, P, & Hamilton, G, 2007, Literature review of cranial nerve injuries during carotid endarterectomy, *Acta Chirurgica Belgica*, vol. 107, no. 1, pp. 25–28.

Sappok, T, Faulstich, A, Stuckert, E, Kruck, H, Marx, P et al., 2001, Compliance with secondary prevention of ischemic stroke: a prospective evaluation, *Stroke*, vol. 32, no. 8, pp. 1884–1889.

Schrader, J, Luders, S, Kulschewski, A, Hammersen, F, Plate, K et al., 2005, Morbidity and mortality after stroke: eprosartan compared with nitrendipine for secondary prevention: principal results of a prospective randomized controlled study (MOSES), *Stroke*, vol. 36, pp. 1218–1226.

Scientific Advisory Committee on Nutrition, 2003, *Salt and Health*, The Stationery Office, London.

Sever, PS, Dahlof, B, Poulter, NR, Wedel, H, Beevers, G et al., 2003, Prevention of coronary and stroke events with atorvastatin in hypertensive patients who have average or lower-than-average cholesterol concentrations, in the Anglo-Scandinavian Cardiac Outcomes Trial–Lipid Lowering Arm (ASCOT-LLA): a multicentre randomised controlled trial, *Lancet*, vol. 361, no. 9364, pp. 1149–1158.

SHEP Cooperative Research Group, 1991, Prevention of stroke by antihypertensive drug treatment in older persons with isolated systolic hypertension: final results of the Systolic Hypertension in the Elderly Program (SHEP), *Journal of the American Medical Association*, vol. 265, pp. 3255–3264.

Shinton, R, & Beevers, G, 1989, Meta-analysis of relation between cigarette smoking and stroke, *British Medical Journal*, vol. 298, no. 6676, pp. 789–794.

Silagy, C, Lancaster, T, Stead, L, Mant, D, & Fowler, G, 2004, Nicotine replacement therapy for smoking cessation, *Cochrane Database of Systematic Reviews* no. 3, CD000146.

Skerrett, PJ, & Hennekens, CH, 2003, Consumption of fish and fish oils and decreased risk of stroke, *Prevention Cardiology*, vol. 6, no. 1, pp. 38–41.

Slavish, LG, Nicholas, GG, & Gee, W, 1984, Review of a community hospital experience with carotid endarterectomy, *Stroke*, vol. 15, no. 6, pp. 956–959.

Stam, J, 2005, Thrombosis of the cerebral veins and sinuses, *New England Journal of Medicine*, vol. 352, no. 17, pp. 1791–1798.

Stern, EB, Berman, M, Thomas, JJ, & Klassen, AC, 1999, Community education for stroke awareness: an efficacy study, *Stroke*, vol. 30, no. 4, pp. 720–723.

Straus, SE, Majumdar, SR, & McAlister, FA, 2002, New evidence for stroke prevention: scientific review, *Journal of the American Medical Association*, vol. 288, no. 11, pp. 1388–1395.

Sudlow, C, 2007, Dipyridamole with aspirin is better than aspirin alone in preventing vascular events after ischaemic stroke or TIA, *British Medical Journal*, vol. 334, no. 7599, p. 901.

The ACTIVE Investigator, 2006, Clopidogrel plus aspirin versus oral anticoagulation for atrial fibrillation in the Atrial Fibrillation Clopidogrel Trial with Irbesartan for Prevention of Vascular Events: a randomised controlled trial, *Lancet*, vol. 367, pp. 1903–1912.

The ESPRIT Study Group, 2006, Aspirin plus dipyridamole versus aspirin alone after cerebral ischaemia of arterial origin (ESPRIT): randomised controlled trial., *Lancet*, vol. 367, no. 9523, pp. 1665–1673.

The European Stroke Initiative Writing Committee for the EUSI Executive Committee, 2006, Recommendations for the management of intracranial haemorrhage – Part I: Spontaneous intracerebral haemorrhage, *Cerebrovascular Diseases*, vol. 22, pp. 294–316.

Tones, K, & Green, J, 2004, *Health Promotion: Planning and Strategies*, Sage, London.

Toole, JF, 2004, Surgery for carotid artery stenosis, *British Medical Journal*, vol. 329, no. 7467, pp. 635–636.

Topol, EJ, 2004, Intensive statin therapy – a sea change in cardiovascular prevention, *New England Journal of Medicine*, vol. 350, no. 15, pp. 1562–1564.

UK Prospective Diabetes Study Group, 1998, Intensive blood-glucose control with sulphonylureas or insulin compared with conventional treatment and risk of complications in patients with type 2 diabetes, *Lancet*, vol. 352, no. 9131, pp. 837–853.

University Group Diabetes Program, 1970, A study of the effects of hypoglycemic agents on vascular complications in patients with adult-onset diabetes. II. Mortality results, *Diabetes*, vol. 19 Suppl, pp. 789–830.

Vascular Society, 2004, *Fourth National Vascular Database Report*, http://www.vascularsociety.org.uk/Docs.nvdr2004.pdf (Accessed 27/12/06), Vascular Society of Great Britain and Ireland; accessed 12 May 2009.

Wardlaw, JM, Chappell, FM, Best, JJ, Wartolowska, K, & Berry, E, 2006, Non-invasive imaging compared with intra-arterial angiography in the diagnosis of symptomatic carotid stenosis: a meta-analysis, *Lancet*, vol. 367, no. 9521, pp. 1503–1512.

Warshafsky, S, Packard, D, Marks, SJ, Sachdeva, N, Terashita, DM et al., 1999, Efficacy of 3-hydroxy-3-methylglutaryl coenzyme A reductase inhibitors for prevention of stroke, *Journal of General Internal Medicine*, vol. 14, no. 12, pp. 763–774.

West, R, McNeill, A, & Raw, M, 2000, Smoking cessation guidelines for professionals: and update, *Thorax*, vol. 55, pp. 987–999.

Wilcox, R, Bousser, MG, Betteridge, DJ, Schernthaner, G, Pirags, V et al., 2007, Effects of pioglitazone in patients with type 2 diabetes with or without previous stroke: results from PROactive (PROspective pioglitAzone Clinical Trial In macroVascular Events 04), *Stroke*, vol. 38, no. 3, pp. 865–873.

Williams, LS, Bruno, A, Rouch, D, & Marriott, DJ, 1997, Stroke patients' knowledge of stroke. Influence on time to presentation, *Stroke*, vol. 28, no. 5, pp. 912–915.

Winslow, CM, Solomon, DH, Chassin, MR, Kosecoff, J, Merrick, NJ et al., 1988, The appropriateness of carotid endarterectomy, *New England Journal of Medicine*, vol. 318, no. 12, pp. 721–727.

Wolf, PA, 1998, Prevention of stroke, *Lancet*, vol. 352 Suppl 3, pp. S1115–S1118.

Wolf, PA, D'Agostino, RB, Kannel, WB, Bonita, R, & Belanger, AJ, 1988, Cigarette smoking as a risk factor for stroke. The Framingham Study, *JAMA*, vol. 259, no. 7, pp. 1025–1029.

Yoon, SS, & Byles, J, 2002, Perceptions of stroke in the general public and patients with stroke: a qualitative study, *British Medical Journal*, vol. 324, no. 7345, pp. 1065–1068.

Yoon, SS, Heller, RF, Levi, C, Wiggers, J, & Fitzgerald, PE, 2001, Knowledge of stroke risk factors, warning symptoms and treatment among an Australian urban population, *Stroke*, vol. 32, pp. 1926–1930.

Young, GR, Sandercock, PA, Slattery, J, Humphrey, PR, Smith, ET et al., 1996, Observer variation in the interpretation of intra-arterial angiograms and the risk of inappropriate decision about carotid endarterectomy, *Journal of Neurology, Neurosurgery and Psychiatry*, vol. 60, pp. 152–157.

Zeiger, HE, Jr, Zampella, EJ, Naftel, DC, McKay, RD, Varner, PD, & Morawetz, RB, 1987, A prospective analysis of 142 carotid endarterectomies for occlusive vascular disease, 1979–1985, *Journal of Neurosurgery*, vol. 67, no. 4, pp. 540–544.

Chapter 14

Longer-term support for survivors and supporters

Louise Brereton and Jill Manthorpe

Key points

- The transition from hospital to home requires meticulous planning, organisation and communication between all agencies, the patient and their supporters.
- Carers' individual needs and circumstances must be assessed and managed, in addition to those of the person with stroke.
- People with stroke and their supporters become expert in the management of their condition and circumstances.
- Rehabilitation and vocational rehabilitation should be considered in keeping with the individual's aspirations.
- Regular reviews are needed to signpost the person with stroke and their supporters to additional services, organisations and information as appropriate.

[...] just sit down and see people as people, not just as stroke victims or stroke survivors which are not terms I particularly like, I've got to be honest [...]. Because I don't feel like I'm a survivor of a stroke, I feel I'm struggling, I'm struggling with the stroke but I don't think I want to be called a struggler either. Just a person. I think sometimes a person is not seen.

c. DIPEx (http://www.healthtalkonline.org)

Introduction

This chapter explores longer-term support and treatment for people who have had a stroke. Whilst in the current climate long-term support frequently refers to the period three to six months after the stroke, which is often the time frame for Early Supported Discharge schemes (see Chapter 11), this chapter will address the 'real' long term. People with stroke, and their carers, experience a wide range of problems affecting their well-being and quality of life for ever, not least because a third of people with stroke are not functionally independent even one year later (Wolfe 1996). It is axiomatic that professionals need to recognise and respond to these problems; ideally, they should also have a major role in preventing the problems developing in the first place.

Whilst many may think that people with stroke require nursing home care, this is rarely the case, with the majority being cared for, or living independently, in their own home (Australian Bureau of Statistics 2003; Office for National Statistics 2003). It is perhaps unsurprising that stroke has been described as a 'family illness' because it is likely to affect the physical, psychological, social and financial well-being of the whole family (Mackenzie et al. 2007).

This chapter first looks at the long-term support or management of stroke survivors' own concerns before highlighting carers' needs and how practitioners can support carers in the long term. This dual focus is important, because carers often report that professionals focus exclusively on the needs of the person with stroke (Low et al. 2004). Planning the discharge from hospital is the first step in delivering long-term support, preparing everyone for the move back home, putting in place what is required and setting up a system for the long term. This is a key transition but it is of course not the only one.

The model of transition or transfer of care (Young & Forster 2007) can be used to think through some principles of wider relevance to long-term support of people with stroke and those affected by stroke. In using the term 'those affected by stroke' we refer to people who are often family members or partners, but they may also include friends and neighbours and wider supporters. There is increasing interest in the diversity of people with, and affected by, stroke and greater recognition that we need to explore what works, and for whom, in practice (Dowswell et al. 2000).

Leaving hospital

Discharge planning

Effective discharge planning is vital to promote well-being and maximum recovery, (Intercollegiate Stroke Working Party 2008). Professionals admit that discharge planning is frequently not done well, with poor preparation, lack of notice of time of discharge, insufficient coordination amongst the health care team and weak communication between hospital and community services (Closs & Tierney 1993; McKenna et al. 2000). There are many challenges for all parties: hospital staff are under pressure to discharge patients promptly; patients and families may overestimate their ability to manage at home; and there is limited availability of community health and social care services (Bull & Roberts 2001).

When it is done well, discharge planning ensures people with stroke move smoothly between services, the quality of support is high, there is continuity of care, and patients' and carers' knowledge and ability develop (Arts et al. 2000; Burton & Gibbon 2005; Dai et al. 2003). Hospital stay may be short-

---

Case example 14.1 Mary (1).

Mary is a 64-year-old single woman, previously independent and living alone, who has been admitted to hospital following a stroke that has resulted in her having considerable right-sided weakness. She has one married stepsister, Natalie, in her late forties, who lives in the same town and works part-time whilst running the home for her husband and three teenage children. As Mary's rehabilitation proceeds, it appears unlikely she will be able to continue living independently at home.

---

ened, and unplanned readmissions may be avoided, potentially reducing costs (Kane et al. 2000; Saposnik et al. 2005).

Discharge planning is a process, rather than a single or one-off event (Shepperd et al. 2004). Typically, it involves pre-discharge assessment, guidance and education, referral for continuing care funding, obtaining equipment, negotiation of primary health, and social care support, coordination of services, and follow-up (Naylor et al. 1999). This interdisciplinary process should start on admission (Dai et al. 2003), but be delivered by a discharge coordinator, or someone taking that role, prior to discharge from hospital (Burton & Gibbon 2005; Haddock 1994; Phillips-Harris 1998). Uncertainty in the time frame for recovery from stroke may make planning from admission difficult, but does not preclude the collection of basic information and identification of key people at any early stage. In the example of Mary (see Case example 14.1), it starts with gathering information from Mary, or her sister if Mary is not able to supply it, about her wishes, her social network, and the nature of her home environment. It is useful to understand issues of access, physical layout, and other relevant matters. The single assessment process, or a shared assessment, avoids duplication of effort and repeated questioning of survivors and supporters.

It is particularly important that potential carers are included as 'partners' in the process (Department of Health 2003) because their opposition to, or reservations about, discharge home is the strongest predictor of entry to long-term care (Zureik et al. 1995). Carers have often felt uninvolved in the discharge process (Brazil et al. 2000). Involving carers in the right way may not be easy: the relationship between survivor and carer may be complicated; professionals may be slow to recognise what carers need; and there may be an assumption that carers will want to, and be able to, cope (Brereton & Nolan 2000). As a result, possible alternative or additional sources of support may not be adequately explored (Bakas et al. 2002; Kerr & Smith 2001).

It is the responsibility of the care team to work with the survivor and their support network about their willingness, and ability, to provide care. In the case of Mary (see Case example 14.1), Natalie may be able to offer some support and may in fact wish to, but her ability to do so may be limited. Conversations with potential carers should take place and their support should not be taken for granted. This applies in the long term as much as early postdischarge. The risk is high of a 'care gap' developing after well-meshed support in hospital and very little support immediately after.

Home assessments

Whilst in hospital, a home visit may be performed, involving an occupational therapy assessment of the patient's ability to manage at home, with or without support (College of Occupational Therapy (COT) 2000). Other members of the care team may attend, depending on circumstances and availability, but will need to be informed of the outcomes of, and issues raised by, the visit. Being able to assess the person's functioning, wishes and environmental risks in their own home may assist in better identification of needs (Welch & Lowes 2005). Such visits take time and money.

Whilst home visits are thought to be effective due to reducing the risk of falls, preventing further disability, and reducing loss of autonomy in the longer term (Cumming et al. 1999; Nuffield Institute for Health & NHS Centre for Reviews and Dissemination (NHSCRD) 1996; Pardessus et al. 2002), overall there is limited evidence to support this (Patterson & Mulley 1999). The limited resources and time in which to provide home visits may even render them detrimental. Time pressure may increase stress for staff, patients and carers, whilst time restrictions may result in a short-term concentration on equipment and adaptations, without the much needed exploration of, and time dedicated to, the person with stroke or their carers' concerns about the future. Further research is required to properly understand the role and contribution of home visits in promoting safe discharge, to explore: optimal timing; who should be present; the effect on outcomes (e.g. patients' quality of life and readmission rates) (Welch & Lowes 2005).

Alternative approaches to improve preparation for going home

Standardised teaching packs for patients and families, adaptation of the Acute Care for Elders (ACE) intervention and model of care for stroke patients, and 'managed care', may be useful, but have not been formally evaluated (Allen et al. 2003; Monane et al. 1996; Reiley et al. 1996). Whilst liaison nurses were thought to improve communication and discharge planning between hospital and home care staff, problems still occurred. Home care workers and medication still arrived later than they should. Moreover, whilst nurses felt that patients were better prepared for discharge, patients disagreed, being less satisfied with discharge preparation after the introduction of the liaison nurses than were the patients pre-intervention (Arts et al. 2000).

In contrast, a patient-generated checklist improved preparedness for discharge, particularly when friends and family were involved (Grimmer et al. 2006), and a professional-partnership model enhanced discharge planning and reduced length of readmission stays by improving continuity of care and service information (Bull et al. 2000). In addition, carers were more positive about care-giving. However, the exact details of the intervention are not provided. A complex intervention focusing on the transition between hospital and home (carers learnt about what was necessary by observing therapy) was compared to a usual care control (Grasel et al. 2005, 2006). The intervention group, in addition to usual care, had a pre-discharge weekend home stay, an individual-ised training course and a psycho-educational seminar for family carers before discharge, followed by telephone counselling three months after discharge. The intervention group had fewer new illnesses, and had fewer falls with subsequent injuries, in the first four weeks post-discharge. However, they needed more outpatient care and community services than the control group in the first six months post-discharge (Grasel et al. 2005). After two and a half years, fewer patients in the intervention group were dead or institutionalised (care home or hospital), and had better quality of life (Grasel et al. 2006).

What is required longer term?

Promoting independence

The long-term consequences of stroke vary considerably. Seventy to eighty-five per cent of people have hemiplegia after their first stroke and of these 60% achieve functional independence in basic activities of living by six months post-stroke. Seventy per cent of people with stroke have significant mobility, activities of daily living, social integration and employment problems (Churchill 1998; Dobkin 2003; Patel et al. 2000). In the US permanent disability affects 15–30% of those with stroke and 20% enter institutional care three months post-stroke (American Heart Association 2003). Half of a sample of people with stroke had not changed disability category between three months and five years after stroke, while the other half had deteriorated (Wilkinson et al. 1997).

People need help with basic activities: bathing, climbing stairs and dressing (Wade & Hewer 1987). In the UK, people get help from public services if they have extensive needs, and many manage with a mixture of family care and domestic support that they arrange and pay for themselves.

Whilst motor impairments are visible, mood and cognitive problems, and perceptual deficits are often only elucidated by specific testing (Edwards et al. 2006). However, adequate cognitive functioning and comprehension are vitally important for independent living, while mood and emotional problems reduce quality of life. Once home, the former problems may become harder to cope with, whilst the latter may only then become apparent. These problems can affect the lives of both the patient and carer. This can be seen with post-stroke incontinence, where both parties find problems difficult to manage, leading to isolation due to the feeling of stigma and embarrassment about smell and leakage (Brittain & Shaw 2007).

Cognitive problems require specific testing, and although they are sometimes identified in hospital, it may be too early to make conclusions about the rela-tionship to the stroke itself or to dementia or depression. Failure to correctly identify and so treat problems may cause a breakdown in relationships, and even premature care home placement (Anderson et al. 1995; Hajek et al. 1997). These issues are discussed further in Chapter 9.

Promoting independence requires attention to the emotional and social consequences of stroke as well as to the physical or medical effects. Stroke

---

Case example 14.2 John (1).

John is a 48-year-old man who had an infarct within the left cerebral hemisphere that affected his right arm function and ability to express himself. He lives in a rural area, is a self-employed carpenter and is married to his second wife, Karen, with an 8-year-old son, Ewan. There is a mortgage on the family home and John is supporting his two children from his first marriage at college. John has returned home with numerous offers of helpful telephone numbers and support groups.

---

rehabilitation should involve combined and coordinated use of medical, social, educational and vocational resources to enable people to reach maximum physical, psychological, social and vocational recovery (Schwamm et al. 2005). Carers' ability to cope is helped by encouraging positive coping strategies and providing them with tailored information on stroke and how to help manage the changes to their lives and those of the survivor (Low et al. 1999). Living with disability can be a lifelong challenge to find ways to compensate or adapt to persisting neurological deficits as well as tackling discrimination and challenging negative attitudes. Many people say that the real work of recovery begins after formal rehabilitation ends when people apply skills in real life situations without professional oversight (Bates et al. 2005). Resuming work is one such transition.

How can people be helped to return to work?

Work is a key defining factor for many people. Although many of those with stroke may have retired, for others return to work can significantly affect emotional, psychological and social well-being (Zerwic et al. 2002). Returning to pre-stroke role and lifestyle is an important goal for the majority (Parker et al. 1997). However, employment rates after stroke have been reported to be from 7–10% (Nai et al. 2006), to 20% (Hofgren et al. 2007), to as high as 78% (Neau et al. 1998).

Loss of employment may entail major financial hardship and worry for the whole family (O'Neill et al. 1998; see Case example 14.2). Not surprisingly, better physical (Hofgren et al. 2007) and communication abilities have been associated with return to work after a stroke (Ramsing et al. 1991), with greater severity of neurological deficits on admission to hospital and greater residual disability associated with subsequent inability to return to work (Hofgren et al. 2007; Neau et al. 1998).

Consequently, people should have the opportunity to work, or volunteer, through timely access to financial support and employment advice (Department of Health 2007a). Although many survivors may not be able to return to work in the short term, this may be possible longer term. They, and their carers, should be able to participate in paid, supported or voluntary work, because work is one of the best forms of rehabilitation (Department of Health 2007a; Waddell 2006). Vocational rehabilitation (VR) refers to the processes involved in enabling disabled people to enter, return to, or remain in work (Nai et al. 2006). For some, this will be a return to their existing job, for others it may involve a period of retraining for new employment. VR interventions post-stroke can help up to two-thirds of those who receive such interventions to return to work (Nai et al. 2006).

People with physical, cognitive and possibly mental health problems face particular difficulties in returning to work. However, UK legislation to support the rights of disabled people in employment, such as the Disability Discrimination Acts 1995 and 2005, underpins people's rights to accommodation and adjustments in the work setting. The Equality and Human Rights Commission, a non-departmental public body (NDPB), was established under the Equality Act 2006; it is accountable for its public funds, but independent of government. It has taken over the functions of the Equal Opportunities Commission, the Commission for Racial Equality, and the Disability Rights Commission as well as oversight of the workings of the Human Rights Act 1998 (see its website http://www.equalityhumanrights.com). The Commission is a source of advice about disabled people's rights, as are other voluntary sector groups (in the UK these include The Stroke Association and Radar).

However, VR services are in short supply, and are often targeted at younger people (Bates et al. 2005). The process of returning to work is extremely individual, and is affected by multiple factors (Saeki 2000) with little specific evidence to guide staff wishing to assist in VR. In addition, staff need to have a clear understanding of employers' obligations and employees' rights in order to prepare survivors for return to work. This information is available from the Department for Work and Pensions (DWP) in the UK. Access to Work, for example, is a scheme that provides support to disabled people at work. This support may come from having funding for a person to accompany the disabled person to work, or in the workplace. In the case of John (see Case example 14.2), early advice about finance might be very helpful to the family, and this could be available from a combination of the DWP, a local specialist advice centre and the Benefits Agency. Family tensions might be more complex than money alone and so those supporting John and his family may find it useful to link them to counselling and other sources of help with family relationships. For Natalie, advice about the implications of caring for her sister might help her to assess whether she is able to take some carer's leave from work.

Stroke review

A key goal of long-term support is to prevent recurrence of stroke and associated complications (Zerwic et al. 2002). People should have their health and support needs reviewed by primary health services within six weeks of their discharge, again before six months and then annually (Department of Health 2007a). As Case example 14.3 demonstrates, situations may change and over time services identified at hospital discharge may not meet needs. These reviews should prompt further specialist review, advice, information, support and rehabilitation where necessary (Department of Health 2007a), and should include

> **Case example 14.3** John (2).
>
> Eight months after John's return home, things are going badly. His wife Karen has had to take up a job in the local meatpacking factory, and arrangements for the after-school care of Ewan are very stressful. The stroke club John went to once seemed to be full of people much older than he was. Ewan is having difficulties at school, John is drinking alcohol in the afternoon, and relationships with his other children have broken down, as they feel abandoned. The family are in debt and thinking of moving to a caravan park to get themselves away from so much financial pressure.

treatment of risk factors and secondary prevention advice (Intercollegiate Stroke Working Party 2008; see Chapter 13). Stroke reviews provide an ideal opportunity for survivors, carers and professionals to consider ongoing needs in partnership.

What do carers want?

The strategic importance of carers is recognised internationally (Pearlin et al. 2001), as needs for services are influenced by the presence or absence of carers (Wilkinson et al. 1997). Professional–carer partnership working is widely advocated (Archbold et al. 1995; Audit Commission 2004; Hanson et al. 2006; Nolan et al. 2003; Stewart et al. 1993). Professionals should adopt a family-centred approach, considering the needs of carers as well as those with stroke (Low et al. 2004; van der Smagt-Duijnstee et al. 2001b). Comprehensive needs should be considered from the outset, in transfer of care from hospital and in the long term (Duncan et al. 2005; Intercollegiate Stroke Working Party 2008; National Stroke Foundation 2005; Scottish Intercollegiate Guidelines Network (SIGN) 2004). There will be a need for information about stroke, and families should be signposted to local and national support services, including those in the voluntary and community sectors. All parties should be involved in planning and decision-making. Carer stress or depression is more likely if the person with stroke has less obvious impairments such as cognitive loss, irritability, depression, personality change and urinary incontinence (Manthorpe & Iliffe 2006). Speech and language problems arising from a stroke (see Chapter 8) may be stressful for carers (Draper & Brocklehurst 2007), and can impact on relationships.

Carer assessments

Carers' needs are not always routinely assessed (Guberman 2005), and this is inconsistent with the recommendation of an assessment of carer needs (Department of Health 1995, 2004, 2006). This is particularly important if they provide regular and/or substantial care, although 'substantial' was not defined, leaving interpretation to professional discretion. Rights to a carer's assessment were established in England and Wales in 1995. Three pieces of legislation underpin carers' rights to be assessed:

- Carers (Recognition and Services) Act 1995
- Carers and Disabled Children Act 2000
- Carers (Equal Opportunities) Act 2004

Carer profiling also features in Australian policy, as is part of Comprehensive Assessment, which is the basis of case management in New South Wales (NSW Department of Ageing 2006).

Assessment should cover the carer's perceptions of the situation; relationship with the person they support; caring tasks; willingness and ability to continue to provide care; other commitments; and their coping strategies. This assessment should lead to a care plan, which not only details services required, but stipulates arrangements for monitoring and review, which necessitates agreed outcomes. Local authorities can delegate their powers of carers' assessment to health service staff, but it will only be performed if the carer's needs meet the local authority's eligibility criteria. However, the Carers (Equal Opportunities) Act 2004 dictates that local authorities inform carers of their rights to an assessment. They must also consider carers' preferences for the balance between caring, employment and leisure, and moreover must involve other sectors in providing support as appropriate.

Nurses working with carers should ensure that they:

- Provide information about carers' assessment if this has not been taken up
- Explain the purpose of carers' assessments so that they seem non-stigmatising and potentially helpful
- Encourage carers to seek an assessment (even if the person they are supporting refuses to be assessed)
- Explain that the carer can be assessed separately and in private, away from the person they are supporting
- Discuss with carers their desired outcomes from such assessments
- Record the existence and conclusions of a carer's assessment
- Are mindful of carers' possible worries about involvement with social services
- Encourage carers to make sure that they receive written copies of their assessment and a care plan
- Recommend carers ask for a review if needs change or circumstances alter
- Ensure carers' assessments are audited

Following a stroke, carers sometimes immediately engage in a range of 'seeking' activities, trying to obtain the best care possible for their relative and themselves by establishing partnerships with professionals (Brereton 2005). Carers' needs are reflected in three key themes:

- What's it all about? – Need for information and to understand the situation
- Up to the job? – Need for skills and resources to provide care
- What about me? – Need for recognition of their own needs, expertise and potential contribution to care

However, needs may change, and whilst some will develop caring expertise, others will choose to give up caring. Some carers report a 'strong sense of partnership' with professionals, feeling that they are 'in it together', whilst those who are dissatisfied feel 'little or no sense of partnership' suggesting they are 'going it alone', and others may be reluctant to develop partnerships with professionals.

Carer assessment tends to focus on stress and burden, perhaps reflecting researchers' views of family care-giving as being mostly about problems. However, this ignores other potentially useful avenues for assessment (Ory 2000). Nolan and his colleagues recognised the limits of existing assessment tools and produced three carer assessment indices: the Carers' Assessment of Difficulties Index (CADI), the Carers' Assessment of Satisfactions Index – CASI (Nolan & Grant 1992) and the Carers' Assessment of Managing Index – CAMI (Nolan et al. 1995). Not stroke specific, these 30-item indices are suitable for use with long-term carers, are quick and easy to administer, have been widely tested and found reliable, and are suggested as valid in a range of care-giving situations in the UK, mainland Europe, North America and Australasia. Nolan et al. (2003) advises professionals to consider their role in assessing carers' needs. He describes current assessment processes as 'allocation' or 'imparting' of services, rather than of exploring ways for professionals to respond to carers' needs, whilst acknowledging their expertise.

Increasingly, carers are gaining recognition as 'experts' (Allen 2000; Department of Health 2006; Nolan et al. 1996). Working in partnership with carers is advocated (Bauer & Nay 2003; Gallant et al. 2002; Hervey & Ramsay 2004; MacIntosh & McCormack 2001), and requires proactive identification of carers (Audit Commission 2004) and the development of improved professional–carer relationships (Nolan et al. 2006).

What is helpful for carers?

It is widely agreed that carers may need information, education, skills training, emotional support and counselling (Audit Commission 2003; Brazil et al. 2000; Smith et al. 2004; van der Smagt-Duijnstee et al. 2001a). However, it is not yet clear how to respond to these needs, what interventions might be suitable, how they should be delivered, or what influences effectiveness. There needs to be recognition of individual characteristics and wishes, as well as an acknowledgement that some carers may know more about some aspects of caring than their professionals.

Information giving and education

Carers may have information needs that equal or exceed those of patients (McLennan et al. 1996). However, despite the Audit Commission's (2004) recommendation that carers should receive clear, concise, relevant information about their rights, benefits and support without having to ask or search for it, there are longstanding inadequacies in the provision of information (Close & Procter 1999; Dai et al. 2003; Forster et al. 2001; Rodgers et al. 2001; Wiles et al. 1998). Carers have complained that insufficient information contributes to their lack of preparedness for their role (Audit Commission 2003; Brazil et al. 2000; Brereton 2005; Smith et al. 2004). Even when professionals provide information for carers, this can be of uncertain relevance and it may lack essential details (Hanger et al. 1998; Hart 1999, 2001; Kelson et al. 1998; O'Connell et al. 2003; Smith et al. 2004). As a result, many carers live with uncertainty (Close & Procter 1999).

Common information needs of survivors and carers (adapted from Young & Forster 2007):

- Risk factors and causes of stroke
- Availability of local services and support groups for stroke and disabled people and carers' groups
- Financial and housing advice
- Guidance on driving and transport
- Medication and secondary prevention
- Understanding of an agreed or shared care plan
- Advice on returning to work, including voluntary and community work, and support for participation in leisure activities
- Discussion of sexual and relationship issues

Carers frequently report being unsure of services and support they should expect, might be offered, or might receive (Brereton 2005; Close & Procter 1999; van Veenendaal et al. 1996). When carers lack knowledge about how systems work, they experience difficulties accessing health and social care services (Brereton 2005; Kelson et al. 1998; Smith et al. 2004; Wiles et al. 1998). This is particularly trying given the diverse and complex problems that many carers face (Dowswell et al. 2000).

Lack of information for patients and carers can lead to dissatisfaction and a failure to comply with professionals' advice (Clark & Smith 1998). However, staff may have difficulties communicating with distressed relatives (Dewar et al. 2003) and may withhold information to avoid creating anxiety, or to avoid overwhelming them (Gladden 2000). However well meaning the motive, this may result in carers not fully understanding their situation. Moreover, such paternalistic behaviour undermines the essence of partnerships, which rely on sharing of resources and interdependent working towards common goals (MacIntosh & McCormack 2001). Information giving should be based on understanding of carers' preferences and needs.

A systematic review of information and education interventions following stroke suggested that combining information giving with educational sessions might be more effective in improving survivors' and carers' knowledge than information giving alone (Forster et al. 2001). A large multicentre trial to test the effectiveness of carer training and information giving is ongoing (see SRN website: http://www.uksrn.ac.uk). Education may overcome the potential inadequacies of information alone, which has been reported as not always being very readable (Eames et al. 2003; Hoffman et al. 2004). These inadequacies may be overcome by using simple language, large font size, colour and diagrams that complement the text (Eames et al. 2003). Web-based interventions may help meet carers' needs by enabling survivors and carers to manipulate font size and style to meet their individual requirements. For example, The Stroke Association website (http://www.stroke.org.uk) is a comprehensive resource, covering frequently asked questions and specialist subjects.

Skills training and resources

People with stroke and their carers often require training in the use of equipment, as well as additional skills, such as assistance with basic activities (Archbold et al. 1995; Bates et al. 2005; Brown et al. 1997; Chesson et al. 1999; Schumacher et al. 1998, 2000). Timely skills-training may enable carers to acquire a range of skills in emotional, cognitive and practical areas (Archbold et al. 1995; Nolan & Grant 1992; Stewart et al. 1993) and will promote well-being (Evans et al. 1994). Direct involvement in rehabilitation, to reinforce learning, and to generalise new behaviours or skills to the home may prove beneficial (Dickens et al. 2005).

Currently, carers report receiving little preparation for caring (Audit Commission 2004; Bakas et al. 2002; Brereton 2005; Dowswell et al. 2000; Hart 1999, 2001; Kerr & Smith 2001; Simon & Kendrick 2002; Smith et al. 2004). Carers have to acquire skills little by little without adequate support, whilst staff are under pressure to deliver care and therapy to patients and reduce length of hospital stay.

Carers' difficulties are compounded by delays in receiving equipment or adaptations at home (Smith et al. 2004). This may be due to a lack of information, or misinformation (Brereton 2005), or may arise from failures or inadequacies within health and social care – 'system induced setbacks' Hart (2001). These are often due to a lack of continuity and delays in provision, particularly common at service interfaces (Kerr & Smith 2001; Schwamm et al. 2005). Professionals frequently underestimated the difficulties faced by carers in getting community services (Brazil et al. 2000) and ignored problems, believing that nothing could be done to remedy the situation (Hart 2001). A review of 23 studies identified health and social care services deficiencies as the second main problem area after the stroke, accounting for 29% of all problems experienced by survivors and carers in the community (Murray et al. 2003).

In England the personalisation policy of the Department of Health (2007b) is an attempt to resolve some of these problems and to provide greater choice for people needing support and care. People will be encouraged to self-assess needs and goals, and be able to choose whether to use resources to provide care themselves rather than purchasing external service providers. Mary and Natalie (see Case example 14.1) might find this helpful (see Case example 14.4). There are suggestions that such personalised budgets may be extended to the NHS for people with long-term conditions (Darzi 2008).

Emotional support and counselling

The contribution of family carers is critical to successful rehabilitation (Bates et al. 2005), and carers should not only be recognised for their contribution but should be provided with support and services (Audit Commission 2004).

Case example 14.4 Mary (2).

Natalie, Mary's sister, begins to realise that if her sister is to stay at home, as she wishes, then she will need considerable help round the home, in going out, and with her personal care. They have a detailed discussion about the various options with the hospital social worker, who helps them to complete an assessment and support plan that gives some idea of the resources that the local council will make available to Mary, combined with her pension and other social security income. The sums available are more than the family are expecting, and Natalie is able to think about the possibility of giving up her part-time job to look after her sister. Both women are very pleased with this. The social worker tells Mary about a local support agency (in the voluntary sector) that will help deal with the financial transactions, and the family decide to use this service to start with, particularly in setting up the contract about employment and self-employment responsibilities and to sort out the payments to Natalie. The family decide that this money from the council can also be used to pay for taxi fares so that Mary can go to church every week, since the bus journey is too difficult for her. The money also pays for an alarm system that enables Mary to call for help in an emergency. Mary decides that she will use part of the money to go on holiday each year to visit her cousin and to give Natalie a break. The social worker keeps in touch to see that the arrangement is working out and helps with modifying the support plan to meet Mary's changing needs.

Support required should be reviewed, and those stroke survivors and carers who wish to return to work should receive help to do so.

New technologies, should they be available or should stroke survivors and families feel physically and mentally able to use them, may have a role to play in providing support; for example, through the telephone and internet, such as the Caring-Web (Pierce et al. 2004) and the ACTION model (Magnusson et al. 2002).

Nurses' emotional support of carers is well recognised as important (Boland & Sims 1996; Davis & Grant 1994). Carers may face specific and diverse problems requiring tailored support, as the case of John and his family illustrates (see Case examples 14.2 and 14.3). Cultural and other characteristics may play a part in what families find accessible and acceptable, requiring nurses to be sensitive to factors such as age (John may feel that he is much younger than other people who have had a stroke and that they have nothing in common), ethnicity and sexuality.

To date few interventions developed specifically for carers have been rigorously tested (Brereton et al. 2007) but this makes it even more important that support for carers is provided, services evaluated and outcomes identified. Reviewing effectiveness of interventions, Brereton et al (2007) explored six complex interventions from the US, UK, Sweden and the Netherlands. Interventions included care-giver training (Kalra et al. 2004), education and counselling (Young & Forster 2007), social problem solving partnerships (Grant 1999; Grant et al. 2002), a psycho-educational telephone group (Hartke & King 2003), a nurse-led support and education programme (Larson et al. 2005) and a support programme delivered either to groups in hospital or individuals during home visits (van den Heuvel et al. 2000, 2002). All reported some benefit for carers; however, the quality of studies was variable. Small wonder that commissioners may find it difficult to work out what they should commission; thus consultation with practitioners and survivors and carers is likely to be important in shaping their decisions.

Community support and support groups

Survivors and carers need support over the short and long term, and contact with other survivors and carers is helpful (Schure et al. 2006). The Department of Health (2007a) recommends lifelong access to rehabilitation and continued support from specialist stroke services if appropriate, and through community-based health and social care services, and the voluntary sector (Department of Health 2007a).

A range of support groups are available, nationally, regionally and locally. These groups are frequently founded by survivors and those caring for them (Zorowitz 1999). In the UK, The Stroke Association, and the Northern Ireland and Scotland branches of the Chest, Heart and Stroke Association, as well as Different Strokes, offer a range of services including stroke clubs, family and carer support services, websites, a stroke helpline and information services. These enable survivors and carers to contact others in similar positions, and specific support is available to stroke survivors with particular problems. For example, AVM Support UK, the InterAct Reading Service, Connect and Speakeasy assist people with communication problems (see Chapter 15 for websites). Hospitals may also run support groups for survivors and carers, sometimes through expert patient and expert carer programmes. Professionals need to have a good knowledge of local stroke support networks and many assist groups with publicity, social events, fundraising and access to resources.

Survivors and carers may also gain support from non-stroke-specific sources such as independent living centres or carer groups. For example, in the UK, carers can get support through Carers UK, The Princess Royal Trust for Carers, Crossroads: caring for carers, Caring Net (Scotland) and Counsel and Care, and access to advice, information and advocacy (see Chapter 15). In the families described in the case examples in this chapter, different approaches are needed. Mary may find it helpful and enjoyable to go to a stroke support group, appreciating the break away from the house, and Natalie may use the time to get some shopping and to go to the hairdresser. John and Karen have been given information about local groups but may feel that they are not for them, and in addition, Karen is working shifts and preoccupied with the family's problems. Help here needs to be coordinated and relationships built up to be able to work with the family to reduce their multiple stressors.

Conclusion

Stroke affects the person with stroke and the caring network. Transitions such as discharge from hospital should not be the end of the story. People with stroke and their carers should be involved as partners in planning, provided with contact numbers for help and advice from knowledgeable and accessible services, and with information about local statutory, private and voluntary services. Home Assessment Visits should be used judiciously and attention needs to be given to long-term support. Consideration and active listening should be given to family relationships and carers' needs. Professionals should avoid assuming that carers can cope in favour of assessment and exploration of all available sources of support and understanding of what people regard as important to their quality of life.

Rehabilitation back to work is challenging but there is increasing interest and resources to enable disabled people to get back to work. Carers too have increased employment rights in the UK (Department of Health 2004) (see Carers UK for information: http://www.carersuk.org/Home).

Clinical guidelines supported by good quality evidence recommend that professionals provide survivors and carers with information, education and skills training but also build up relationships and mutual understandings. Professionals should be alert to stress and family dynamics, and should consider ways of enhancing the satisfaction of caring and strategies used to manage day-to-day care-giving. Professionals need to develop and recognise survivors' and carers' expertise if they are to work in partnership with them.

There is growing research to guide services for long-term support after stroke, and the management of long-term conditions is a national priority in the UK. Interventions for survivors and carers should be implemented and evaluated in the longer term rather than assuming that those implemented in the early rehabilitation phase will successfully meet people's needs over time.

References

Allen, D, 2000, Negotiating the role of expert carers on an adult hospital ward, *Sociology of Health and Illness*, vol. 22, no. 2, pp. 149–171.

Allen, KR, Hazelett, SE, Palmer, RR, Jarjoura, DG, Wickstrom, GC et al., 2003, Developing a stroke unit using the acute care for elders intervention and model of care, *Journal of American Geriatrics Society*, vol. 51, no. 11, pp. 1660–1667.

American Heart Association, 2003, *Heart Disease and Stroke Statistics – 2004 – Update*, American Heart Association, Dallas Texas.

Anderson, CS, Linto, J, & Stewart-Wynne, EG, 1995, A population-based assessment of the impact and burden of caregiving for long-term stroke survivors, *Stroke*, vol. 26, no. 5, pp. 843–849.

Archbold, PG, Stewart, BJ, Miller, LL, Harvath, TA, Greenlick, MR et al., 1995, The PREP system of nursing interventions: a pilot test with families caring for older members. Preparedness (PR), enrichment (E) and predictability (P), *Research in Nursing and Health*, vol. 18, no. 1, pp. 3–16.

Arts, SE, Francke, AL, & Hutten, JB, 2000, Liaison nursing for stroke patients: results of a Dutch evaluation study, *Journal of Advanced Nursing*, vol. 32, no. 2, pp. 292–300.

Audit Commission, 2003, *What Seems To Be the Matter? Communication Between Hospitals and Patients*, HMSO, London.

Audit Commission, 2004, *Support for Carers of Older People. Independence and Well-being*, HMSO, London.

Australian Bureau of Statistics, 2003, *Disability, Ageing and Carers, Australia: Caring in the Community*, http://www.abs.gov.au/ausstats/abs@.nsf/0/c258c88a7aa5a87eca2568a9001393e8?OpenDocument; accessed 12 May 2009.

Bakas, T, Austin, JK, Okonkwo, KF, Lewis, RR, & Chadwick, L, 2002, Needs, concerns, strategies, and advice of stroke caregivers the first 6 months after discharge, *Journal of Neuroscience Nursing*, vol. 34, no. 5, pp. 242–251.

Bates, B, Duncan, PW, Glasberg, JJ, Graham, GD, Katz, RC et al., 2005, Clinical Practice Guideline for the Management of Adult Stroke Rehabilitation, *Stroke*, vol. 36, p. 2049.

Bauer, M, & Nay, R, 2003, Family and staff partnerships in long-term care. A review of the literature, *Journal of Gerontological Nursing*, vol. 29, no. 10, pp. 46–53.

Boland, DL, & Sims, SL, 1996, Family care giving at home as a solitary journey, *Image: Journal of Nursing Scholarship*, vol. 28, no. 1, pp. 55–58.

Brazil, K, Roberts, J, Hode, M, & Vanderbent, SD, 2000, Managing the transition from hospital to home from family carers of stroke survivors, *National Academies of Practice Forum*, vol. 2, no. 4, pp. 259–266.

Brereton, ML, 2005, *The needs of 'new' family carers following stroke: A constructivist study*, University of Sheffield, Sheffield.

Brereton, L, & Nolan, M, 2000, 'You do know he's had a stroke, don't you?' Preparation for family care-giving – the neglected dimension, *Journal of Clinical Nursing*, vol. 9, no. 4, pp. 498–506.

Brereton, L, Carroll, C, & Barnston, S, 2007, Interventions for adult family carers of people who have had a stroke: a systematic review, *Clinical Rehabilitation*, vol. 21, no. 10, pp. 867–884.

Brittain, KR, & Shaw, C, 2007, The social consequences of living with and dealing with incontinence – a carer's perspective, *Social Science and Medicine*, vol. 65, no. 6, pp. 1274–1283.

Brown, SM, Humphry, R, & Taylor, E, 1997, A model of the nature of family-therapist relationships: implications for education, *American Journal of Occupational Therapy*, vol. 51, no. 7, pp. 597–603.

Bull, MJ, & Roberts, J, 2001, Components of a proper hospital discharge for elders, *Journal of Advanced Nursing*, vol. 35, no. 4, pp. 571–581.

Bull, MJ, Hansen, HE, & Gross, CR, 2000, A professional-patient partnership model of discharge planning with elders hospitalized with heart failure, *Applied Nursing Research*, vol. 13, no. 1, pp. 19–28.

Burton, C, & Gibbon, B, 2005, Expanding the role of the stroke nurse: a pragmatic clinical trial, *Journal of Advanced Nursing*, vol. 52, no. 6, pp. 640–650.

Chesson, R, Massie, S, & Reid, A, 1999, Carers' perceptions of rehabilitation in a stroke unit, *British Journal of Therapy and Rehabilitation*, vol. 6, no. 1, pp. 32–37.

Churchill, C, 1998, Social problems post acute stroke, *Physical Medicine and Rehabilitation: State of the Art Reviews*, vol. 7, pp. 213–214.

Clark, MS, & Smith, DS, 1998, Factors contributing to patient satisfaction with rehabilitation following stroke, *International Journal of Rehabilitation Research*, vol. 21, no. 2, pp. 143–154.

Close, H, & Procter, S, 1999, Coping strategies used by hospitalized stroke patients: implications for continuity and management of care, *Journal of Advanced Nursing*, vol. 29, no. 1, pp. 138–144.

Closs, SJ, & Tierney, AJ, 1993, The complexities of using a structure, process and outcome framework: the case of an evaluation of discharge planning for elderly patients, *Journal of Advanced Nursing*, vol. 18, no. 8, pp. 1279–1287.

College of Occupational Therapy (COT), 2000, *Standards for Practice: Home Assessment with Hospital Inpatients*, COT, London.

Cumming, RG, Thomas, M, Szonyi, G, Salkeld, G, O'Neill, E et al., 1999, Home visits by an occupational therapist for assessment and modification of environmental hazards: a randomized trial of falls prevention, *Journal of the American Geriatrics Society*, vol. 47, no. 12, pp. 1397–1402.

Dai, YT, Chang, Y, Hsieh, CY, & Tai, TY, 2003, Effectiveness of a pilot project of discharge planning in Taiwan, *Research in Nursing and Health*, vol. 26, no. 1, pp. 53–63.

Darzi, 2008, *High Quality Care for All – NHS Next Stage Review Final Report*, Department of Health, London.

Davis, LL, & Grant, JS, 1994, Constructing the reality of recovery: family home care management strategies, *Advances in Nursing Science*, vol. 17, no. 2, pp. 66–76.

Department of Health, 1995, *The Carers (Recognition and Services) Act*, HMSO, London.

Department of Health, 2003, *The Community Care (Delayed Discharges) Act*, The Stationery Office, London.

Department of Health, 2007a, *A New Ambition for Stroke: A Consultation on a National Strategy*, The Stationery Office, London.

Department of Health, 2007b, *Putting People First*, Department of Health, London.

Department of Health, 2004, *Carers Equal Opportunities Act*, The Stationery Office, London.

Department of Health, 2006, *Our Health, Our Care, Our Say: A New Direction for Community Services*, The Stationery Office, London.

Dewar, B, Tocher, R, & Watson, W, 2003, Enhancing partnerships with relatives in care settings, *Nursing Standard*, vol. 17, no. 40, pp. 33–39.

Dickens, J, McAdam, J, Leathley, MJ, Watkins, CL, Jack, CIA, & Crighton, M, 2005, A pilot study of rehabilitation support: improving outcome after discharge following an acute stroke, *Clinical Rehabilitation*, vol. 19, pp. 572–578,

Dobkin, BH, 2003, *The Clinical Science of Neurologic Rehabilitation*, Oxford University Press, New York.

Dowswell, G, Lawler, J, Dowswell, T, Young, J, Forster, A et al., 2000, Investigating recovery from stroke: a qualitative study, *Journal of Clinical Nursing*, vol. 9, no. 4, pp. 507–515.

Draper, P, & Brocklehurst, H, 2007, The impact of stroke on the well-being of the patient's spouse: an exploratory study, *Journal of Clinical Nursing*, vol. 16, no. 2, pp. 264–271.

Duncan, PW, Zorowitz, R, Bates, B, Choi, JY, Glasberg, JJ et al., 2005, Management of Adult Stroke Rehabilitation Care: a clinical practice guideline, *Stroke*, vol. 36, no. 9, pp. e100–e143.

Eames, S, McKenna, K, Worrall, L, & Read, S, 2003, The suitability of written education materials for stroke survivors and their carers, *Topics in Stroke Rehabilitation*, vol. 10, no. 3, pp. 70–83.

Edwards, DF, Hahn, MG, Baum, CM, Perlmutter, MS, Sheedy, C et al., 2006, Screening patients with stroke for rehabilitation needs: validation of the post-stroke rehabilitation guidelines, *Neurorehabilitation and Neural Repair*, vol. 20, no. 1, pp. 42–48.

Evans, RL, Connis, RT, Bishop, DS, Hendricks, RD, & Haselkorn, JK, 1994, Stroke: a family dilemma, *Disability and Rehabilitation*, vol. 16, no. 3, pp. 110–118.

Forster, A, Smith, J, Young, J, Knapp, P, House, A, & Wright, J, 2001, Information provision for stroke patients and their caregivers, *Cochrane Database of Systematic Reviews*, CD001919.

Gallant, MH, Beaulieu, MC, & Carnevale, FA, 2002, Partnership: an analysis of the concept within the nurse-client relationship, *Journal of Advanced Nursing*, vol. 40, no. 2, pp. 149–157.

Gladden, JC, 2000, Information exchange: critical connections to older adult decision-making during health care transitions, *Geriatric Nursing*, vol. 21, no. 4, pp. 213–218.

Grant, JS, 1999, Social problem-solving partnerships with family caregivers, *Rehabilitation Nursing*, vol. 24, no. 6, pp. 254–260.

Grant, JS, Elliott, TR, Weaver, M, Bartolucci, AA, & Giger, JN, 2002, Telephone intervention with family caregivers of stroke survivors after rehabilitation, *Stroke*, vol. 33, no. 8, pp. 2060–2065.

Grasel, E, Biehler, J, Schmidt, R, & Schupp, W, 2005, Intensification of the transition between inpatient neurological rehabilitation and home care of stroke patients. Controlled clinical trial with follow-up assessment six months after discharge, *Clinical Rehabilitation*, vol. 19, no. 7, pp. 725–736.

Grasel, E, Schmidt, R, Biehler, J, & Schupp, W, 2006, Long-term effects of the intensification of the transition between inpatient neurological rehabilitation and home care of stroke patients, *Clinical Rehabilitation*, vol. 20, no. 7, pp. 577–583.

Grimmer, KA, Dryden, LR, Puntumetakul, R, Young, AF, Guerin, M et al., 2006, Incorporating patient concerns into discharge plans: evaluation of a patient-generated checklist, *The Internet Journal of Allied Health Services and Practice*, vol. 4, no. 2.

Guberman, N, 2005, *Caregiver Assessment: What's new and where do we go from here? Symposium at 18th Congress of the International Association of Gerontology*, IAG, Rio de Janeiro, Brazil.

Haddock, KS, 1994, Collaborative discharge planning: nursing and social services, *Clinical Nurse Specialist*, vol. 8, no. 5, pp. 248–252.

Hajek, VE, Gagnon, S, & Ruderman, JE, 1997, Cognitive and functional assessments of stroke patients: an analysis of their relation, *Archives of Physical Medicine and Rehabilitation*, vol. 78, no. 12, pp. 1331–1337.

Hanger, HC, Walker, G, Paterson, LA, McBride, S, & Sainsbury, R, 1998, What do patients and their carers want to know about stroke? A two-year follow-up study, *Clinical Rehabilitation*, vol. 12, no. 1, pp. 45–52.

Hanson, E, Nolan, J, Magnusson, L, Sennemark, E, Johansson, L, & Nolan, M, 2006, *COAT: The Carer Outcome Agreement Tool: A new approach to working with family carers*, University College of Boras, Sweden: AldreVast Sjuharad Research Centre.

Hart, E, 1999, The use of pluralistic evaluation to explore people's experiences of stroke services in the community, *Health and Social Care in the Community*, vol. 7, no. 4, pp. 248–256.

Hart, E, 2001, System induced setbacks in stroke recovery, *Sociology of Health and Illness*, vol. 3, no. 1, pp. 101–123.

Hartke, RJ, & King, RB, 2003, Telephone group intervention for older stroke caregivers, *Topics in Stroke Rehabilitation*, vol. 9, no. 4, pp. 65–81.

Hervey, N, & Ramsay, R, 2004, Carers as partners in care, *Advances in Psychiatric Treatment*, vol. 10, pp. 81–84.

Hoffman, T, McKenna, K, Worral, L, & Read, SJ, 2004, Evaluating current practice in the provision of written information to stroke patients and their carers, *International Journal of Therapy and Rehabilitation*, vol. 11, no. 7, pp. 303–310.

Hofgren, C, Bjorkdahl, A, Esbjornsson, E, & Sunnerhagen, KS, 2007, Recovery after stroke: cognition, ADL function and return to work, *Acta Neurologica Scandinavica*, vol. 115, no. 2, pp. 73–80.

Intercollegiate Stroke Working Party, 2008, *National Clinical Guidelines for Stroke*, 3rd edn, Royal College of Physicians, London.

Kalra, L, Evans, A, Perez, I, Melbourn, A, Patel, A, Knapp, M, & Donaldson, N, 2004, Training carers of stroke patients: randomised controlled trial, *British Medical Journal*, vol. 328, no. 7448, p. 1099.

Kane, RL, Chen, Q, Finch, M, Blewett, L, Burns, R et al., 2000, The optimal outcomes of post-hospital care under Medicare, *Health Services Research*, vol. 35, no. 3, pp. 615–661.

Kelson, M, Ford, C, & Rigge, M, 1998, *Stroke Rehabilitation: Patient and Carer Views. A Report by the College of Health for the Intercollegiate Working Party for Stroke*, Royal College of Physicians, London.

Kerr, SM, & Smith, LN, 2001, Stroke: an exploration of the experience of informal caregiving, *Clinical Rehabilitation*, vol. 15, no. 4, pp. 428–436.

Larson, J, Franzen-Dahlin, A, Billing, E, Arbin, M, Murray, V, & Wredling, R, 2005, The impact of a nurse-led support and education programme for spouses of stroke patients: a randomized controlled trial, *Journal of Clinical Nursing*, vol. 14, no. 8, pp. 995–1003.

Low, JT, Payne, S, & Roderick, P, 1999, The impact of stroke on informal carers: a literature review, *Social Science and Medicine*, vol. 49, no. 6, pp. 711–725.

Low, JT, Roderick, P, & Payne, S, 2004, An exploration looking at the impact of domiciliary and day hospital delivery of stroke rehabilitation on informal carers, *Clinical Rehabilitation*, vol. 18, no. 7, pp. 776–784.

MacIntosh, J, & McCormack, D, 2001, Partnerships identified within primary health care literature, *International Journal of Nursing Studies*, vol. 38, no. 5, pp. 547–555.

Mackenzie, A, Perry, L, Lockhart, E, Cottee, M, Cloud, G et al., 2007, Family carers of stroke survivors: needs, knowledge, satisfaction and competence in caring, *Disability and Rehabilitation*, vol. 29, no. 2, pp. 111–121.

Magnusson, L, Hanson, E, & Nolan, M, 2002, Assisting carers using the ACTION model for working with family carers, *British Journal of Nursing*, vol. 11, no. 11, pp. 759–763.

Manthorpe, J, & Iliffe, S, 2006, *Depression in Later Life*, Jessica Kingsley, London.

McKenna, H, Keeney, S, Glenn, A, & Gordon, P, 2000, Discharge planning: an exploratory study, *Journal of Clinical Nursing*, vol. 9, no. 4, pp. 594–601.

McLennan, M, Anderson, GS, & Pain, K, 1996, Rehabilitation learning needs: patient and family perceptions, *Patient Education and Counselling*, vol. 27, no. 2, pp. 191–199.

Monane, M, Kanter, DS, Glynn, RJ, & Avorn, J, 1996, Variability in length of hospitalization for stroke. The role of managed care in an elderly population, *Archives of Neurology*, vol. 53, no. 9, pp. 875–880.

Murray, J, Ashworth, R, Forster, A, & Young, J, 2003, Developing a primary care-based stroke service: a review of the qualitative literature, *British Journal of General Practice*, vol. 53, no. 487, pp. 137–142.

Nai, A, Turner-Stokes, L, & Tyerman, A, 2006, Vocational rehabilitation for acquired brain injury in adults (protocol), *Cochrane Database of Systematic Reviews*, CD006021.

National Stroke Foundation, 2005, *Clinical Guidelines for Stroke Rehabilitation and Recovery*, National Stroke Foundation, Melbourne.

Naylor, MD, Brooten, D, Campbell, R, Jacobsen, BS, Mezey, MD et al., 1999, Comprehensive discharge planning and home follow-up of hospitalized elders: a randomized clinical trial, *Journal of American Medical Association*, vol. 281, no. 7, pp. 613–620.

Neau, JP, Ingrand, P, Mouille-Brachet, C, Rosier, MP, Couderq, C et al., 1998, Functional recovery and social outcome after cerebral infarction in young adults, *Cerebrovascular Diseases*, vol. 8, no. 5, pp. 296–302.

Nolan, MR, & Grant, G, 1992, *Regular Respite: An Evaluation of a Hospital Rota Bed Scheme for Elderly People*, Age Concern, London.

Nolan, M, Keady, J, & Grant, G, 1995, CAMI: a basis for assessment and support with family carers, *British Journal of Nursing*, vol. 4, no. 14, pp. 822–826.

Nolan, M, Grant, G, & Keady, J, 1996, *Understanding Family Care*, Open University Press, Buckingham.

Nolan, MR, Grant, G, Keady, J, & Lundh, U, 2003, New directions for partnerships: relationship centred care, in *Partnerships in Family Care: Understanding the Caregiving Career*, MR Nolan et al., eds., Open University Press, Maidenhead.

Nolan, MR, Brown, J, Davies, S, Nolan, J, & Keady, J, 2006, *The Senses Framework: Improving Care for Older People Through a Relationship-Centred Approach. Getting Research into Practice (GRiP)*, University of Sheffield, Report No. 2.

NSW Department of Ageing, Disability and Home Care (DADHC), 2006, *Good Practice Guide for HACC Funded Case Management Projects*, http://www.dadhc. nsw.gov.au/NR/rdonlyres/39C1876A-27F6-4C70-ABAD-CAD56D4F64E1/2094/ GoodPracticeGuidefinal.pdf; accessed 13 May 2009.

Nuffield Institute for Health, NHS Centre for Reviews and Dissemination (NHSCRD), 1996, Preventing falls and subsequent injury in older people, *Effective Health Care*, vol. 2, no. 4, pp. 1–16.

O'Connell, B, Baker, L, & Prosser, A, 2003, The educational needs of caregivers of stroke survivors in acute and community settings, *Journal of Neuroscience Nursing*, vol. 35, no. 1, pp. 21–28.

Office for National Statistics, 2003, *Carers*, http://www.statistics.gov.uk/cci/nugget. asp?id=347; accessed 12 May 2009.

O'Neill, J, Hibbard, MR, Brown, M, Jaffe, M, Sliwinski, M et al., 1998, The effect of employment on quality of life and community integration after traumatic brain injury, *Journal of Head Trauma Rehabilitation*, vol. 13, no. 4, pp. 68–79.

Ory, MG, 2000, Dementia caregiving at the end of the 20th Century, in *Interventions in Dementia Care: Towards Improving Quality of Life*, MP Lawton & RL Rubinstein, eds., Springer Publishing Company, New York.

Pardessus, V, Puisieux, F, Di, PC, Gaudefroy, C, Thevenon, A et al., 2002, Benefits of home visits for falls and autonomy in the elderly: a randomized trial study, *American Journal of Physical Medicine and Rehabilitation*, vol. 81, no. 4, pp. 247–252.

Parker, CJ, Gladman, JR, & Drummond, AE, 1997, The role of leisure in stroke rehabilitation, *Disability and Rehabilitation*, vol. 19, no. 1, pp. 1–5.

Patel, AT, Duncan, PW, Lai, SM, & Studenski, S, 2000, The relation between impairments and functional outcomes poststroke, *Archives of Physical Medicine and Rehabilitation*, vol. 81, no. 10, pp. 1357–1363.

Patterson, CJ, & Mulley, GP, 1999, The effectiveness of predischarge home assessment visits: a systematic review, *Clinical Rehabilitation*, vol. 13, no. 2, pp. 101–104.

Pearlin, LI, Harrington, C, Lawton, MP, Montgomery, RJ, & Zarit, SH, 2001, An overview of the social and behavioral consequences of Alzheimer's disease, *Aging and Mental Health*, vol. 5 Suppl 1, pp. S3–S6.

Phillips-Harris, C, 1998, Case management: high-intensity care for frail patients with complex needs, *Geriatrics*, vol. 53, no. 2, pp. 62–68.

Pierce, LL, Steiner, V, Govoni, AL, Hicks, B, Cervantez Thompson, TL et al., 2004, Internet-based support for rural caregivers of persons with stroke shows promise, *Rehabilitation Nursing*, vol. 29, no. 3, pp. 95–99, 103.

Ramsing, S, Blomstrand, C, & Sullivan, M, 1991, Prognostic factors for return to work in stroke patients with aphasia, *Aphasiology*, vol. 5, pp. 583–588.

Reiley, P, Pike, A, Phipps, M, Weiner, M, Miller, N et al., 1996, Learning from patients: a discharge planning improvement project, *Joint Commission Journal on Quality Improvement*, vol. 22, no. 5, pp. 311–322.

Rodgers, H, Bond, S, & Curless, R, 2001, Inadequacies in the provision of information to stroke patients and their families, *Age and Ageing*, vol. 30, no. 2, pp. 129–133.

Saeki, S, 2000, Disability management after stroke: its medical aspects for workplace accommodation, *Disability and Rehabilitation*, vol. 22, no. 13–14, pp. 578–582.

Saposnik, G, Webster, F, O'Callaghan, C, & Hachinski, V, 2005, Optimizing discharge planning: clinical predictors of longer stay after recombinant tissue plasminogen activator for acute stroke, *Stroke*, vol. 36, no. 1, pp. 147–150.

Schumacher, KL, Stewart, BJ, & Archbold, PG, 1998, Conceptualization and measurement of doing family caregiving well, *Image: Journal of Nursing Scholarship*, vol. 30, no. 1, pp. 63–69.

Schumacher, KL, Stewart, BJ, Archbold, PG, Dodd, MJ, & Dibble, SL, 2000, Family caregiving skill: development of the concept, *Research in Nursing and Health*, vol. 23, no. 3, pp. 191–203.

Schure, LM, van den Heuvel, ET, Stewart, RE, Sanderman, R, de Witte, LP et al., 2006, Beyond stroke: description and evaluation of an effective intervention to support family caregivers of stroke patients, *Patient Education and Counselling*, vol. 62, no. 1, pp. 46–55.

Schwamm, LH, Pancioli, A, Acker, JE, III, Goldstein, LB, Zorowitz, RD et al., 2005, Recommendations for the establishment of stroke systems of care: recommendations from the American Stroke Association's Task Force on the Development of Stroke Systems, *Stroke*, vol. 36, no. 3, pp. 690–703.

Scottish Intercollegiate Guidelines Network (SIGN), 2004, *Management of Patients with Stroke part III: Identification and Management of Dysphagia No. 78.*, Scottish Intercollegiate Guidelines Network, Edinburgh.

Shepperd, S, Parkes, J, McClaren, J, & Phillips, C, 2004, Discharge planning from hospital to home, *Cochrane Database of Systematic Reviews*, CD000313.

Simon, C, & Kendrick, T, 2002, Community provision for informal live-in carers of stroke patients, *British Journal of Community Nursing*, vol. 7, no. 6, pp. 292–298.

Smith, LN, Lawrence, M, Kerr, SM, Langhorne, P, & Lees, KR, 2004, Informal carers' experience of caring for stroke survivors, *Journal of Advanced Nursing*, vol. 46, no. 3, pp. 235–244.

Stewart, BJ, Archbold, PG, Harvath, TA, & Nkongho, NO, 1993, Role acquisition in family caregivers of older people who have been discharged from hospital, in *Key Aspects of Caring for the Chronically Ill: Hospital and Home*, SG Funk et al., eds., Springer, New York.

van den Heuvel, ET, de Witte, LP, Nooyen-Haazen, I, Sanderman, R, & Meyboom-de, JB, 2000, Short-term effects of a group support program and an individual support program for caregivers of stroke patients, *Patient Education and Counselling*, vol. 40, no. 2, pp. 109–120.

van den Heuvel, ET, Witte, LP, Stewart, RE, Schure, LM, Sanderman, R, & Meyboom-de, JB, 2002, Long-term effects of a group support program and an individual support program for informal caregivers of stroke patients: which caregivers benefit the most? *Patient Education and Counselling*, vol. 47, no. 4, pp. 291–299.

van der Smagt-Duijnstee ME, Hamers, JP, bu-Saad, HH, & Zuidhof, A, 2001a, Relatives of hospitalized stroke patients: their needs for information, counselling and accessibility, *Journal of Advanced Nursing*, vol. 33, no. 3, pp. 307–315.

van der Smagt-Duijnstee ME, Hamers, JP, bu-Saad, HH, & Zuidhof, A, 2001b, Relatives of hospitalized stroke patients: their needs for information, counselling and accessibility, *Journal of Advanced Nursing*, vol. 33, no. 3, pp. 307–315.

van Veenendaal, H, Grinspun, DR, & Adriaanse, HP, 1996, Educational needs of stroke survivors and their family members, as perceived by themselves and by health professionals, *Patient Education and Counselling*, vol. 28, no. 3, pp. 265–276.

Waddell, G, 2006, *Is Work Good for Your Health and Wellbeing*, The Stationery Office, London.

Wade, DT, & Hewer, RL, 1987, Functional abilities after stroke: measurement, natural history and prognosis, *Journal of Neurology, Neurosurgery and Psychiatry*, vol. 50, no. 2, pp. 177–182.

Welch, A, & Lowes, S, 2005, home assessment visits within the acute setting: a discussion and literature review, *British Journal of Occupational Therapy*, vol. 68, no. 4, pp. 158–164.

Wiles, R, Pain, H, Buckland, S, & McLellan, L, 1998, Providing appropriate information to patients and carers following a stroke, *Journal of Advanced Nursing*, vol. 28, no. 4, pp. 794–801.

Wilkinson, PR, Wolfe, CD, Warburton, FG, Rudd, AG, Howard, RS et al., 1997, A long-term follow-up of stroke patients, *Stroke*, vol. 28, no. 3, pp. 507–512.

Wolfe, C, 1996, *Stroke Services and Research: An Overview with Recommendations for Future Research*, The Stroke Association, London.

Young, J, & Forster, A, 2007, Review of stroke rehabilitation, *British Medical Journal*, vol. 334, no. 7584, pp. 86–90.

Zerwic, JJ, Ennen, K, & DeVon, HA, 2002, Stroke. Risks, recognition, and return to work, *Official Journal of the American Association of Occupational Health Nurses*, vol. 50, no. 8, pp. 354–359.

Zorowitz, RD, 1999, Returning to life. Stroke survivor community and Internet resources, *Physical Medicine and Rehabilitation Clinics of North America*, vol. 10, no. 4, pp. 967–985, x.

Zureik, M, Lang, T, Trouillet, JL, Davido, A, Tran, B et al., 1995, Returning home after acute hospitalization in two French teaching hospitals: predictive value of patients' and relatives' wishes, *Age and Ageing*, vol. 24, no. 3, pp. 227–234.

Chapter 15

Stroke resources for professionals, patients and carers

Graham Williamson

This chapter is divided into eight sections. A final additional section supplies links for references in the preceding chapters. Much of the information contained in the websites listed is relevant to professionals, to patients and to carers, so whilst some section headings may reflect this division, the resources that they contain may usefully be read by all. Resources are presented under the headings:

- National associations
- Resources for patients and carers
- Other resources and organisations
- Specialist international journals
- Non-specialist journals' stroke collections
- Clinical practice guidelines
- Finding current stroke research
- Evidence-based practice resources

Resources within each section are presented in alphabetical order. No claims are made as to the veracity of information contained in these sites and no responsibility can be taken for information given by them.

National associations

These websites contain lots of useful information and resources, particularly on research, fundraising, services and contacts for professionals, patients and carers.

American Speech-Language-Hearing Association (ASHA).
http://www.asha.org/public/speech/disorders/dysarthria.htm

American Stroke Association, National Centre, 7272 Greenville Avenue Dallas TX 75231; tel.: 1-888-478-7653.
http://www.strokeassociation.org/presenter.jhtml?identifier=1200037

Australia: National Stroke Foundation. Stroke Helpline 1800 787 653.
http://www.strokefoundation.com.au/

National Institute for Health and Clinical Excellence. See documents:
   Ischaemic stroke (acute): Alteplase Technological Appraisal 2007,
   Acute stroke and TIA: clinical guidelines July 2008.
http://www.nice.org.uk

National Institute of Neurological Disorders and Stroke.
http://www.ninds.nih.gov/disorders/stroke/stroke.htm
Information about stroke and subtypes including locked-in-syndrome.
http://www.ninds.nih.gov/disorders/lockedinsyndrome/lockedinsyndrome.htm

National Stroke Association UK. Stroke Information Service, The Stroke Association, 240 City Road, London, EC1V 2PR. Stroke helpline 0845 3033 100 (open Monday to Friday, 9 am to 5 pm).
http://www.stroke.org.uk/
E-mail info@stroke.org.uk

National Stroke Association USA. 9707 E. Easter Lane, Centennial, CO 80112. 1-800-787-6537.
http://www.stroke.org/site/PageServer?pagename=HOME

Royal Hospital for Neuro-disability: web-based resources for locked in syndrome and other neurological conditions.
http://www.rhn.org.uk/institute/cat.asp?catid=1296

Resources for patients and carers

Aphasia Now: an aphasia-friendly website and a weekly support group in Gloucestershire, UK.
http://www.aphasianow.org

AVM Support, a unique group working throughout the UK offering free, patient-friendly information and support to all whose lives have been affected by the rare condition arteriovenous malformation.
http://www.avmsupport.org.uk/

Carers UK.
http://www.carersuk.org/Home

Connect and Speakeasy, communication disability networks.
http://www.ukconnect.org/index.aspx
http://www.buryspeakeasy.org.uk/

Different Strokes: provides free services to younger stroke survivors throughout the UK.
http://www.differentstrokes.co.uk/

Directgov.
http://www.direct.gov.uk/en/CaringForSomeone/index.htm

Electronic Quality Information for Patients (EQUIP) gateway for quality health and social care information for UK patients carers and families.
http://www.equip.nhs.uk/index.html#top

Locked-in syndrome resources:
http://www.club-internet.fr/alis – click on 'Alis in English' tab on left-hand side of the page
http://www.locked-in-syndrom.org/englisch/index.htm
http://www.marykoch.com/locked-in_syndrome.htm
http://www.mikeydee.com/strokeinfo.html

National Women's Health Information Centre: US Federal government women's health site.
http://www.4women.gov/faq/stroke.htm

National Women's Health Resource Centre: aims to provide up-to-date and objective women's health information based on the latest advances in medical research and practice.
http://www.healthywomen.org/aboutnwhrc

Princess Royal Trust for Carers.
http://www.carers.org/

Stanford Stroke Center: explains different types of stroke, warning signs and risk factors and recommends steps to reduce stroke risks, provides an overview of the advanced techniques for diagnosis and treatment available at the Stanford Stroke Center.
http://strokecenter.stanford.edu/guide/

Stroke (Brain Attack): various patient resources.
http://www.doctorscorner.net/healthinfocenter/medical-conditions/
cardiovascular/cardiac-conditions/untitled-folder/stroke.html

Stroke Survivor: a resource based on the experiences of a man affected by stroke.
http://www.positivepowerpublishing.com/index.html
   Includes stroke and aphasia resources.
http://www.positivepowerpublishing.com/stroke_aphasia.html

Stroke Survivor International: international links list.
http://strokesurvivors.org/International/index.html

Other resources and organisations

Association of Rehabilitation Nurses: to promote and advance professional rehabilitation nursing practice through education, advocacy, collaboration, and research to enhance the quality of life for those affected by disability and chronic illness.
http://www.rehabnurse.org/

Boehringer-Ingelheim Stroke Corporate website. Lots of useful and relevant information including links to related journals. Some areas require sign-up.
http://www.boehringer-ingelheim.com/stroke/links/generalb.htm

British Association of Stroke Physicians: to promote the advancement of Stroke Medicine in the UK. Contains useful information and links to other associations and resources.
http://www.basp.ac.uk/

British Association of Stroke Physicians CT scan Training Series.
http://www.dcn.ed.ac.uk/ist3/20031205_BASP%20CT%20Sampler_files/frame.htm

Chest, Heart and Stroke Scotland: aims to improve the quality of life for people in Scotland affected by chest, heart and stroke illness through medical research, advice and information, and support in the community. Also has good range of educational resources for professionals.
http://www.chss.org.uk

Department of Health stroke resources.
http://www.dh.gov.uk/stroke

Evidence Based Review of Stroke Rehabilitation: aims to maintain timely and accurate information on effective stroke rehabilitation, identifying ideas for further research, supporting continuous peer review and encouraging improved evidence-based practice. The 11th edition is available.
http://www.ebrsr.com

Expert Patient Programme: a self-management course giving people the confidence, skills and knowledge to manage their condition better and be more in control of their lives.
http://www.expertpatients.co.uk

National Stroke Nursing Forum: UK forum for any professional with an interest in stroke nursing.
http://uclan.ac.uk/nsnf

National Stroke Research Institute: Australian research foundation.
http://www.nsri.org.au/

NHS Evidence Health Information Resources (formerly National Library for Health): stroke specialist library.
http://www.library.nhs.uk/stroke/

Rural Nurse Organisation Digital Resources on stroke.
http://ruralnurseorganization-dl.slis.ua.edu/clinical/neurology/cerebrovascular/ischemicstroke.htm

Stroke-information.net website on stroke: dedicated to the improvement of medical information and fostering of stroke information in developed and developing countries. http://www.stroke-information.net
Includes World-Stroke Mailing List (World-stroke@jiscmail.ac.uk).

SAFE (Stroke Awareness for Everyone, Inc.): an international internet coalition of stroke survivors and their families, doctors, nurses and therapists involved with stroke.
http://www.strokesafe.org/

Safe Implementation of Thrombolysis in Stroke (SITS) registry: register here to enter all thrombolysis cases into an international database. Contains other useful links and resources.
http://www.acutestroke.org/modules.php?op=modload&name=News&file=article&sid=82

Safe Stroke Developments email list.
http://www.lsoft.com/scripts/wl.exe?SL1=SAFE-STROKE_DEVELOPMENTS&H=LISTSERV.TBINET.ORG

Skills for Health: National Occupational Standards including in stroke care.
www.skillsforhealth.org.uk

STARS project: has developed a set of core competencies for professionals working with people with stroke and coronary heart disease (CHD) conditions.
http://www.strokecorecompetencies.org/

Stepping Out Project: a stroke self-management programme enabling individuals to take control of their daily lives.
http://www.steppingoutuk.org.uk

Stroke Forum: brings together the multidisciplinary stroke community to improve stroke care in the UK.
http://www.ukstrokeforum.org/

Stroke Improvement Programme: set up to provide national support for local improvement of stroke and TIA services. It is an NHS initiative to support the development of Stroke Care Networks and the implementation of the National Stroke Strategy.
http://www.improvement.nhs.uk/stroke/

The Brain Attack Coalition: US professional, voluntary and governmental coalition aimed at reducing stroke incidence, disability and death.
http://www.stroke-site.org/index.html

The Internet Stroke Center: stroke information for health professionals. US site with subsections including resources, basic science, diagnosis, management and news.
http://www.strokecenter.org/prof/organizations_prof.htm

United Kingdom Stroke Research Network: A topic specific network of the UK Clinical Research Network.
https://www.uksrn.ac.uk

World Health Organisation classification: International Classification of Functioning, Disability and Health (ICF).
www.who.int/classification/icf

Specialist international journals

Cerebrovascular Diseases: international forum for sophisticated scientific information on clinical data, diagnostic testing, and therapeutic issues, dealing with all aspects of stroke and cerebrovascular diseases.
http://content.karger.com/ProdukteDB/produkte.asp?Aktion=JournalHome& ProduktNr=224153

International Journal of Stroke: concentrates on clinical aspects of stroke with basic science contributions.
http://www.blackwellpublishing.com/journal.asp?ref=1747-4930&site=1

Journal of Stroke and Cerebrovascular Diseases: publishes original papers on aspects of basic and clinical science related to the fields of stroke and cerebrovascular diseases. http://www.strokejournal.org/

Stroke: journal on cerebrovascular diseases (American Heart Association).
http://stroke.ahajournals.org/

Non-specialist journals' stroke collections

American Journal of Psychiatry stroke collection.
http://ajp.psychiatryonline.org/cgi/collection/stroke

Archives of Surgery stroke collection.
http://archsurg.ama-assn.org/cgi/collection/stroke

British Medical Journal stroke collection.
http://bmj.bmjjournals.com/cgi/collection/stroke

Circulation: acute stroke syndromes.
http://circ.ahajournals.org/cgi/collection/stroke_syndromes

Circulation: embolic stroke collection.
http://circ.ahajournals.org/cgi/collection/embol_str?notjournal=ahajournals& page=9

Journal of the American Medical Association and archives stroke collection.
http://pubs.ama-assn.org/cgi/collection/stroke?page=18

Journal of Neuropsychology and Neurosciences stroke collection.
http://neuro.psychiatryonline.org/cgi/collection/stroke?page=2

New England Journal of Medicine stroke collection.
http://content.nejm.org/cgi/collection/stroke

Psychosomatics stroke collection.
http://psy.psychiatryonline.org/cgi/collection/stroke?notjournal=psy&page=4

Clinical practice guidelines

A large number of guidelines are available, and these sites should be searched with discrimination.

Australia and New Zealand

Australian guidelines can be accessed at the National Stroke Foundation website at http://www.strokefoundation.com.au/component/option,com_docman/task, cat_view/gid,76/dir,DESC/order,date/limit,5/limitstart,5/

New Zealand guidelines can be accessed at the Stroke Foundation website at http://www.nzgg.org.nz/guidelines/dsp_guideline_popup.cfm?guidelineID=37

UK

Department of Health National Service Framework for Older People lists these good practice examples and case studies relating to Standard Five (strokes).
http://www.dh.gov.uk/PolicyAndGuidance/HealthAndSocialCareTopics/
OlderPeoplesServices/OlderPeoplePromotionProject/
OlderPeoplePromotionProjectArticle/fs/en?CONTENT_ID=4002291&chk=
zrxP%2BG

National Service Framework for Older People. Standard Five: Stroke.
http://www.dh.gov.uk/assetRoot/04/07/12/83/04071283.pdf

Royal College of Physicians: National Clinical Guidelines for Stroke.
http://www.rcplondon.ac.uk/pubs/books/stroke/

Scottish Intercollegiate Guidelines Network. Management of Patients with Stroke.
http://www.sign.ac.uk/pdf/sign64.pdf

US

American Academy of Neurology: current AAN clinical practice guidelines and related tools, including patient and physician summaries of selected guidelines can be found here.
http://www.aan.com/professionals/practice/guideline/index.cfm?fuseaction=
home.welcome&Topics=20&Submit=Search

American Heart Association.
http://www.americanheart.org/presenter.jhtml?identifier=3004586
    For free on-line National Institutes for Health Stroke Scale (NIHSS) training, following links from this site or go to:
http://learn.heart.org/ihtml/application/student/interface.heart2/index2.html?
searchstring=583

National Guideline Clearinghouse™ is a public resource for evidence-based clinical practice guidelines.
http://www.guideline.gov/

The Internet Stroke Center: stroke information for professionals, provides a full list of guidelines on prevention, management and recovery in relation to stroke.
http://www.strokecenter.org/prof/guidelines.htm

Finding current stroke research

Australia and New Zealand
Australian clinical trials registry.
http://www.actr.org.au/

UK
Current Controlled Trials: allows users to search, register and share information about randomised controlled trials.
http://www.controlled-trials.com/

Stroke Research Network (SRN): provides a world-class health service infrastructure to support clinical stroke research and remove barriers to its conduct (UK).
http://www.ukcrn.org.uk/index/networks/stroke.html

US
ClinicalTrials.gov: provides regularly updated information about federally and privately supported clinical research in human volunteers.
http://www.clinicaltrials.gov/

Stroke Trials Registry: a continuously updated registry of randomised clinical trials in stroke and cerebrovascular disease.
http://www.strokecenter.org/trials/

Evidence-based practice resources

BMJ Clinical Evidence: medical resource for informing treatment decisions and improving patient care.
http://www.clinicalevidence.com/ceweb/conditions/index.jsp

Evidence Based Nursing: A journal of quality appraised abstracted research relevant to nursing practice.
http://ebn.bmj.com/

Joanna Briggs Institute: provides a collaborative approach to the evaluation of evidence derived from a diverse range of sources, including experience, exper-

tise and all forms of rigorous research and the translation, transfer and utilisation of the 'best available' evidence into health care practice.
http://www.joannabriggs.edu.au/about/home.php

The Cochrane Library and The Cochrane Collaboration: evidence-based health care databases and systematic reviews.
http://www.cochrane.org/index.htm

Chapter links

Chapter 1

Meeting the recommendations in the NSS will challenge not just the NHS but also other health, social and voluntary care services. To deliver this, the NSS proposed the establishment of Stroke Care Networks, supported by a national Stroke Improvement Programme (http://www.improvement.nhs.uk/stroke).'
(p. 7)

Participation in clinical trials is promoted via the national Stroke Research Network (SRN;
http://www.uksrn.ac.uk). (p. 8)

Chapter 2

A pragmatic approach was adopted by the British Association of Stroke Physicians in 2005 (see http://www.basp.ac.uk/LinkClick.aspx?fileticket= h6zszwmXQfk%3D&tabid=653&mid=1053&language=en-GB) in designation of three levels of stroke unit, differentiated by the availability of specialist staff and resources to deliver aspects of acute stroke care. (p. 24)

For nursing, profession-specific guidelines are available from the National Stroke Nursing Forum (http://uclan.ac.uk/nsnf) and can be downloaded at http://www.rcplondon.ac.uk/pubs/contents/0bcf7680-7e4b-4cd1-a863-6080efde9a12.pdf. (p. 26)

Much of the development in stroke care appears to be focused on the 'stroke pathway': what should happen and when, and who should have the competences to do it. For example, the UK organisation Skills for Health provides six competences for stroke care (http://www.skillsforhealth.org.uk/). (p. 27)

... intended to re-focus the organisation and delivery of health services closer to the needs and aspirations of patients. In stroke, there are a wide range of sources of information about the experiences and expectations of patients. These include an extensive qualitative research literature (e.g. Murray et al. 2003) and internet-based sources such as http://www.dipex.org. (p. 28)

Development priorities were identified through a synthesis of work-based learning activities designed to critically evaluate stroke policy, patient and carer priorities, team working, and personal leadership skills and resources to facilitate change (http://uclan.ac.uk/nsnf). (p. 30)

Chapter 4

This is one part of a major international trial (the CLOTS trial: http://www.
dcn.ed.ac.uk/clots/), an earlier component of which demonstrated that compression stockings alone are ineffective (The CLOTS Trial Collaboration 2009).
(p. 82)

Chapter 5

Recent focus on hospital food in the UK has resulted in national standards
(Department of Health 2004) and the Better Hospital Food programme focused
on recipes, snack-provision and the mealtime environment on wards
(http://195.92.246.148/nhsestates/better_hospital_food/bhf_content/
protected_mealtimes/overview.asp). (p. 103)

Reliance upon clinical signs for nutritional screening may not be effective; use
of screening tools with demonstrated validity and reliability is recommended
(National Institute for Health and Clinical Excellence 2006); for example, the
Malnutrition Universal Screening Tool (see http://www.bapen.org.uk/pdfs/
must/must_full.pdf). (p. 93)

In 2006 the National Institute for Health and Clinical Excellence (NICE) issued
a clinical guideline to help UK health care staff identify patients who are malnourished or at risk of malnutrition (National Institute for Health and Clinical
Excellence 2006) and similar recommendations were issued from the Council
of Europe (http://www.bapen.org.uk/res_council.html). (p. 105)

The UK Mental Capacity Act (2005) provides guidance on establishing whether
and to what extent someone can contribute to decisions about their care, and
when Lasting Power of Attorney can be used or a deputy appointed (http://
www.opsi.gov.uk/ACTS/acts2005/ukpga_20050009_en_1). (p. 107)

For all patients with neurological damage who have nothing orally, oral stimulation programmes are essential in order to prevent hypersensitive oral defensive patterns becoming established, which may make oral hygiene routines
difficult to maintain (http://www.fott.co.uk). (p. 113)

Chapter 6

Desmopressin nasal spray is no longer available for nocturnal enuresis in the
UK (http://www.mhra.gov.uk). Blood pressure and blood electrolytes should
be monitored regularly since desmopressin action also leads to sodium retention. (p. 141)

Chapter 8

Useful resources are: The Stroke and Aphasia Handbook (Parr et al. 2004) and
the Stroke Talk manual (Cottrell & Davies 2006), both available from Connect
(http://www.ukconnect.org). (p. 191)

There are personal accounts in the literature of individuals with long term aphasia who have achieved new and satisfying lives (see (Hinckley 2006) and Aphasia Now website: http://www.aphasianow.org. (p. 201)

Chapter 11

The model (ICF) was endorsed by the World Health Assembly in 2001 and can be found at http://www.who.int/classification/icf. (p. 242)

Comparison of models of stroke care and collaboration in research will enhance the identification of important and effective components of stroke care. In the UK, high grade evidence will be facilitated through the newly formed UK Stroke Research Network (see http://www.uksrn.ac.uk). (p. 253)

There are many interesting and insightful stories from stroke survivors that can be accessed on http://www.healthtalkonline.org (Health talk online 2009). (p. 256)

Chapter 13

More recently introduced, varenicline (http://www.nps.org.au/_data/assets/ pdf_file/0012/17031/varenicline.pdf) is showing promise but long-term evaluation has yet to be undertaken. (p. 278)

Chapter 14

'Because I don't feel like I'm a survivor of a stroke, I feel I'm struggling, I'm struggling with the stroke but I don't think I want to be called a struggler either. Just a person. I think sometimes a person is not seen' (http://www. healthtalkonline.org). (p. 309)

A large multicentre trial to test the effectiveness of carer training and information giving is ongoing (see SRN website: http://www.uksrn.ac.uk). (p. 319)

For example, The Stroke Association website (http://www.stroke.org.uk) is a comprehensive resource, covering frequently asked questions and specialist subjects. (p. 320)

The Equality and Human Rights Commission is a source of advice about disabled people's rights (http://www.equalityhumanrights.com) (p. 315)

Index

Page numbers in *italics* represent figures, those in **bold** represent tables.